SOCIAL AND REHABILITATION SERVICES FOR THE BLIND

Publication Number 846

AMERICAN LECTURE SERIES®

A Publication in

The BANNERSTONE DIVISION *of*

AMERICAN LECTURES IN SOCIAL AND REHABILITATION PSYCHOLOGY

Consulting Editors

JOHN G. CULL, Ph.D.

Director, Regional Counselor Training Program
Department of Rehabilitation Counseling
Virginia Commonwealth University
Fishersville, Virginia

and

RICHARD E. HARDY, Ed.D.

Chairman, Department of Rehabilitation Counseling
Virginia Commonwealth University
Richmond, Virginia

The following books have appeared thus far in this Series:

Vocational Rehabilitation: Profession and Process—John G. Cull, Jr., and Richard E. Hardy

Contemporary Field Work Practices in Rehabilitation—John G. Cull, Jr., and Craig R. Colvin

The American Lecture Series in Social and Rehabilitation Psychology offers books which are concerned with man's role in his milieu. Emphasis is placed on how this role can be made more effective in a time of social conflict and a deteriorating physical environment. The books are oriented toward descriptions of what future roles should be and are not concerned exclusively with the delineation and definition of contemporary behavior. Contributors are concerned to a considerable extent with prediction through the use of a functional view of man as opposed to a descriptive, anatomical point of view.

Books in this series are written mainly for the professional practitioner; however, academicians will find them of considerable value in both graduate and undergraduate courses in the helping services.

SOCIAL AND REHABILITATION SERVICES FOR THE BLIND

RICHARD E. HARDY, Ed.D.

Chairman, Department of Rehabilitation Counseling
Virginia Commonwealth University
Richmond, Virginia

and

JOHN G. CULL, Ph.D.

Director, Regional Counselor Training Program
Department of Rehabilitation Counseling
Virginia Commonwealth University
Fishersville, Virginia

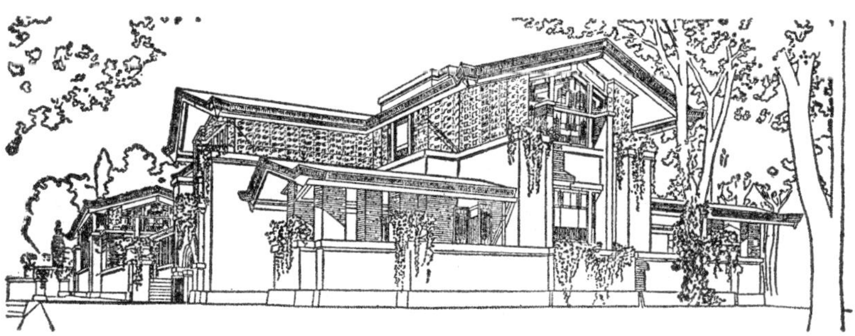

CHARLES C THOMAS · PUBLISHER

Springfield · Illinois · U.S.A.

Published and Distributed Throughout the World by

CHARLES C THOMAS • PUBLISHER
BANNERSTONE HOUSE
301-327 East Lawrence Avenue, Springfield, Illinois, U.S.A.

ISBN 0-398-02309-3
Library of Congress Catalog Card Number: 70-184599

With THOMAS BOOKS *careful attention is given to all details of manufacturing and design. It is the Publisher's desire to present books that are satisfactory as to their physical qualities and artistic possibilities and appropriate for their particular use.* THOMAS BOOKS *will be true to those laws of quality that assure a good name and good will.*

Printed in the United States of America
HH-11

Contributors

Mary K. Bauman, M.S.: Diplomate in Counseling, ABEPP, Director, Personnel Research Center, Philadelphia, Pennsylvania. Consultant to agencies for the blind and visually handicapped in Pennsylvania, New Jersey, Maryland, Deleware, and South Carolina, formerly also Virginia. Researcher in psychological evaluation of blind persons, nature of employment, effects of blindness, social competency, and other psychological characteristics of the visually handicapped. Author of numerous books and articles in the professional literature.

Donald Blasch: Director, Institute of Blind Rehabilitation, Western Michigan University, B.E. degree Northern Illinois University, M.A. degree University of Chicago. Formerly operational assistant and acting chief and counselor, Central Blind Rehabilitation Section, VA Hospital, Hines, Illinois; former psychologist, Illinois State Training School. Member of various professional organizations including executive board member of American Association of Workers for the Blind.

Warren Bledsoe: Consultant to U.S. Department of Health, Education and Welfare, Social and Rehabilitation Services Administration, Office for the Blind and Visually Handicapped. Advisor to various public organizations on the subject of blindness and adjustment to disability. Former chief, Blind Rehabilitation, Physical Medicine and Rehabilitation Services, Veterans Administration. Former consultant to VA Department of Medicine and Surgery on Blindness. Former coordinator of blinded veterans affairs in the Veterans Administration. Former editor of the *New Outlook for the Blind.* Mr. Bledsoe has also taught at the Maryland School for the Blind. He is a graduate of Princeton University and a graduate of the Harvard course for teachers of the blind. He has published widely in the field of rehabilitation of blind persons and is the author of *War Blinded Veterans in A Post-War Setting.*

Robert S. Bray: Chief, Division for the Blind and Physically Handicapped, Library of Congress, Washington, D. C. Member: Board of Trustees, American Foundation for the Blind; Board of Directors, National Accreditation Council for Agencies Serving the Blind and Visually Handicapped. Member of numerous professional associations and contributor of articles to professional literature. Numerous awards for outstanding contributions to work for the blind.

William T. Coppage: Director of the Virginia Commission for the Visually Handicapped, M.Ed. degree from the University of Virginia and M.S. degree in Rehabilitation Counseling from Virginia Commonwealth University. Formerly an area supervisor of the vending stand program, Virginia Commission for the Visually Handicapped and assistant superintendent of the Virginia Workshop for the Blind. Former supervisor of the rehabilitation evaluation and training program for the blind in Virginia and assistant director of the Commission for the Visually Handicapped. Member of a number of rehabilitation related associations and board member of six associations concerning blindness.

John G. Cull, Jr., Ph.D.: Director, Regional Counselor Training Program and Associate Professor, Department of Rehabilitation Counseling, Virginia Commonwealth University. Former rehabilitation counselor, Texas Commission for the Blind and Texas Education Agency, Division of Vocational Rehabilitation. Former staff psychologist, South Plains Adult Mental Health Clinic, Lubbock, Texas, and Director, Division of Research and Program Development, Department of Vocational Rehabilitation, Richmond, Virginia. Author of numerous articles and several books on vocational rehabilitation and consultant to various rehabilitation agencies and organizations.

William F. Gallagher, M.S.W.: Director of Rehabilitation Services, New York Association for the Blind; formerly director of Rehabilitation Center, Greater Pittsburgh Guild for the Blind; chief of professional services at Catholic Guild for all the Blind, Newton, Massachusetts; instructor at the University of Pittsburgh; contributor of numerous articles to professional literature.

Margaret Bowers Gill, M.Ed.: Executive Director, Virginia Society for the Prevention of Blindness, Inc., an affiliate of the National Society for the Prevention of Blindness; formerly with the American National Red Cross as executive secretary, Henrico County, Virginia Chapter; field representative, Eastern area; and director of recruitment, Blood Program, Baltimore chapter.

Richard E. Hardy, Ed.D.: Chairman, Department of Rehabilitation Counseling, Virginia Commonwealth University. Formerly a rehabilitation counselor in Virginia; rehabilitation advisor, Rehabilitation Services Administration, Department of Health, Education, and Welfare, Washington, D.C. Former chief psychologist and supervisor of professional training, South Carolina Department of Vocational Rehabilitation and member of South Carolina State Board of Examiners in Psychology. Author of numerous articles published in national journals and co-author of *Vocational Rehabilitation: Profession and Process,* and *The Unfit Majority.*

Dennis L. Holmes: Principal, Department for the Blind, Virginia School for the Deaf and Blind; formerly director of Education Services Department, Virginia Commission for the Visually Handicapped; trustee, American Printing House for the Blind; lecturer, Virginia Commonwealth University, University of Virginia, Old Dominion University, Norfolk State College, Madison College, Medical College of Virginia and University of Virginia Medical School.

Douglas C. Mac Farland, Ph.D.: Director, Office for the Blind and Visually Handicapped, Rehabilitation Services Administration, Department of Health, Education, and Welfare, Washington, D.C. Former director, Virginia Commission for the Visually Handicapped. He has also served as assistant director of the Virginia Commission for the Visually Handicapped, as vocational counselor and supervisor for the Delaware Commission for the Blind, and as a rehabilitation counselor with the New Jersey Commission for the Blind. He is past president of American Association of Workers for the Blind and is a member of the Commission on Accreditation and the Board. He served as a trustee of the Board of Directors of the American Foundation for the Blind, and is co-chairman of the Committee on Industrial and Rural Employment of the World Council for the Welfare of the Blind.

George A. Magers, M.S.: Assistant Director, Office for the Blind and Visually Handicapped, RSA, SRS, Department of Health, Education, and Welfare, Washington, D. C. Former rehabilitation specialist with the Division of Services to the Blind of the Rehabilitation Services Administration. Formerly chief, Bureau of Services to the Blind, Nevada State Welfare Department and counselor for the Illinois Division of Vocational Rehabilitation. Author of a number of articles in rehabilitation journals.

Robert L. Pogorelc: Vocational Rehabilitation Program Specialist, Office for the Blind and Visually Handicapped, Rehabilitation Services Administration, Department of Health, Education, and Welfare; formerly assistant regional representative, Region V, Rehabilitation Services Administration, Department of Health, Education, and Welfare. Previously served as project supervisor, Wood County Special Demonstration Project, Wisconsin Division of Vocational Rehabilitation.

Louis H. Rives, Jr., J.D.: Director, Operations Division, Office for Civil Rights, Health Education and Welfare; former chief of the Social Welfare and Related Programs Division and assistant director for State Agency Compliance, Office for Civil Rights; former special assistant to the Commissioner of Vocational Rehabilitation, RSA; former chief, Division of Services to the Blind, RSA, HEW. Former assistant regional representative in RSA Dallas regional office; past president of the American Association of Workers for the Blind and former member of the Board of Directors of the American Foundation for the Blind. Mr. Rives has received numerous awards including the Distinguished Service Award from the Department of HEW.

William D. Rusher, M.D.: Assistant Clinical Professor, Department of Ophthalmology, Virginia Commonwealth University; supervising ophthalmologist, Virginia Commission for the Visually Handicapped; lecturer, Virginia Commonwealth University, Regional Counselor Training Program, Woodrow Wilson Rehabilitation Center.

Stanley Suterko: Assistant Director, Orientation and Mobility Program, Institute of Blind Rehabilitation, Western Michigan University. B.S. degree University of Illinois, M.A. degree Western Michigan University. Guest lecturer in various universities and author of numerous articles on orientation and mobility. Member of various professional organizations and committees. Chairman of the Certfication Committee of Mobility Instructors of American Association of Workers for the Blind.

Louis Vieceli: Assistant Professor, Rehabilitation Institute, Southern Illinois University, Carbondale, Illinois; formerly a rehabilitation counselor for the Illinois Division of Vocational Rehabilitation; American Association of Workers for the Blind's 1969 winner of the John H. McCauley Award for outstanding achievement in the placement of blind persons; treasurer and member of Executive Committee American Association of Workers for the Blind during 1969-1971.

John H. Wallace, Ph.D.: Assistant Professor of Rehabilitation Counseling at Virginia Commonwealth University; vocational consultant with the Bureau of Hearings and Appeals, Social Security Administration. He earned his doctoral degree from the American University in Washington, D.C. and holds a M.S. degree in rehabilitation counseling from Virginia Commonwealth University.

Allan L. Ward, Ph.D.: Director of Research and Staff Development, Arkansas Enterprises for the Blind, and director of the program for training professional workers with the blind, International Services for the Blind; formerly dean of instruction, Philander Smith College; board member, American National Institutes for Social Advancement; Baha'i Lecturer; contributor of a variety of published articles.

Roy J. Ward, M.S.: Supervisor of rehabilitation teachers, Virginia Commission for the Visually Handicapped. Former home teacher, orientation and mobility specialist and assistant supervisor of training, New York Association for the Blind. Previously teacher, Maryland School for the Blind. Member of National Rehabilitation Association, the American Association of Workers for the Blind, the Eastern Conference of Rehabilitation Teachers, and the Virginia Chapter, American Association of Workers for the Blind; past president of the Eastern Conference of Rehabilitation Teachers; formerly chairman of the Special Interest Group for Rehabilitation Teachers in the American Association for Workers for the Blind, and past member of the Board of Directors of the American Association of Workers for the Blind; presently secretary of the Virginia Chapter, American Association of Workers for the Blind. Coordinator of Low Vision Aids Services, Virginia Commission for the Visually Handicapped.

Russell C. Williams: Chief of Blind Rehabilitation in the Department of Medicine and Surgery, Veterans Administration, Washington, D.C. Formerly in charge of the Veterans Administration, Blind Rehabilitation Center, Hines, Illinois. Former counselor-instructor in the blind rehabilitation program, Army Valley Forge General Hospital. Guest lecturer and consultant in many universities. Mr. Williams holds a D.Hu. degree from Western Michigan University.

Keith C. Wright: Professor, Department of Rehabilitation Counseling, School of Community Services, Virginia Commonwealth University. Former research analyst, West Virginia Division of Vocational Rehabilitation; counselor and research analyst, United States Public Health Service; past president Virginia Rehabilitation Association; past president Virginia Association of Workers for the Blind; coordinator, short-term in-service training institutes in rehabilitation. Contributor of various articles to the professional literature.

This book is dedicated
to our parents

MR. AND MRS. CLIFFORD E. HARDY

Victoria, Virginia

and

MR. AND MRS. JOHN G. CULL

San Angelo, Texas

Preface

Social service and rehabilitation workers employed in the field of work for the blind have long needed comprehensive materials which would be useful to them as professional persons in self-directed study and as textbooks in college courses. The field of work for the blind has had a special need for a collection of works such as those which appear in this book.

The ever-increasing complexity of social and rehabilitation services requires that educational materials be developed. This book is an effort to bring together some of the important information which is necessary for effective social and rehabilitation work. It is not all inclusive but is intended to provide a type of basic pool of information.

Preparation of the papers contained herein was made with careful consideration of the whole field of social and rehabilitation services as these are related to blindness. The various chapters have been designed to help the newly employed professional person explore basic concepts concerning these services.

Without the support, cooperation, and encouragement of the various contributors, the development of the book would have been impossible. We express our special gratitude to each of them who have taken time from various pursuits to prepare the manuscripts.

We owe much to Warren Bledsoe and George Magers of RSA for their continued support and diligent efforts. Special thanks also go to Sharon C. Kelley for her patience and outstanding secretarial work.

RICHARD E. HARDY
JOHN G. CULL

Richmond, Virginia

Contents

PART FOUR
SOCIAL AND EDUCATIONAL SERVICES FOR THE BLIND

SOCIAL AND REHABILITATION SERVICES FOR THE BLIND

Part One
Introduction

1

History and Philosophy of Work for the Blind

Warren Bledsoe

Of late years there has been a great fad of challenging the usefulness of this or that by saying that it is irrelevant. And though a purist about words may demand a specific to which the irrelevant entity is irrelevant, we may as well accept the term as meaning "insignificant, out-of-date, unimportant." Not merely those who are young today, but many great innovators down through the ages have expressed scorn for history in terms like these. Yet sometimes we find that they have sneaked off and read history like thieves in the night, hoping thereby to gain an advantage over the rest of us.

A good rule of the game in all academic pursuits is the disclosure of bias, especially in work which is basically an art based on sciences, rather than a science. This I believe work for the blind to be. In such a realm cold, scientific objectivity is too much to hope for; the most we can expect is an enlightened subjectivity. For the disclosure of my bias, I would like to say that some of my friends tell me I am the victim of what they call the "great man fallacy." In other words, I believe that within limits, human events are shaped by individuals. Approaching the history and philosophy of work for the blind from this angle, I find a procession of men and women in whose lives and work practices have been tried and validated. When they have been especially significant, institutions and laws have evolved from them, sometimes after their originators have passed out of the world. These take root in the minds of new generations, enduring with an effect which may be benign but may also be malignant. Wherefore all of us should hold our pride in leash a little when something we have had a hand in starting shows signs of becoming a social fixture, bearing in mind Bertram Russell's dictum, "It is the fate of radicals to found a new orthodoxy."

There is a stitch of verse by Clarence Day which says:

> When eras die, their legacies
> Are left to strange police.
> Professors in New England guard
> The glory that was Greece.

HISTORY

I would first like to bring before you some word portraits of individuals who in my opinion have had a significant influence on the world's thought and action with respect to blindness. And I am going to take the liberty of selecting lives which on the whole have left a benign residue.

It will give my inventory a little more meaning if we consider the men and women cited as playing certain classic roles in the field of work for the blind (which I have described elsewhere and thereby found durable). Six distinct parts stand out, according to my observation:

1. Status figures or cynosures.
2. Counselors of state.
3. Hewers and haulers, fetchers and carriers.
4. Inventors.
5. Shining examples.
6. Stormy petrels or agitators.

The actions and ideas of people playing these parts account for a great deal of what we know as work for the blind. Someone has told me that this may also be said of other areas. That may be, but I would hazard one great difference: namely, the relative importance of the various functions, if not in the eyes of the world, certainly to those who are intimately familiar with life as it is lived by people without sight.

A simple chart will illustrate human beings performing in the manner described in behalf of blind people. Some are so famous you will undoubtedly be familiar with their careers; others will be introduced to you for the first time, and more will be said of them as our discussion continues.

Status Figure or Cynosure Outside Work For Blind	*Counselor of State on Blindness*	*Doers, Hewers, Haulers, Fetchers, Carriers*	*Inventors*	*Shining Examples*	*Stormy Petrel Agitator for Blind People*
Homer (850 B.C.)				Homer	
Louis IX (St. Louis) (1214-1270)					
John Milton (1608-1674)				John Milton	
Denis Diderot (1713-1781)	Denis Diderot				Denis Diderot
	Valentin Haüy (1745-1822)	Valentin Haüy	Valentin Haüy		
		Louis Braille (1809-1854)	Louis Braille	Louis Braille	Louis Braille
			Thomas Edison (1847-1931)		
Helen Keller (1880-1968)	Helen Keller			Helen Keller	Helen Keller

With this framework in mind, let us go through a listing of worthies in the field of work for the blind. I will not categorize these by the above scheme, but will leave that to you. I will simply give their chronology, their role in specific terms (such as scholar, writer, scientist), and what their contribution has been to work for the blind or the evolving image of blindness.

Miss Mary Switzer has pointed out that one of the most important things she has learned about blindness during her career is the influence of "the visible handicap" of blindness. Nothing before kings and parliaments, presidents and legislatures has ever gotten more mileage than the gifted blind individual. An equally high value should be assigned to the hewers and haulers, fetchers and carriers who give these shining examples the skills with which to shine. Certain individuals play more than one of these roles. One or two seem to have played all six parts. The opening wedge of many programs has been a combination of the status figure and the shining example. But the hewer and hauler, fetcher and carrier role is indispensible.

PERSONS WHOSE LIVES HAVE BEEN SIGNIFICANT WITH RESPECT TO DEVELOPMENT OF WORK FOR THE BLIND OR THE IMAGE OF BLINDNESS

HOMER (originally named Melesigenes) (850 B.C.—?)
Believed to have lost sight as an adult.
Poet.
He was to embed in the consciousness of the civilized world the image of the blind poetic genius, by creating the difficult epic form, which few poets have since mastered. The fact that John Milton, also blind, was one of these poets has led to occasional scholarly comment suggesting that the isolation of blindness, following an active life, acted similarly on the powers of the two poets.

CONFUCIUS (551-479 B.C.)
Sighted.
Teacher, philosopher.
The *Analects* show Confucius carefully guiding his sightless music teacher down a flight of steps, seating him on his mat, and telling him who were present in the room. To a visitor who inquired, "Is it the

rule to tell these things to the music master?" Confucius replied, "This is certainly the rule for those who lead the blind."

DEMOCRITUS (450 B.C.)
Lost sight as an adult.
Philosopher.
He projected the image of the blind intellectual genius in ancient Greece. He had a wide knowledge of the material sciences, mathematics, music and grammar. He advanced the theory that the world was formed by the concourse of atoms, confirmed and developed by recent scientific discovery. His cheerfulness, undisturbed even in blindness, led to his being called the laughing philosopher.

APPIUS CLAUDIUS CAECUS (4th century B.C.)
Blind in early manhood.
Statesman.
In ancient Rome, he demonstrated that a statesman could continue to function after losing his sight. Blinded about the time he was censor in 312 B.C. he was later consul in 307, 298 and 296 B.C. As censor he brought about reforms which gave added privileges to the plebians. A powerful orator and writer, his speech against peace with Pyrrhus is the first in Roman history to have been handed down in writing. He was an author of legal treatises, aphorisms and verse.

DIDYMUS OF ALEXANDRIA (313-398 A.D.)
Blinded at age of five.
Teacher.
Demonstrated to the early Christian church fathers in Alexandria that such subjects as geometry and astronomy could be mastered by a blind person. Also showed that a blind individual could be a great teacher. St. Jerome was his admiring pupil and left a clear cut picture of his learned tutor, who by voracious curiosity and by making the most of sighted readers, became one of the most thoroughly educated men of his time. Living about as long after Christ as the present time is distant from the Reformation, Didymus was the head of the catechetical school supported by the Council of Nicea and the moderator of fierce battles over the creed, his dissertations being considered masterpieces of logic and rhetoric. St. Anthony came out of the wilderness for the purpose of seeing him and attempted to convince him that it was better to have wisdom such as his than eyesight. To this Didymus took acrimonious exception. Most of his books were condemned in partisan religious wars after his death.

HITOYASU, PRINCE OF JAPAN (853)

Lost sight at 28.

Prince, organizer, philanthropist.

When he lost his sight, he established a kind of order for the blind, making them members of his household and dividing his income among them. This was afterwards greatly augmented and given to all the blind in the country. At his death, in his memory, some blind officers were appointed to look after the welfare of the blind throughout the country. The chief officer was appointed in Kyoto, then the capital of Japan, while others were allotted a province each.

LOUIS IX, KING OF FRANCE (St. Louis) (1214-1270)

Sighted.

Monarch, organizer philanthropist.

In 1260, he reorganized and confirmed by letters patent the charity for the care of the blind called the Quinze-Vingts, which is still in existence, having survived a long and turbulent history. As the name implies, it was designed to provide for 300 blind individuals, and according to legend, St. Louis's interest in it stemmed from his concern for men blinded in his crusade. The special privileges granted to the order seem to substantiate this. The conduct of the house lay in the hands of a "master," appointed by the king, and important questions were decided by the chapter in full assembly. Members were permitted to marry and have children. Women were admitted as members. In return for making soup for the poor and performing religious functions daily, important privileges were granted: freedom from taxation, the right to asylum, the right to beg in the churches. The Quinze-Vingts set a pattern for similar orders at Chartres, Tournai and Strasbourg. Others followed outside France at Bruges, Ghent, Padua, Palemo, Hanover, Swansea and London. None equalled the Quinze-Vingts, which in the centuries immediately following its founding enjoyed great prestige. The king attended the church yearly. Famous orators preached in its pulpit. People of consequence flocked to it and endowed it handsomely in recompense for prayers for their souls said by the members. The order became extremely rich and put its roots deep into the Paris community, though in actual fact it was a community for the blind itself, having a number of small businesses, a church, a cemetery and even a fire engine of its own. In 1777 it changed its location in a real estate transaction, which was the beginning of a long, tortuous series of financial difficulties during which the order was the victim first of the unethical schemes of Cardinal de

Rohan and later of the turbulent days of the revolution. During this time the members of the order are said to have come into disrepute, descending through lower forms of begging to cynical burlesquing exhibits of their blindness and to thievery. When France put its house in order, first by the actions of Napoleon and next by the Restoration, the Quinze-Vingts returned to its original purpose of providing for 300 blind individuals.

Luigi Groto (1541-1584)
Totally blind at one week.
Writer, musician, philosopher.
Demonstrated competence in literature and philosophy.

Galileo (1564-1642)
Blinded late in life.
Scientist.
One of the gifted people blinded well along in life, who continued his work and is not thought of as blind.

Prospero Fagnani (1587-1677)
Lost sight at age 44.
Doctor of civil and canon law.
Author of commentaries on canon law, pointing out that there should be no bending of the canon law because of blindness per se, but rather that the effect of blindness in an individual life should be taken into account.

John Milton (1608-1674)
Slow loss of sight in late youth and early middle age.
Epic poet, political pamphleteer.
Demonstrated ability to write with epic sweep after losing sight.

Nicholas Saunderson (1682-1739)
Blinded at one year.
Mathematician, Lucasian professor of mathematics at Cambridge University.
Demonstrated capacity of blind individual to excel among the first mathematicians of the time. Recommended for professorship by Isaac Newton. Devised "palpable arithmetic," a ciphering board, forerunner of mathematical equipment for the blind. Authored algebra textbook.

MARQUISE DU DEFFAND (1697-1780)

Lost sight, probably in late middle age, totally in old age.

Hostess of a salon frequented by the French "enlightenment."

Brought together the French "philosophes," including Diderot, out of whose interest in blindness education of the blind was to grow. Probably focused their attention on blindness, and functioned very well as a blind person herself.

LEONHARD EULER (1707-1783)

Lost sight of one eye at 28, the other at 59.

Mathematician.

Demonstrated to the world ability to function as a mathematician after losing sight. Is credited with evolving the calculus of variations. Some of his most important work done after total loss of sight.

DENIS DIDEROT (1713-1784)

Sighted.

Encyclopedist, philosopher.

Made an in-depth study, based largely on the observation and conversation of one blind man, first published as a "Letter on the Blind" and later a part of his great encyclopedia, which related every subject to the ideals of the French "enlightenment" and Revolution. Diderot anticipated modern thought about blindness with a number of apperceptions: that the senses of the blind are not especially sharpened by the loss of sight, but that the loss of sight compels increased use of the remaining senses; that education ought to be built on what the blind man has rather than on what he has lost; and above all else that he should keep active all possible contacts with the objective world. Diderot also suggested that a deaf-blind individual could be educated. Though virtually the thinking of an "armchair psychologist," Diderot's essay continues as one of the masterpieces of the literature of blindness.

JOHN METCALF (1717-1810)

Lost sight at age six.

Road builder, entrepreneur.

One of the most positive and picturesque contributors to the "image of blindness." Became independently mobile through own determination. Peddler, horse trader. Set up stagecoach service. To improve roads, studied road engineering, bidding successfully for government contracts amounting to 65,000 pounds.

THOMAS BLACKLOCK (1721-1791)

Lost sight at six months.

Scholar, poet, and writer.

Propagandized exposure of blind people to common experiences of life, even though dangerous. Wrote article on blindness which appeared in the *Encyclopedia Britannica* 1783.

JOHN FIELDING (1722-1780)

Blinded by accident at age 19.

Magistrate and police chief.

Demonstrated ability of blind individual to function as a magistrate and administrator. In charge of London police force 1754-80. Made public aware of blind person's ability to recognize a large number of individuals' voices. Knighted in 1761 for services.

VALENTIN HAÜY (1745-1822)

Sighted.

Teacher, propagandist, "counselor of state."

Called "The Father of the Blind"; developed raised letter method of reading, established first school for the blind in the world, "L'Institution Nationale des Jeunes Aveugles"; adviser to old French monarchy, "Societé Philanthropic" of the old regime, The National Assembly of the Revolution, Robespierre, the First Empire (by which he was rejected), Frederick William III of Prussia, Czar Alexander. Spread the idea that blind children could be educated widely in Europe, from which it was spread to other parts of the world.

FRANCOIS HUBER (1750-1831)

Lost sight totally at 16.

Naturalist, apiarist.

Demonstrated ability of blind individual to function as a naturalist. Wrote classic, *New Observations of the Bees.* With his wife and manservant acting as his eyes, he was able to draw revolutionary conclusions regarding the habits of bees; his conclusions gained universal acceptance.

EDWARD RUSHTON (1755-1814)

Lost sight at age of 19, regained it in 1807 as a result of an operation.

Sailor, bookseller publisher.

Was the prime mover in the second school for the blind, opened in 1790 at Liverpool, England. No literary subjects were taught in the beginning; trades were taught to blind children, and they were also taught to sing in churches and play the organ. Rushton himself put before the community a positive image of blindness. A rugged sailor who had a compassionate and grateful temperament, he befriended a Negro shipmate on one occasion, who, when they were both shipwrecked at a later date, sacrificed his own life to save Rushton. On a later voyage in a slaver, when malignant ophthalmia broke out among the slaves in the hold and the officers refused to tend them, he lost his sight in trying to help them. As a blind individual he had a long fight against poverty, but eventually rose to a position of comfort and influence. He advocated all measures of progress and reform: freedom of the slaves, relief for sailors who were seized by the press gang, help for the Irish and sympathy for the French and American Revolutions. He reproved the Americans for slave trading and wrote a letter to George Washington on the subject. A letter circulated by him through the Liverpool Literary and Philosophic Society led to the founding of the Liverpool school.

MARIA THERESA VON PARADIS (1759-1824)

Partially sighted, diagnosis and eye handicap debated. At one time a subject of Mesmer. Indications of hysterical blindness.

Musician, singer, concert performer, teacher.

As a gifted musician and protege of the Empress Maria Theresa of Austria, and as a concert artist, she attracted wide attention through her intelligence and charm. She is often credited with calling the attention of Haüy and others to the potentialities of blind children. Eager to share the devices by which she dealt with blindness, she had extensive conversations with Haüy about such implements as a music board with raised lines to indicate staff, and words spelled out with pins on a pincushion.

JOHANN WILHELM KLEIN (1765-1848)

Sighted.

Educator, author (Before growing interested in education of the blind, he had been an administrator of aid to the poor, serving gratuitously for 23 years; previous to that a lawyer.)

In 1804 founded school for the blind in Vienna on broad educational principles which distinguished the ends of a school from those of a charity. Author of "Description of an Attempt to Educate Blind Children" which had an immense public effect, drawing blind children to his school in large numbers, leading to imperial status and support in 1816. Author of widely used *Teacher's Manual for the Education of the Blind.* He tried to make provision for the education of the blind in schools for the sighted. His careful study of the problems of the blind established the tradition of learning at the imperial school which was to prevail for the entire 19th century and into the 20th. Klein was also the inventor of the Stacheltypenapparat, an apparatus for point writing.

FRANCOIS LESUEUR (1767-?)
Lost sight at six weeks.
None.
The pupil with whom Valentin Haüy experimented in developing a reading method for the blind. Accidentally discovered that he could read engraving with unusually thick lettering. Of average intelligence, he was an excellent subject with whom to demonstrate that blind people can be made literate. He was also the victim of Haüy's failure to realize that education without vocational training and placement avails the blind person little in most cases. Well motivated, he worked hard at the tasks Haüy set for him, but never secured any other means of livelihood, and ended as a pensioner of the Quinze-Vingts.

AUGUST ZEUNE (1778-1853)
Sighted.
Educator, geographer.
Chosen by Valentin Haüy, and recommended to the King of Prussia (Frederick William III) to activate the first German school for the blind at Steglitz, near Berlin. He studied the methods of others with care, in Paris particularly, and, weathering the turbulence of the Napoleonic Wars, established an enduring school over which he presided from 1806 until he died. He is often credited with the most practical working out of Haüy's concept.

JOHANN G. KNIE (1794-1869)
Blinded at age 10.
Educator, author.
Director of School for the Blind at Breslau, the first blind director of such an institution. Graduate of the University of Breslau. At his school, he emphasized the tactile and the practical. His school "a mélange of bells, rattles, drums, models of animals, machines, buildings." Author of "A Guide to the Proper Management of Blind Children," said to have been "gospel reading" in the world of the blind.

SEBASTIAN GUILLE (?-1851)
Sighted.
Educator, physician.
Under the restoration of the Bourbon monarchy in 1815, he became

director of the reconstituted Paris school for blind youth, renamed the Royal Institution for the Blind. Both imaginative and practical, he made exceptional use of student-teachers, and developed the teaching of music to a high degree. Wrote a discerning treatise on the "Instruction and Amusements of the Blind" (1819). However, he was chiefly remembered for having experimented with Braille and rejected it, and for having repudiated Haüy for his compromises with revolutionaries.

W. H. PRESCOTT (1796-1859)

Partially seeing, due to an injury while a junior at Harvard.

Historian.

As an historian of the first rank, had so little use of his eyes that he demonstrated the feasibility of practicing his profession largely by the methods of a blind person, using readers extensively and developing phenomenal use of his memory. Author of the *Conquest of Mexico.* In the 1830's, published unsigned articles on blindness in "The American Review." Thereby helped to shape intellectual thought of the New England Community and prepared it for manipulation by Howe for the advantage of blind people.

SAMUEL GRIDLEY HOWE (1801-1876)

Sighted.

Physician, philospher, administrator, teacher, educator.

By many, thought to have been the strongest influence ever exerted in the field of work for the blind, as well as the most discerning observer of the effects of society's efforts in their behalf. His thought was permeated by an awareness of the hazards of segregating mechanisms. The first director of the Perkins School for the Blind in Massachusetts, he also admitted to having appealed to legislatures to found "a dozen other" schools for the blind; he laid the cornerstone of one with misgivings lest he had perpetrated a system which deprived the blind of social contacts with the seeing. He pioneered the education of the deaf-blind, penetrating the consciousness of Laura Bridgman with a means of communication (the manual alphabet) and keeping exact and elaborate records of his progress and procedures. His exceptional capacity enabled him to make substantial contributions to the alleviation of virtually every salient human disadvantage. Said to have "driven the charities four abreast," he gave his home base, the Perkins School, a unique contact with the progress of the world at large. His basic writings form the classic theory of work for the blind in America, though they still must be searched out in annual reports of the Perkins School. His negative influence lay in a stubborn and dogmatic refusal to abandon raised letters in favor of a dot system.

JOHN DENNISON RUSS (Active 1832-35; Died 1881)
Sighted.
Physician, administrator, teacher.
With Howe of Massachusetts and Friedlander of Pennsylvania, is cited as a pioneering head of schools for the blind in America. Had previously been associated with Howe in Greece, administering relief, but acted independently in 1832 when he initiated the instruction of the blind in America by taking three pupils, and thus began what was to become the New York Institute for the Blind. The director of the school for two years only, he nevertheless devised an arithmetic slate which endured.

JULIUS FRIEDLANDER (1803-1839)
Sighted.
Educator, teacher.
The third of the three pioneering heads of schools for the blind in the United States in the 1830's. He had taught blind children for three years in Germany when in 1833 he took charge of activating a school in Philadelphia, which was subsequently to become the Overbrook School for the Blind. His six years as head of the infant endeavor defined it as an educational institution and mustered the support of the community. He is credited with exceptional moral influence on his pupils, one of whom (William Churchman) was to become the first visually handicapped head of a school for the blind in the United States.

HANNIBAL HAMLYN (1809-1891)
Sighted.
Statesman, Vice-President of United States.
Sponsored first public demonstration of vocational performance of blind people by Francis Campbell in Bangor, Maine.

LOUIS BRAILLE (1809-1854)
Lost sight totally at age three.
Teacher of the blind in music, history, geometry, and algebra.
He gave the world the universally adopted system of dot reading. He credited Major Barbier, a French army intelligence officer, with the invention of a code of raised dots. His own contribution was the six dot arrangement and alphabet which bears his name. In perfecting this, he persisted in the face of enduring opposition from older teach-

ers of the blind committed to raised letters. The braille system was complete by 1834, but obtained no real acceptance until 1854. (See statement by Lewis W. Rodenberg (1893-1967).

EDWARD VON JAEGER (1818-1884)
Sighted.
Scientist.
Produced 20 sizes of reading type which are still used for vision testing at short distances. (For long distances, modern adaptations correlate with those of Snellen.)

WILLIAM CHURCHMAN (1818-1882)
Lost sight totally at age 17.
Teacher, educator.
The first blind head of a school for the blind in the United States, he was the first principal of the Tennessee School for the Blind, and later head of the schools for the blind in Indiana and Wisconsin. Among his first handful of pupils in Tennessee was Francis Campbell, one day to become an outstanding and picturesque educator of blind youth, and who credited much of his success to Churchman's example and tutelage.

WILLIAM MOON (1818-1894)
Lost sight of one eye at four—the other totally at 21.
Philanthropist, inventor.
Originator of a system of tactile reading which bears his name. Designed for the aged and rough-handed, it is the most easily perceived of all embossed type, each letter simplified for easy recognition. Moon used no contractions, nor in any other way demanded sophistication. Allied with religious missionary work, the system was widely popular, and ultimately in use in 419 languages and dialects.

QUEEN VICTORIA OF GREAT BRITAIN (1819-1901)
Slow loss of sight in old age.
Monarch, moral and philanthropic leader.
She insisted that her family should never give their names to causes without also giving money and time. This provided systematic philanthropic leadership to the Royal Normal College year in and year out during her reign, and during that of her successor, King Edward VII.

W. HANKS LEVY (?-1874)
Blinded at an early age.
Social worker, author.
An associate of Elizabeth Gilbert, he assisted her in most of her under-

takings from 1851 until he died. Through him she sounded out the blind beggars of London to decide whether it was feasible to establish a work program. He was manager of her workshop (known as "The Repository"). A hard worker, largely self-taught, it was his deep conviction that the blind must work alone and that the seeing knew nothing of their problems. Both were opposed to all forms of charity and committed to the idea that blind people could and must work. With Miss Gilbert's help, Levy wrote a discerning book, *Blindness and the Blind.*

FANNY CROSBY (1820-1915)
Lost sight totally at six weeks.
Hymn writer, teacher.
One of the most widely known and popular hymn writers of the 19th century evangelical revivals. As a pupil and teacher at the New York Institute, she drew unusual attention to herself by a phenomenal memory coupled with personal magnetism. At the age of 45, wrote her hymn, "Safe in the Arms of Jesus," the first of many similar hymns which brought her great popularity and increased an already wide circle of friends, including prominent and influential people, to whom she became the image of blindness.

THOMAS RHODES ARMITAGE (1824-1890)
Slowly lost sight as an adult.
Physician specializing in ophthalmology, author, philanthropist.
The key figure in middle and late 19th century progress in work for the blind in Great Britain. A rare diplomat in behalf of the blind, he spent his life and his fortune on promotion of various kinds of educational and rehabilitation programs. He sponsored the British and Foreign Association for the Blind in 1868. Also was the link between the rich and powerful British establishment and the American innovations of Francis Campbell which strongly influenced concepts of work for the blind through first British and then American philanthropy.

HUGH LUPUS, DUKE OF WESTMINSTER (1825-1899)
Sighted.
Hereditary manager of wealth, peer of Great Britain.
Financial sponsor of the Royal Normal College for the Blind and its patronage by the British Establishment. The personal link between Campbell as an entrepreneur and Queen Victoria's family.

Elizabeth Gilbert (1826-1885)

Blinded totally in infancy.

Philanthropist, social worker, publicist.

An extremely gifted individual, daughter of an English bishop, she used her social connections to call attention to the need for blind people to have the dignity of work. First having mastered skills herself (jointly with W. Hanks Levy), she studied the crafts which seemed feasible for blind people, initiated work in the home and later a workshop which furnished blind people opportunities to earn through handwork. Baskets and brooms, then not regarded as a stereotype of blindness, were two major products. She secured Royal and Parliamentary backing for her undertakings and started the Association for Promoting the General Welfare of the Blind in 1855. She attempted to get mention of the blind into the Education Act of 1870, thereby calling attention to the needs of blind children, and paving the way for their admission to schools for the seeing in the 1890's.

Mary Caroline Greene (1829-1908)

Sighted.

Teacher.

In 1879 was chosen to superintend the education of blind children in schools with the seeing in London. From 1864 to 1872, she had taught at Perkins; from 1872 to 1879, at the Royal Normal College for the Blind outside London. Her experiment with educating the blind in schools for the seeing flourished in her time. In 1901, with the help of 12 young blind women whom she supervised, 200 children were attending schools for the seeing despite their visual handicap.

Laura Bridgman (1829-1889)

Blind and deaf from her third year.

Subject of an educational experiment.

The first totally blind and deaf individual to emerge as a full-fledged member of the human family with a means of communication (the manual alphabet), skill in self-management for common social functions, strong personal affections, moral sense, and a realistic awareness of the world. With Howe as her teacher at Perkins, she attracted wide attention and was graphically described by Charles Dickens in his *American Notes.* It was through this book that the family of Helen Keller became aware of the potentialities of a deaf-blind child and made contact with the Perkins School. Though Miss Bridgman made visits to her family, she never effectively returned to the community outside Perkins, where she remained as an example, with appropriate routines of activity.

SIR FRANCIS JOSEPH CAMPBELL LL.D.Kt. (1832-1914)
Lost sight at five years due to accident.
Teacher, educator, musician.

The character and personality on which modern work for the blind hinged. After Howe, he was the undoubted champion of the capabilities of blind people, both by his own example, his demands on himself and what he asked of other blind people and society. As a boy on a Tennessee farm, when relegated to inactivity by his father, he got hold of an axe in the absence of his family, and, when they returned, presented them with a stack of kindling. At the Tennessee School for the Blind, when diagnosed as lacking musical aptitude, he paid another pupil to give him lessons surreptitiously, eventually astonishing his teacher with his performance in piano exercises, the beginning of his distinguished career in which the teaching of music was to figure prominently. Also while at the Tennessee School for the Blind he procured the dismissal of its principal for supplying the students with pauper fare while living off the fat of the land himself. Few blind men have overcome the pity of the community to the point of being threatened with lynching, but Campbell achieved this by teaching a sighted Negro to read during the turbulent period preceding the Civil War. An impassioned abolitionist, he left Tennessee, first for Wisconsin, then for Boston where Howe's young Perkins School was flourishing. Campbell arrested Howe's attention by telling him the Perkins School was not making the blind truly independent. This led to an 11-year experiment with Campbell in full charge of a selected group of 20 children to be trained as musicians. The project was based on Campbell's theory that competence in music was related to competence in mathematics. Nineteen of the twenty subjects were afterwards gainfully employed, but their employment was the beginning of a difference between Howe and Campbell. Campbell insisted that a condition for their success was a placement program, and when Howe held that this would prolong the graduate's dependence, Campbell sought the patronage of Vice-President Hamlyn over Howe's head. In other ways his success and temperament had contributed to divisiveness at Perkins, and Howe resorted to giving him a leave of absence for advanced music study in Berlin. From this study, Campbell never returned permanently to the United States. Stopping in Britain on the way home, he captured the imagination first of Dr. T. R. Armitage, then of the Duke of Westminster and Queen Victoria, who opened the way to the establishment of a school according to his principles and design. This became the Royal Normal College and Academy of Music for the Blind at Upper Norwood, a suburb of London. This "college" was founded with British capital and American teachers, 44 of whom crossed the Atlantic in relays, many of them generously loaned by Howe, who never lost faith in Campbell's personal capability as a teacher and galvanizer of blind youth, though he termed the Royal Normal College an "exotic," and was cool toward Campbell in his last years. Campbell thought of the Royal Normal College as a temporary assignment to demonstrate a method of training teachers, intending after it took root to return to the United States. But it absorbed the rest of his life and in its time was the fountainhead of progress in education and rehabilitation of the blind. Its patterns of theory and practice were to recross the Atlantic in the person of Campbell's son, Charles, in the early 1900's when American work for the blind stood in need of renaissance. One of Campbell's major contributions was to assume responsibility for the employment of his graduates, 80 percent of whom were said to have been gainfully employed. He was also a past master at obtaining support for his program from people of standing. This he did on his own terms. One of his star pupils was Prince Alexander of Hesse, who on applying for admission was told he must give up his valet and wait on himself. Campbell had the enduring good will of Queen Victoria's family, as well as republican-minded Britons. As an old man he was reluctantly persuaded to be naturalized as a British subject, in order to be knighted. It was represented to him that this honor would crystallize his achievements as a blind person in the minds of the public as well as his colleagues. This proved to be the case. Even the most democratic-minded of his contemporaries in the field of work for the blind felt pride in the redoubtable old "Sir Francis." He died with the era in which he lived in June 1914 within a few days of the assassination which precipitated World War I. An international conference of blindness, which had just been terminated in London, had engulfed him with assurance that his dynamic example had infected his fellow workers for the blind.

STEPHEN BABCOCK (1832-1916)

An eye accident at 16, lost sight totally at 19.

Teacher.

Produced the Babcock system of mental arithmetic, which was to become a part of the curriculum of residential schools with high standards, and in certain respects resembling the "new math" of the present time. Babcock also designed the first dissected raised maps. Was teacher at New York Institute for the Blind from 1855 till 1904 (Principal-teacher from 1857). With William Wait, he designed an arithmetic slate which was to have universal acceptance.

HENRY FAWCETT (1833-1884)
Blinded at age 25.
Political economist, member of Parliament, administrator.
Demonstrated effectiveness as an administrator. Postmaster General of England. Originated parcel post and postal money orders. He identified with the cause of blind people, supported the work of Francis Campbell and worked for the appointment of a royal commission to study blindness, which was appointed after his death and which led to an act passed in 1889 which made education of the blind compulsory.

HERMAN SNELLEN (1834-1908)
Sighted.
Ophthalmologist.
His Snellen eye chart, which made practical application of the brilliant formulas of Dr. Cornelius Donders which separated errors of refraction from those of accommodation. Dr. Donders' formulas were said to use every symbol in the Greek alphabet, and it was from these that Snellen developed a practical way to determine not only a patient's visual acuity, but also to find corrective lenses to compensate for refractive errors. The chart which he developed for this purpose became the basic instrument for fitting glasses all over the world.

BENJAMIN F. HUNTOON (1836-1919)
Sighted.
Educator, inventor, publisher.
As superintendent of the Kentucky School for the Blind and the American Printing House for the Blind, he was a unique practical worker in both education and publishing as well as a potent diplomat between them and also with the public and Congress. Was designer not only of the administration of the American Printing House for the Blind, but inventor of many mechanisms for the production of embossed books. Devised the first cylinder embossing press. In 1879 he helped to secure legislation which provided the first federal appropriation for the Printing House, and continued to govern the growth of such appropriations until his death.

Michael Anagnos (1837-1906)

Sighted.

Teacher, educator.

Succeeded his father-in-law, Howe, as director of the Perkins School. A consolidator of gains, he was said to be the greatest money collector for blind people of his own, or any, time. For the lower school at Perkins, called in its time, the kindergarten, he amassed one million dollars. A native of Greece, he was a picturesque figure, an arresting conversationalist. He put his personality fully into the promotion of Perkins. His unusual rapport with small children was exceptionally warm, and he did not hesitate to use it in bringing their cause before the public. His most dramatic feat as an educator was choosing Anne Sullivan to be the teacher of Helen Keller and instructing Anne Sullivan in how to go about her task, based on the notes of Dr. Howe with respect to Laura Bridgman.

Joel W. Smith (1837-1924)

Blinded by accident at the age of 25.

Teacher of piano tuning.

Contrived many devices to overcome handicap of blindness, including the first braille "typewriter." One of the American teachers "loaned" by Howe from Perkins to aid in the founding of the Royal Normal College. Said to be the first to teach the "touch" system of typewriting, which he developed for his blind students. A teacher at Perkins for 30 years. He developed "American braille." Also was founder of the first magazine in the United States devoted to the interests of the blind (1891-1894). A charter member of the American Association of Workers for the Blind.

David Duffle Wood (1838-1910)

Blinded as a child, totally by the age of four.

Musician, teacher.

A preeminent organist, he was director of music at the School for the Blind in Philadelphia, now called Overbrook. As an accomplished concert performer, he gave a positive image of blindness; in his teaching he brought his pupils to a high degree of perfection in performance of oratorios of Handel, Haydn, Mendelssohn. A close contemporary of Sir Francis Campbell, he strongly contrasted with him both in personality and experience. Enrolled as a pupil in the Philadelphia School, Wood grew up with it, spending all his life in that environment, backed by the stable community of Philadelphia. Like Sir Francis Campbell he was a brilliant mathematician, but unlike him he was a natural and inspired musical artist. He had better teachers and was in a more sophisticated musical setting; he did not have to fight to master music by sheer force of intellect and determination as Campbell did. Campbell charmed important segments of society as a fascinating zealot and rebel in behalf of the blind. Wood enchanted them with pure music. The last time he played, by an improvisation, he caused a lady taking communion to think of the pipes of Pan in Mrs. Browning's lines:

> Blinding sweet, O great God Pan!
> The sun on the hill forgot to die,
> And the lilies revived and the dragon-fly
> Came back to dream by the river.

He was given an honorary doctorate of music by Temple University.

William Wait (1839-1916)
Sighted.
Educator, inventor.

Principal of the New York Institute for the Blind (1863-1905), he raised the standards of the school from asylum level to those of schools for the sighted in New York State. Wait was the redoubtable protagonist for a raised dot system known as New York Point, which is still regarded by many authorities as more scientific than braille. Only two dots vertically, it could be extended in base forms of two, four, six, eight dots. It also took into account the frequency with which letters occur, using simpler forms for most frequently encountered letters. It was pitted against braille in many battles between educators of the blind. Many books were printed in it. But it was ultimately defeated by braille in the Uniform Type Conference of 1917.

Emile Javal (1839-1907)
Blinded late in life.
Ophthalmologist.

Author of an unusually perceptive book on the problems of the newly blinded entitled, *On Becoming Blind.*

Mathilda Ziegler (1841-1932)
Sighted.
Philanthropist.

Paid for the publication of a free magazine *(The Mathilda Ziegler Magazine)* in braille and New York Point type from 1907 till 1929, at which time she endowed it with $600,000. Distributed free to 15,000 readers, it has been an enduring standby for information, inspiration and entertainment, especially in the years before aural media were so pervasive. It continues to enjoy popularity.

FRANK H. HALL (1841-1911)
Sighted.
Teacher, educator, inventor.
The inventor of the Hall braille writer, sterotypemaker and mapmaker, he used two relatively short terms as superintendent of the Illinois School for the Blind (1890-93) and (1897-1902) to study techniques of educating blind children and produce instruments which were to gain wide acceptance. He was also innovative with respect to curriculum, making revisions to fuse the "literary" and the "practical." Among those who early favored the education of blind children in public schools, he furnished the Chicago public schools with a plan for organizing such a program, which was used when the first class of this type was inaugurated in Chicago in 1900. A political appointee, in and out at the pleasure of incumbent governors, he acquired great enthusiasm for the cause of blind people, and made the most of a checkered, but rich, background in behalf of his pupils.

SOPHIA FAULKNER (Lady Francis Campbell) (1848-1933)
Sighted.
Teacher, social leader.
One of the Perkins staff, "loaned" to the Royal Normal College. An excellent teacher and intrepid intellectual, upon her marriage to Francis Campbell she turned her talents to creating and governing the social environment of the Royal Normal College for the Blind. Exceptionally perceptive with respect to the social disadvantages of blind people, she contrived for the people surrounding her an atmosphere in which all sorts of people who passed through it were able to feel at ease with blind people. Based on many years of experience with those she had helped, she wrote a treatise on the subject *(Outlook for the Blind, 1911).* She also authored essays documenting the development of the Royal Normal College for the Blind and the philanthropic work for the blind of Great Britain.

ALEXANDER MELL (1850-1931)
Sighted.
Teacher, educator, encyclopedist.
The author of the only encyclopedia concerning blindness so far published, *Encyklopadisches Handbuch des Blindenwesens,* a work of almost 1,000 pages, published in 1900. Mell was for half a century the central figure in work for the blind in Austria. As director of the

then Imperial-Royal Institution for the Education of the Blind in Vienna from the year 1886, he took over the school and began his administration with vigorous reorganization. Later he became the originator of a movement for special training of teachers of the blind in Austria in 1889 (with a ten weeks' summer course.) He foresaw the possibilities of introducing courses on blindness in the general pedagogical courses and attempted to have such training introduced to normal schools, though without success. His most notable achievement beside his encyclopedia was the organization and expansion of the professional library of his school, which served as an inspiration to development of a similar collection by Michael Anagnos at the Perkins School. Acting upon a standing order, Mell made double purchases routinely, the second item coming to America and helping to form a considerable part of the unique Perkins collection.

AMBROSE M. SHOTWELL (1853-1930)
Partially seeing from infancy, slow loss to near total as an adult.
Teacher, organizer benign "agitator," librarian.

Was key leader in organization of blind people to make known their problems and needs, according to their experience and point of view with respect to services offered them by society. One of the founders of the American Blind Peoples' Higher Improvement Association in 1895, which was converted into the American Association of Workers for the Blind in 1905. He functioned at many levels in work for the blind, was an expert on braille, operated a sterotype machine himself, functioning for many years at the "Saginaw Center" for which he had lobbied in the Michigan legislature. In Wisconsin, he had pressed for a school for the blind separate from the school for the deaf, but was excluded from the institution resulting therefrom. An idea ahead of its time which he especially cherished was subsidized higher education for the blind, a bill for which he succeeded in having introduced to the U. S. Congress in 1902 but which failed to pass. Later, he favored "outdoor relief" or pensions for certain groups of blind individuals, for which ideas he was branded a radical. However, his ultimate standing in the field is indicated by the Ambrose M. Shotwell Award (conferred by the American Association of Workers for the Blind).

F. PARK LEWIS, M.D. (1855-1940)
Sighted.
Ophthalmologist.

Prime mover in prevention of blindness movement in the United States. In 1903 and 1906 he chaired commissions in New York State to investigate blindness and its prevention. Reports of these commissions led to the formation of the New York State Committee for the Prevention of Blindness, from which emerged the National Society for Prevention of Blindness. He was credited with having played the leading role in securing legislation requiring the use of a silver nitrate solution in babies' eyes at birth in order to eliminate the danger of infection from ophthalmia neonatorum. His interest in prevention of blindness was motivated by his association with the New York School for the Blind at Batavia of which he was a board member for 47 years and president for 40 years until his death. This interest extended beyond medical knowledge, and in addition to writing a large number of medical articles, he translated from the French, Maurice de La Sizeranne's *The Blind as Seen through Blind Eyes.*

HANNAH A. BABCOCK (185?-1931)
Sighted.
Teacher, hostess.

The niece of William B. Wait and also of Stephen Babcock, she was a teacher of music at the New York Institute for the Blind for 30 years from 1872. She developed a system of musical notation in New York Point type and oversaw the transcription of a vast quantity of compositions which she was able to make useful as one of the ablest teachers of her day. Of equal importance was the role she played in the social training of the pupils at the New York Institute, which was similar to that of Lady Campbell at the Royal Normal College for the Blind. Her warmth and grace were said to be infectious and pervasive, dominating the environment without overwhelming the people she undertook to influence. Part of her success was due to her own interest in civic and public questions, which brought the world outside into the school.

MAURICE DE LA SIZERANNE (1857-1924)
Blinded by accident at the age of 11.
Editor, author, propagandist, organizer.

One of the ablest propagandists for the blind of his own (or any other) time. With a background of wealth and prestige, when he lost his sight he was sent to the school for the blind in Paris, where he was thrown with all classes of pupils. This resulted in his developing a keen awareness of the limitations of work for the blind at the time, especially what was available for the artisan class. He founded the Association Valentin Haüy, which, in addition to other activities, established workshops for the blind. He also established the magazine called the *Louis Braille,* and authored a book entitled *The Blind as Seen through Blind Eyes* (translated into English by Dr. F. Park Lewis.) In addition to his interest in the working class blind of France La Sizeranne promoted the interests of blind musicians and teachers, already intrenched through earlier work for the blind. The Association Valentin Haüy developed a large library of braille books, and embarked on a variety of other activities, even including legal services for the blind.

WILLIAM A. HADLEY (1860-1941)
Sighted.
Educator, teacher.
Founder in 1922 of the Hadley Correspondence School for the Blind at Winnetka, Illinois, which he headed until his retirement in 1936. A unique institution, it was founded on the supposition that "blind people might welcome an opportunity to devote leisure hours to cultural pursuits." It was to serve thousands of blind individuals and offer a wide variety of courses on a number of subjects.

WALTER G. HOLMES (1862-1946)
Sighted.
Editor.
He suggested to Mathilda Ziegler the establishment of the *Mathilda Ziegler Magazine,* and as its editor for 39 years, became the most popular sighted friend of the blind of his time. Having made a success of a career in journalism he set himself the task of editing a publication which would fill in a measure the needs of all the reading blind people of the United States and Canada. Stories, scientific articles, general information material were all aimed at the "average" blind individual in modest circumstances, but had a quality which earned the respect of the gifted blind person as well. Tributes to him upon his death clearly demonstrate that a high grade of diplomacy is a prime factor in giving service to blind people. *(Outlook for the Blind, March, 1946.)*

PRINCE ALEXANDER, LANDGRAF OF HESSE-CASSEL (1863-1945)
Partially seeing in early youth, slowly lost sight in later life.
Musician.
An extremely gifted musician, he attended the Royal Normal College for the Blind shortly after it was founded, submitted to the regime prescribed for him by Francis Campbell (the first item of which was dispensing with his valet) and became in certain respects Campbell's

primary exhibit. Closely related to the monarchs of Great Britian, Russia, Denmark, Germany and Greece, he undoubtedly influenced them toward a positive image of blindness at a time when even those who had little political influence were powerful in directing philanthropic enterprises. He was an accomplished pianist, organist, and composer, and even on occasion conducted a symphony orchestra. His house in Hamburg was a resort for musicians and music lovers.

EDWARD J. NOLAN (1864-1939)
Blinded in childhood.
Lawyer, organizer.
As a blind leader of the blind, capable and well-educated, he used inherited wealth to promote their welfare. In 1895 he was a moving force in establishing the Illinois Industrial Home for the Blind; in 1896, the American Blind People's Higher Education and Improvement Association, which in 1905 became the American Association of Workers for the Blind. From 1907 till 1917 he was a member of the Uniform Type Committee. He had also promoted the first library of embossed books outside a residential school, which in time led to the creation of the Chicago Public Library's Department for the Blind. He was the prime organizer of the Social and Mutual Advancement Association of the Blind of Chicago in 1900, one of the first social agencies anywhere in the world to be formed of, for and by the blind themselves. Through him this organization sponsored the first law for blind relief in the state of Illinois.

ALFRED HOLLINS (1866-1942)
Blind from birth.
Organist.
A pupil of Francis Campbell, he became one of the greatest organists of his time, toured the world giving recitals. His memoirs, *A Blind Musician Looks Back,* are a detailed description of his education and career, describing the problems of musical education without sight and giving candid estimates of the possibilities of musical careers for blind people.

SIR ARTHUR PEARSON, BART (1866-1921)
Lost sight as an adult.
Newspaper man and organizer.
Before losing sight, a successful newspaper and magazine publisher. In 1914, he became Chairman of the National Institute for the Blind, Great Britain; in that same year, planned and organized what was

later known as St. Dunstan's Hostel for servicemen blinded in the Great War. From this institution his influence spread to various parts of the British empire. As in other war blind programs, the newly blinded military men redirected attention to the basic training required when adults lose sight. Pearson's influence and methods gave equal emphasis to morale building and the practical in an unusually astute combination, giving life to the undoubtedly valid and well-publicized "St. Dunstan's Spirit," which was synonomous with a courageous and affirmative approach to blindness.

ANNE SULLIVAN MACY (1866-1937)
Very limited partial sight.
Teacher.
The teacher of Helen Keller. Under the guidance of Michael Anagnos, who studied Perkins records concerning Laura Bridgman, Anne Sullivan performed her well-known feat of teaching spoken communication to Helen Keller, the first and most publicized accomplishment of its kind. From the dynamic personality which she thus enabled to function, she was never able wholly to liberate herself, remaining a large part of her life in association with Helen Keller, whose achievements she had constantly to deny were actually hers, and who proved she could function brilliantly without Anne Sullivan Macy when death finally separated them. Undoubtedly one of the greatest teachers of her time though her methods were unorthodox, she was not actually an intellectual but had the satisfaction of seeing her deaf-blind pupil excel in levels of achievement to which she did not aspire.

MOSES CHARLES MIGEL (1866-1958)
Sighted.
Business man, financier, philanthropist and executive.
Mainstay financially of the American Foundation for the Blind. Undoubtedly the most practical and generous American philanthropist to work for the blind, his interest in blind people was thoroughgoing and ubiquitous, implemented by the foundation from its establishment in 1921. As a young man he was a regular reader to groups of blind people, and continued all his life to show a personal skill in his relationships with those he encountered. An accomplished lobbyist, he had a hand in the passage of almost every law passed by the Federal Government to help blind people in the first half of this century. The New York Commission for the Blind came into existence through his

influence; but, more than that, when no money was appropriated to activate it, he paid the salary for the staff the first year. Similarly he financed the meeting which led to the establishment of the international braille system, including the World Conference in 1931.

EDWARD E. ALLEN (1867-1950)
Sighted.
Educator, teacher, writer.
The most scholarly of the third generation of educators of the blind in the United States, his writing must be relied on for both the philosophy and history of education in his time, his most enduring contribution as a writer having been his survey of schools for the blind in Europe, published in the *Outlook for the Blind* in 1910. One of the Perkins teachers, who had had previous training as a novice under the tutelage of Francis Campbell, he became head of the Overbrook School for the Blind at an early age and became its renovator, both physically and academically. From there he returned to Perkins as its third director, succeeding Michael Anagnos, who had left the institution in excellent financial condition, but in need of a change of neighborhood and new architecture. Allen made the most of this opportunity to create the present school at Watertown. Like Anagnos, he made the professional library his particular responsibility. This went hand in hand with his training of teachers, leading to the establishment of the so-called "Harvard Class" in 1920. He was also a promoter of sight-saving classes in public schools.

FLORENCE W. BIRCHARD (1867-1950)
Sighted.
Placement specialist.
Single-hearted determination to place blind people in employment, starting in 1899 and continuing for 50 years. Indefatigable, she once placed a retarded blind girl 12 times before she was satisfactorily employed. She worked in the Massachusetts Commission for the Blind after it was established, but her pioneering efforts antedated it.

JOHN FRANCIS BLEDSOE (1869-1946)
Sighted.
Teacher, educator.
The first to reorganize and rebuild an institution-type school for the blind as an all cottage-family plan school, completed in 1911. Superintendent of the Maryland School for the Blind, 1906-1941. Strongly

opposed to the exploitation of blindness through emotional appeal, he was considered by many the perfect pattern of an educator of blind youth.

THOMAS S. MCALONEY (1869-1932)
Sighted.
Educator, teacher.
One of the few successful administrators of a dual school (blind and deaf). A member of the first national efficiency committee, which undertook to introduce modern concepts of administration in schools for the blind. Chaired the Committee on Uniform Type of the American Association of Instructors of the Blind which adopted uniform type for the United States.

WINIFRED HOLT MATHER (1870-1945)
Sighted.
Philanthropist.
Variegated international action in behalf of the blind. The originator of the "Lighthouse for the Blind" concept, she was one of the most colorful figures of her time. The daughter of Henry Holt, the publisher, she used her inherited wealth to publicize the cause of blind people, and her unusual social and linguistic agility to make personal contact with influential people throughout the world. The heterogeneity of the people she tapped may be illustrated by the fact that they included President Taft, Mussolini, and France's much beloved wizard ambassador to the United States, M. Jusserand, whom she persuaded to allow her to go to France during World War 1 in behalf of the blind. Her base was the New York Lighthouse for the Blind, which she founded in 1905, hoping the term *lighthouse* would spread and promote a positive image of blindness. Her extremely sanguine cast of thought would have been incapable of seeing latter-day sophisticated objections to the word. Unquestionably a masterful lady bountiful, she was nonetheless extremely popular with the blind people who frequented the New York Lighthouse, now the New York Association for the Blind, and a flourishing agency.

COBRUN L. BROUN (1870-1943)
Blinded as an adult.
Placement specialist.
A pioneer in the vending stand movement, 100 of which he opened up in New York, as an employee of the New York Commission for the

Blind. He also persuaded the New York civil services commission to employ blind dictaphone operators.

CLARENCE HAWKES (1870-1954)

Lost his sight at 13.

Naturalist, author.

Author of *Hitting the Dark Trail, The Light That Never Failed* and 52 other books, he lectured on the Chautauqua circuit for 25 years, putting the image of capability before audiences, both with an affirmative point of view and competent and exact knowledge of nature study.

WINIFRED HATHAWAY (1870-1954)

Sighted.

Educator, publicist.

With Dr. F. Park Lewis, an indefatigable campaigner for prevention of blindness. A highly educated woman, she abandoned a university teaching career in history at the age of 36 to become a member of the staff of the National Society for Prevention of Blindness. She was Associate Director for 24 years, during which time she traveled widely in Europe, the United States and Canada surveying facilities and assisting educators. She initiated the Society's campaign for professional education. She was the author of *Education and Health of the Partially Seeing* and *American Standard Practice for School Lighting.*

JOHN B. CURTIS (1871-1951)

Lost sight at age of 10.

Teacher, educator.

With Frank Hall, was implementer of public school education for the blind in Chicago in 1900. From 1897 to 1900, a high school teacher in the Illinois School for the Blind. He was then put in charge of classes in public school by the Chicago Board of Education. The procedure which he worked out was copied, almost without change, by other cities of the country which adopted the day school plan of educating blind children. The Curtis plan was also followed in 1913 when so-called sight-saving classes for partially seeing children were started. An authority on braille as used in educational textbooks, he was one of the American representatives on the Commission on Mathematical and Chemical Notation for the International Conference on the Blind for 1933 in Europe, and author of *Braille Mathematical Notation.* Invented and put into use the plastic braille number slate and plastic number cubes.

Wilhelmina Dranga Campbell (1871-1911)

Sighted.

Art teacher, editor.

As co-editor of the *Outlook for the Blind,* she was (1970-11) credited with the technical excellence of its beginnings, implementing the concepts of the editor, Charles Campbell, the son of Sir Francis Campbell. She was also active in various other phases of her husband's multiple endeavors for blind people, especially in promoting quality production in blind-made products, which she insisted must not "look blind" and must meet the standards of good taste current at the time. Exhibits of weaving resulting therefrom attracted wide attention at the Jamestown Exposition. Her influence was such that her early death produced a seriously depressing effect on morale in the field of work for the blind.

Thomas P. Gore (1871-1938)

Lost sight totally in early childhood.

Legislator.

The first blind man to become a United States senator, "with a bright mind, a ready wit and a remarkably retentive memory" which enabled him to digest the details of legislation as they were being read to him, he projected a positive image of blindness in the Senate during his three terms. He sponsored much legislation dealing with farm credits and Indian affairs.

Henry Randolph Latimer (1871-1944)

Slow loss of sight ending in total blindness as an adult.

Teacher, educator, rehabilitation administrator.

A passionate and constant searcher for right ways of educating blind children and placing young adults in gainful employment which made full use of their intellectual potential. For 30 years a teacher at the Maryland School for the Blind, he transferred into the adult field in Pennsylvania. As one of the third generation of workers for the blind in the United States, he suffered the disenchantment of the time with respect to results obtained from residential school education of that day. The adult programs he developed emphasized special, individual remedial training. He was especially interested in tutoring high school students to enter college, took great pride in the fact that one of his blind pupils became a tutor herself and prepared 200 other blind pupils to enter college. Latimer took a leading role in establishing the AAWB and the American Foundation for the Blind.

JESSICA LANGWORTH (1872-1938)
Sighted.
Teacher and teacher of teachers.
She taught at Perkins for 44 years, during World War I becoming the "Boys' Principal." The type of teacher who could "teach any high school subject," she was chosen by Dr. Edward Allen to be "tutorial guide" to the Harvard Class of teacher training which was established at Perkins in 1925. She continued in this role until 1936, an exacting but beloved martinet.

LYDIA Y. HAYES (1872-1943)
Blinded totally by accident as a child.
Teacher, administrator.
Educated at Perkins. As a novice, taught seeing children. She was then a pioneer of the home teaching movement for blind adults as a volunteer in the 1890's. In 1900 was chosen to be the first official home teacher supported by the state of Massachusetts. In 1909 was chosen by the state of New Jersey to organize the N. J. Commission for the Blind. Continued until 1937, when she became educational consultant, prior to retirement in 1942. Julia Ward Howe charged her to "establish the rights of the blind" in New Jersey, and her administration was shaped to emphasize these rights which she defined as the right to "health, to an education, and to an opportunity to serve." She also emphasized the obligations of blind people toward society. Her policy was conspicuous for its nondependence on an institutional program. This included a scheme of braille classes in public schools which she assiduously fostered. She gave strong emphasis to a program of prevention of blindness.

NEWELL PERRY, PH.D. (1873-1961)
Blinded at the age of 10.
Teacher, lobbyist, organizer.
One of the most brilliant blind people of his time, he made of his own education a cause célèbre, agitating for a college education first for himself, then for other blind individuals. At 10 newly blinded and fatherless, he hitchhiked his way to the California School for the Blind, from which institution he was admitted to the University of California; he later got a Ph.D. at Munich, *summa cum laude,* in 1901. Meanwhile he had organized the alumni of the California School for the Blind with three aims: college education of the blind, aid to the needy blind, and work for those able to work. He traveled extensively to study conditions in the lives of blind people. A brilliant tutor,

he coached sighted students to earn his way through Germany, Austria, Switzerland, Italy and France, finally settling in New York, where he established himself with a clientele of private pupils. He took the cause of blind students to Charles Evans Hughes, then governor-elect of New York, and was able thereby to secure a law to appropriate money to secure readers for blind college students. In 1912 he returned to California where he became head teacher at the California School for the Blind and spent the next 36 years up to his retirement preparing blind boys and girls for college.

CAROLINE O'DAY (1875-1943)

Sighted.

Artist, social worker, legislator.

Introduced in the House of Representatives the bill which became the Wagner-O'Day Act, 1938. (See contribution of Robert F. Wagner for specifics.)

SAMUEL P. HAYES, PH.D. (1875-1958)

Sighted.

Psychologist.

A lifelong student of psychology related to blindness, he was the first formally trained psychologist to produce a long series of studies and monographs. These he summed up in 1941 in a book entitled *Contributions to Psychology of Blindness.* This put into permanent form a wealth of material which serves as a point of departure for students. His method was first to give literature of opinion, and then to follow it with what had been proved by experimentation. All his studies sustained the theory that compensation for loss of sight was not a gift but a reward of effort. He was particularly concerned with the administration and interpretation of intelligence tests for blind children, and wrote many articles on the subject for encyclopedias and professional journals. His adaptation of the Stanford-Binet test as an intelligence test for the blind was widely accepted in schools for the blind. From 1909 till 1940 he was a professor of psychology at Mt. Holyoke College; for the next 14 years he was director of teacher training and research at the Perkins School for the Blind. His doctor's degree was from Cornell University. A graduate of Amherst College, he also had a bachelor of divinity degree from Union College and an M.A. in sociology from Columbia (1902). He was a perfectly agreeable but altogether firm intellectual watchdog, religiously devoted to keeping pseudoscience away from the premises of education of the blind.

MORRIS SHEPPARD (1875-1941)

Sighted.

Legislator.

Sponsored in the U.S. Senate the Randolph-Sheppard Act, jointly with Senator Jennings Randolph, then sponsored the act in the House of Representatives. (See Senator Randolph.)

CHARLES F. F. CAMPBELL (1876-1935)

Sighted.

Educator and publicist.

Brought back to the United States the concepts of his father Francis Campbell, specifically the expectation that blind people could be genuine, rather than fictional, participants in economic and social life of communities. The child of the Royal Normal College in its heyday, he saw Queen Victoria as "a kind old grandmother," and the British Establishment as a fountain of resources for the blind. He was sent to the United States to be educated at the Massachusetts Institute of Technology (and for renewal of his family's political philosophy). This was a brief sojourn outside work for the blind, after which he was to be its catalyst for three decades, starting out as a "lantern slide lecturer," who captivated audiences in Massachusetts with a lecture on the capabilities of blind people. His persuasiveness led to the establishment in 1904 of an "experiment station" to train and place blind workers in industry, and of the Massachusetts Commission for the Blind in 1906, which he served as a member of its council and as superintendent of industries. He successfully encouraged the underwriting by the commission of a professional journal, which became the *Outlook for the Blind;* he edited this without remnueration for 15 years, assisted by his wife. From 1910 until 1923 he worked in Pennsylvania, Ohio (as superintendent of the Ohio School for the Blind) and in the World War I war blind program. Increasingly he became the promoter of a national organization for the blind on the platform with Helen Keller, who pointed up his strongest asset in work for the blind when she said he was the "perfect sighted companion" and when he stepped on a platform with her "all nervousness and apprehension vanished." His generation credited him with having been the chief and most successful advocate for what became the American Foundation for the Blind, citing particularly a speech he made at a convention of the American Association of the Blind in 1919. He was excluded or excluded himself, from the staff of the Foundation, probably because it was thought that the infant organization must bear itself more solemnly than his temperament would allow. At this time he extended his interest to include all the handicapped as director of the Detroit League for the Handicapped, with which agency he continued to assist work for the blind both locally and nationally. He was a key figure in the World Conference of Work for the Blind in 1931. He died in 1935 and the next issue of the *Outlook for the Blind* carried the euphoric praise of practical persons who cannot bring themselves to openly praise men such as Campbell while they are alive.

MARY DRANGA CAMPBELL (1876-1957)
Sighted.
Social worker.
She was the second wife of Charles Campbell, sister of his first wife. Assistant editor of the *Outlook for the Blind,* 1912-19, she brought to it experience of a trained librarian and social worker. From then on, her many services to the blind included heading the Ohio School for the Blind during World War I, serving as first executive director of the Pennsylvania State Commission for the Blind (1926), reorganizing the Missouri State Commission for the Blind (1929-33), coordinating the blind and the crippled program of the Brooklyn (N.Y.) Bureau of Charities. In 1934, she joined the staff of the newly established Seeing Eye School at Morristown, where she remained for 12 years, bringing to the innovation what was required in knowledge of existing practices and serving as field representative. Following her retirement, she was re-enlisted in work for the blind as archivist of the American Foundation for the Blind, where she sorted thousands of items into accessible historical material. She also assisted the Library of Congress in assembling the papers of Sir Francis Campbell, a large collection which is in the rare manuscript room.

ROBERT F. WAGNER (1877-1953)
Sighted.
Lawyer, legislator.
Sponsored the Social Security Act, which gave the needly blind monthly grants. Also the Wagner-O'Day Act, passed in 1938, providing that the Federal Government purchase its brooms, mops, and "other suitable commodities" which can be manufactured by the blind, from non-profit-making agencies for the blind, except when such products can be supplied by federal prison industries. The bill further provided

for the setting up of a committee of representatives of the various government departments concerned, and one private citizen conversant with work for the blind, charged with the duty of fixing fair prices for such commodities and having the power to set up regulations and procedures by which the government orders were to be handled. Upon the death of Senator Wagner 15 years later, M. C. Miget said, "The blind have earned millions of dollars through this industry, and as citizens and taxpayers, hold their heads high and their minds free to believe in the America which is so largely of his making."

Harry Best, Ph.D. (1878-1971)
Sighted.
Socioligist.

Author of the sociologically definitive *The Blind* (1919) and a revision and expansion of the work entitled *Blindness and the Blind in the United States* (1934). This represented 25 years of research and is a repository of facts and statistics not available elsewhere, particularly with respect to legal citations concerning blindness and the chronology of agency establishment. The social value of the book in its time was chiefly in the emphasis it placed on prevention of blindness, pointing out that "75 percent of blindness was preventable." In pressing this point, the author took what appeared to be a lugubrious view of the lot of those permanently and totally blind.

Lucy Goldthwaite (1879-1957)
Sighted.
Librarian.

From 1905-1942, was in charge of books for the blind at the New York Public Library, New York City, where she assembled the largest and best organized collection of embossed books in the U.S., including especially braille music and textbooks, which through interlibrary loan served the whole country. She trained an expert corps of braille transcribers, whereby single copies of rarely needed books were made available to exceptional students. Editor of the *Braille Book Review,* for which she raised supporting funds, this periodical kept braille readers aware of books available with conciseness and perception. She was a promoter of the talking-book in the latter part of her career. From 1942 until 1944 she was editor of the *Outlook for the Blind.* Her liaison with other than library aspects of work for the blind was exceptional. She served as one of the Board of Managers of the New York State Commission for the Blind for several terms.

HELEN KELLER (1880-1968)

Blinded and deafened at 19 months by an illness still undiagnosed. Philosopher, diplomat, publicist.

Undoubtedly the most widely known and publicized blind individual of her own (or any) time, first because her mastery of language seemed, and continues to seem, tinged with the miraculous, later (and less widely) because it became clear that she was exceptionally brilliant and had keen moral sense, as well as a dynamic personality. As recently shown in the stage play and film, *The Miracle Worker,* she was the first deaf-blind child to master speech, this having been accomplished by Anne Sullivan Macy under the direction of Michael Anagnos, by correspondence. Anne Sullivan Macy continued as her teacher first at Perkins, later in conjunction with other private tutors and finally at Radcliffe College from which Helen Keller graduated *cum laude* in 1904. Years of asserting herself and defining her own personality followed as described in her books: *The Story of My Life* (1902); *The World I Live In* (1908); *Out of the Dark* (1913); *My Religion* (1927); *Midstream—My Later Life* (1931). She was one of the first young people of the century to be deeply concerned about social justice and was essentially a socialist all her life. This was without encouragement from the people who had educated her and one of the most clear indications that she was a personality in her own right and an independent thinker. She early outstripped her teacher in understanding the languages which Mrs. Macy faithfully spelled into her hand from foreign texts. In the ultraliberal camp of her youth, she was atypical inasmuch as she remained impervious to atheism, with a deep spirituality which was remarkably free from superstition. Notables who sought her out through interest in how she functioned discovered a knowing consciousness and intellect which made them her friends as equals. These included Alexander Graham Bell, Mark Twain and Andrew Carnegie. Her greatest friend after Mrs. Macy was M. C. Migel, who recognized her potential for publicizing the cause of the blind and persuaded her to be the international representative of the American Foundation for the Overseas Blind. In this role she lectured in behalf of the blind in Australia, Canada, Egypt, France, Great Britain, Greece, Ireland, Israel, Jordan, Lebanon, Syria, Italy, Japan, Yugoslavia, Korea, Manchukuo, New Zealand, and Scotland. She received honorary doctor's degrees from Temple University, the University of Glasgow, the University of Berlin, and Harvard. France made her a Chevalier of the Legion of Honor and she was given the first Alumni Achievement Award of

Radcliffe. In the 1930's she collected 34 million yen (17 million dollars) for the blind of Japan. Although she never mastered a clear and pleasing articulation, and to some extent relied on the manual alphabet all her life, her written style and thought were faultless expressions of a mature and penetrating philosophy. Her bill of particulars with regard to poverty and social justice in 1929 was 30 years creeping onto the editorial pages of the United States. She early recognized without conceit that her capacity was not ordinarily to be found in deaf-blind individuals and had great concern late in life, lest she put them at a disadvantage by setting a standard which they could not match. Her last years were spent in trying to secure suitable education and rehabilitation for those with this double handicap.

LIBORIO DELFINO (1880?-1937)
Blinded by a mining accident at the age of 19.
Placement specialist.
A pioneer placement specialist in the State of Pennsylvania, his indomitable technique in getting jobs for blind people earned admiration amounting to reverence in the workers for the blind who were his contemporaries. He had an ingratiating charm, combined with sincerity and courage in the management of his blindness as well as the additional handicap of the loss of an arm in the same accident which had taken his sight. An immigrant from Italy, he made his way in rehabilitation not only for himself, but for hundreds of other blind people, starting in 1904 and working first as field representative of the Overbrook School for the Blind. His rapport with his field and the community enabled him to follow the progress of individual clients over many years. By 1926 it was estimated that he had enabled blind people to earn what was then the large sum of $720,000. This was for a group to whom he had given personal attention to the point of making more than 20 calls on factories and writing 126 letters to secure one placement. On one occasion, during a survey of his program, he described from memory the success of 125 clients, his facts matching written records when they were sought out. He retired when he realized his methods were out of date. An excellent manager of his own affairs, his will was a masterpiece of appreciation of the help he had received from others.

ROBERTA A. GRIFFITH (188?-1941)
Totally blind from early childhood.
Organizer, philanthropist.
Said to have been the first blind woman to graduate from an institu-

tion of higher learning not intended especially for the blind (Western Reserve). She brought to her city (Grand Rapids) the most forward-looking innovations of the time, through the Grand Rapids Association for the Blind, which she organized, and on which she used her own financial resources. Her special interest was in prevention of blindness and braille classes in public schools. State legislation requiring prophylaxis in the eyes of newly born infants was sponsored in the Michigan legislature, and she was vigilant in promoting its enforcement. She was one of the organizers of the American Association of Workers for the Blind.

GRACE HARPER (1882-1964)
Sighted.
Social worker, administrator.
As director of the New York State Commission from 1919 to 1951, her administrative skill amounted to innovation in work for the blind. Beauty, brains, strength and finesse all went into her formula. She made things smooth for people from the "world of affairs" when it came to implementing their good intentions. One of a group taken to France by M. C. Migel to give early rehabilitation to the war-blinded of World War I, she served with the Red Cross, for which she was decorated; thereafter, she touched virtually every phase of work for the blind when she succeeded Migel as director of the New York State Commission. Her particular thrusts were in the prevention and employment area. She was said to have organized a "network of prevention" which was a pattern copied nationally.

CHARLES B. HAYES (1882-1936)
Sighted.
Social worker, teacher, promoter.
Credited, along with M. C. Migel, Robert B. Irwin and Evelyn McKay, with setting the pattern of the American Foundation for the Blind, where he served from 1923 until 1936 as its Director of Information, Field Director and Editor of the *Outlook for the Blind.* He was one of the first trained social workers to enter the field. He was trained at the New York School of Social Work, and then (in 1913) at the School of Philanthropy. He showed a flair for public education when he organized the Brooklyn Exchange and Training School for the Blind in 1913, and initiated exhibits known as "Weeks for the Blind." He was executive director of the Massachusetts Commission for the Blind from 1917 to 1923. Blind people thought he had an exceptional understanding of their social problems. One of his apperceptions was:

"To look into the face of a friend is a great privilege. Likewise to look upon the countenance of one's opponent is a great protection. Not to be able to use this power is one of the greatest handicaps of blindness. This faculty of observation and interpretation is one of the secrets of personality. The blind should use every resource to possess it." He used his powers to the full in helping them to do this.

WILLI H. EBELING (1882-1961)
Sighted.
Teacher, administrator, philosopher.
With Dorothy Harrison Eustis, he was one of the founders of the first guide-dog school for the blind in the United States, Seeing Eye, Inc., of which he became executive vice-president in 1934. Known to students as "Uncle Willi" he was active in the training program of the school for two decades, and continued as a member of the board upon his retirement in 1954. He was thought by many to have all the better attributes of a trained psychologist without having made an academic approach. An avoider of organizations and publicity, he had widespread respect. His advice to a sighted worker for the blind was, "Don't try to be a big shot, and don't crystallize resistance."

ROBERT B. IRWIN (1883-1951)
Blinded totally at the age of six.
Administrator, executive, publicist, teacher.
The foremost blind leader of the blind of his time, he championed a national and finally an international approach to problems of blindness, often in contest with local policies and jurisdictions. The American Foundation for the Blind and the American Foundation for Overseas Blind were as much his creations as they were M. C. Migel's. He was a staff member from 1923 until 1949 when he retired, becoming the executive director in 1929. He began his career in education of the blind after receiving a master's degree from Harvard. He collaborated on adaptation of the Binet intelligence tests, which later became the Hayes-Binet tests. He was then active in the organization and supervision of classes for the blind in the public schools of Ohio which laid the foundation for one of his lifelong loyalties. As a national leader he adroitly put his influence in balance against the authority and power of the residential schools as time went on to hold them in check rather than to supplant them. With M. C. Migel, he took leadership in fostering much of the legislation which is the backbone of many of the benefits the blind now enjoy and accept as their unquestioned right. Notable among these is the program of Aid

to the Needy Blind under the Social Security Act, which provides for Federal grants-in-aid to the state for the needy blind. He also did much of the work which led to the passage of the Wagner-O'Day Act. (See Senator Robert F. Wagner.) He was also active in securing the $600 exemption which the blind are permitted in computing their income tax. The Barden-La Follette Act, the Randolph Sheppard Act, and "Public Law 309" which supplied mechanical and electronic devices to blinded veterans all had his active support, and the last of these he originated. His lifelong interest in punctography resulted in numerous conferences to secure an international agreement on a uniform system. The World Conference of Workers for the Blind, which he organized in 1931, led to the international agreement on standard revised braille in 1932. However, his favorite project was the talking-book, which he persuaded the Works Progress Administration to develop and make available to blind people. A talking-book department became a part of the regular program of the American Foundation for the Blind. A man of strong opinions, having been a young radical, in middle life he became a skillful diplomat in dealing with his opponent, curbing both a keen sense of humor and a sharp wit in order to make effective compromises. One of his most important observations was the need to develop different methods of teaching for the partially seeing and the blind, and he promoted the production of large type books by the Cleartype Publishing Company. In the last decade of his life he was much preoccupied with international reconstruction of work for the blind in the aftermath of World War II. For this, the French government made him a Chevalier of the Legion of Honor. He attempted without success to persuade Pope Pius IX to establish an order devoted to the deaf-blind. A resilient individual, Irwin was proud of the fact that the braille dots of his name spelled Irwin rightside up or upside down, which he equated with the family motto: "The same in sunshine and shadow." He was by nature a man of business and left the American Foundation for the Blind in excellent financial condition.

RICHARD S. FRENCH, PH.D. (1883-)
Sighted.
Teacher, educator, author.

He wrote *From Homer to Helen Keller,* the first historical treatment of blindness down through the ages, with an educator's analysis of strengths and weakness of workers and their efforts. Preceding Ishbell Ross's *Journey into Light,* Gabriel Farrell's *The Story of Blindness,* it is not so rich in historical fact as either of these. However, as the work of a teacher, scholar, university professor of special education, and principal of a residential school for the blind (California), it excelled in grasp and enunciation of theory, as well as in analysis of programs. Of a sanguine temperament, he listed at the end a bill of particulars showing progress (in 1932), including the opinion:

> Open beggary has practically ceased in all civilized countries . . . reading has become simple and easy, books have multiplied, and the poorest blind can have a wide selection for the slight trouble of asking . . . the point systems have made possible the intercommunication of the blind, while the standard typewriter brings within their power free written communication with those who see . . . through maps, models and other objective material, the world of phenomenal reality has become very largely their own, while through books, the world of the intellect may be theirs to a degree inconceivable 100 years ago . . . trades and occupations are better understood than ever before; and, though the limitations of the blind are reluctantly acknowledged, we are surer of their possibilities than ever before. . . . From being virtual outcasts the blind have come to be accepted as an integral part of society; one no longer pities them as poor dependents; one must often respect them as bread winners and highly cultivated men and women.

DOROTHY HARRISON EUSTIS (1886-1946)
Sighted.
Philanthropist, guide-dog trainer.

Founder and president of Seeing Eye, Inc., in 1929. Previously, she was founder of "Fortunate Fields," a dog-breeding experimental establishment in Switzerland for study of the mental capacity and working potential of dogs in relation to their service to men. In 1927, having studied European instruction of guide-dogs, she contributed an aritcle to the *Saturday Evening Post* which attracted Morris Frank, a young blind man who went to Fortunate Fields to be trained. Subsequently, they returned to America and working with Jack Humphrey, a geneticist, and Willi Ebeling, developed the policy and training methods of Seeing Eye. A unique feature of its early organization was the insistence by Mrs. Harrison that financial support come only from persons who understood the philosophy and policy of the school. This was rigidly oriented to the concept that the dog was a working dog working for a working human being who must, at however moderate a rate, ultimately pay the school for the animal. Her cautious and thoroughgoing approach to financial backing was such unorthodox fund-raising that it had a reverse effect from that which professional fund-raisers might have predicted, partly because of the unique personality of Mrs. Eustis. Her commanding sincerity of purpose had a charisma which bordered on mystique. On one occasion she declined an award, asking that it be given to her guidedogs and thereby offending the donor. In her turn, she showed dudgeon that the donor should have been offended. The legend concerning her includes her having withdrawn from the organization for a year to be certain it could operate without her. This has proved to be the case on a long-term basis.

GABRIEL FARRELL (1886-1968)
Sighted.
Minister, journalist, educator.
The fourth director of Perkins School from 1931-1951, he revitalized the deaf-blind department, raising large sums of money for it by public appeals, chiefly through a yearly Christmas brochure or leaflet entitled "Children of the Silent Night." He also wrote *The Story of Blindness* 1956), along with French's *From Homer to Helen Keller* and Ishbell Ross' *Journey into Light,* one of the three books which has attempted to treat the subject of blindness historically. A "canon" in the Episcopal church, he was brought into the field as an "outsider" to head the Perkins School making his way against the skepticism of his own staff and those in the field of work for the blind. Organizing ability and experience in journalism sustained him. One of his major interests was prevention of blindness, especially finding the cause of retrolental fibroplasia, in which he played a part, securing money through the Foundation for Vision for a study at the Massachusetts Eye and Ear Infirmary.

PHILIP HARRISON (1887-1969)
Blinded in World War 1 (1918).
Agency director.
A community organizer. As executive director of the Pennsylvania Association for the Blind, he opened 17 new branch offices, paving the way for extensive, statewide coverage of problems of blindness, for which purpose he established a mobile eye clinic. He was a great believer in the leadership of the blind by the blind and placed a blind executive in each of the offices he established.

ERNEST A. WHITFIELD (BARON KENSWOOD) (1887-1963)
Lost sight at age of 22.
Diplomat, newspaper correspondent, musician, economist.
An exceptional example of resilience and adaptability, he became a musician when he was blinded in 1909. When he had exhausted him-

self as a concert violinist, and was "ordered to rest," he took a Ph.D. at the London School of Economics. He returned to the concert stage until 1935. When a damaged hand put an end to his musical career in 1935, he became increasingly interested in work for the blind, with which he had been involved since 1928 as a member of the council of the National Institute for the Blind, taking the role of economist in various studies. He was among the representatives of Britain in the final parleys concerning an international code of braille at Louisville, and was credited by some of the participants with the diplomatic skill which finally produced international agreement. He twice unsuccessfully sought election to parliament as a labor candidate. From 1946 to 1950 he served as a governor of the British Broadcasting Company, was created a baron in 1951. He was president of the National Federation of the Blind from 1951-55, and was an inveterate council and committee member for educational and medical causes. His major success lay in his managing himself in so "normal" a manner that he could not be described as a shining example of the blind individual; blindness was not the prime factor in his life. His wife, a descendant of the ducal house of Norfolk, put the security and social skill derived therefrom to practical use, making her husband's associates comfortable in the presence of blindness; her warmth and grace were eminent.

THOMAS CUTSFORTH, PH.D. (1893-1962)
Lost sight at age 11.
Psychologist, author.
He was the author of a scholarly, blistering psychological study and commentary, *The Blind in School and Society,* the most discussed book in the field of work for the blind in the 1930's and from time to time since. With methods and point of view almost diametrically opposed to Dr. French in *From Homer to Helen Keller,* he relentlessly assailed institutions for the blind in all their weakest points. He saw Howe as the only original thinker which work for the blind had ever produced; to him, Helen Keller was an unreal being who did not understand her own words. To him, residential schools were emotional deserts which were natural hotbeds for wickedness and vice. From 1936 to 1959, Cutsforth was a successful practicing psychologist in Los Angeles. As time went on, he came to be considered a kind of dean of stormy petrels in the field of work for the blind, looked on with a certain amount of affection by the school people he had lambasted (who believed they had corrected the faults of which he spoke in so far as they could be corrected). This Cutsforth never was willing to

grant, and late in his life, participating in a panel discussion, declared, "If I had to choose between letting my blind child go without an education or attending a residential school, I would let him "go without an education." He was author of a paper "Blindness as an Adequate Expression of Anxiety." For his direct antithesis, see Richard French, 1893-1902.

LEWIS W. RODENBERG (1893-1967)
Lost sight at age of 10.
Printer, punctographer, author.

An authority on raised dots of every description, he played a key role in securing the international use of revised braille in 1932. For 50 years the superintendent of the braille print shop of the Illinois School for the Blind, he was one of the few participants in the so-called "War of the Dots" who lived to see the resolution of the conflict. He combined the most complete technical knowledge of all the various dot systems with an intellectual viewpoint and skill as an author. He wrote many technical articles, beginning in 1917 with the publication of his "Key to Braille Music Notation." He also occasionally ventured into social and philosophical observation and analysis, exemplified by his summary of the evolution of braille immediately after the Oxford Conference in 1932 which brought about international agreement. This contained the animadversion:

> In no other land have there been such colossal, such costly, such convincing, experiments in finger-reading as in the United States. The blind of this country have paid in full. In some instances the experiments imposed on them were sheer theoretical projects devised by seeing workers. In other cases experiments were projected on them by persons who were themselves without sight. The superior legibility of obsolete American Braille and of surviving Standard English Braille may be traced to the fact that they originated in blindness—which is proof that efficiency in solving problems of human suffering comes first from identity with that suffering. . . . It will not be necessary for us to review one hundred years of experimentation inflicted on American finger-readers who were yearning for and needing more literature and receiving less than they might have been—an appalling history of costly libraries built up, duplicated, and destroyed. The acceptance of Standard English Braille throughout the English-speaking world meant this long and extravagant experimentation has come to an end, has resulted in a definite idea, has the vast significance of establishing the universality of the braille principle; and all of this signifies the final triumph of the son of the harness maker of Coupvray. The name and fame of Louis Braille will now endure. Never, on entering a cathedral, did I have more strongly the sense of treading on holy ground than when I stopped to pass through the low doorway of the stone hut on the stony hillside of Coupvray beyond the Marne. From that lowly

cradle came one whose idea was to have such singular value that, a century after its conception, it would be taken by determined men to the hilltops of the world as a perpetual boon to unfortunate people.

Col. E. A. Baker O.B.E.M.C. Croix de Guerre (1893-1968)
Blinded in military action in World War I.
Executive.

Credited by many with having established the most rational, cohesive and complete national program for the blind in the world in the Canadian National Institute for the Blind. He was one of the St. Dunstan's trained war-blinded of World War I. Like Sir Clutha Mackenzie in New Zealand, he returned to his country to find very little provision for severely handicapped returning veterans. A born leader, he was soon recognized as such by Charles W. Holmes, who was director of the Canadian National Institute for the Blind, and who was struggling to get the organization on its feet. Baker succeeded Holmes as managing director, in which position he continued throughout his active career, blueprinting and implementing the national program for the blind for which he was to receive worldwide respect. In all classes he commanded an extraordinary inclination to fall in with his plans and programs, his personality combining an unusual combination of warmth and aloofness, resting on undoubted conventional strength and virtues. He fused the war and civilian programs for the blind at an early stage and also established cooperation with workers for the blind from the United States, getting his vending stand and placement program under way through Clunk from the United States. Taking advantage of the fact that Canada had very little in the way of a program for the blind, he was able to build a modern and central agency without the difficulties encountered by those who must deal with a tangled network inherited from another generation. Of this freedom he was able to make the most, establishing a system of voluntary local committees which dealt with the widespread isolation of the blind of Canada, and building a strong program including a workshop at headquarters and a prevention of blindness program. Totally blind, he was the only member of the Canadian Ophthalmological Association, which upon his retirement in 1962 established the E. A. Baker Foundation for Prevention of Blindness. He was an always welcome, though sometimes piercingly frank, adviser and critic of work for the blind in the United States. His article "Some Thoughts on an Integrated Program for the Blind" in the 1943 *Outlook for the Blind* was and continues to be a penetrating analysis of the dilemmas faced in making the most of federal, state and private agencies in the United States. He declined knighthood from his monarchs.

JOSEPH F. CLUNK (1895-)
Lost sight in 1919.
Promoter, placement specialist, executive.

He spearheaded selective placement in Canada and the United States during the 1920's and 1930's. He was the first chief of Services to the Blind in the Federal Government, following the passage of the Randolph-Sheppard Act in 1936. (See Senator Jennings Randolph.) Clunk was the undoubted creator of the role of the blind selective placement specialist in the official programs of the United States and Canada. His followers and their followers formed a consortium which was to become one of the strongest influences in work for the blind. One important aspect of his method was testing processes personally with the cooperation of the industrial foreman of a particular factory and in this manner finding operations which could be safely performed by blind persons on a par with sighted workers. Beginning in Ohio not long after losing his sight, he developed an effective sales technique for convincing employers that they should hire blind workers. Seemingly unorthodox because his approach was informal, familiar and jocular (and these qualities were combined with blindness), in actual fact he used conventional high pressure methods. These were closely akin beneath the surface to the high pressure with which employers identified and sympathized, and which they hoped to find in blind employees after they had seen it in Clunk. In 1928 he was invited by the Canadian government to demonstrate his ways in that country. He remained for nine years with great success, earning the undying respect of Canadian workers for the blind. He returned to the United States in 1936 to undertake the implementation of the Randolph-Sheppard Act, which provided not merely for the licensing of vending stands but the surveying of employment opportunities. Financial provision for this was somewhat vague, but Clunk was able gradually to gather some staff under the aegis and budget of the Office of Education. Leonard Robinson, who had played a role in securing passage of the act was one of his assistants. In 1943 the passage of the Barden-Lafollette Act brought the rehabilitation services for the blind into the public program of vocational rehabilitation, and its financial provisions permitted more extensive promotion on which Clunk capitalized to train groups of blind selective placement specialists. His own staff included Maurice Tynan, who was widely experienced both in education and rehabilitation of the blind, Hiram

Chappell, a specialist on farming without sight and John McCauley, who was an expert on the use of power tools by the blind. Clunk's training program eventually carried his methods to all the states and accounted for a dramatic increase in placements which has never abated in the years since. Often restive with bureaucracy, Clunk retired from government in 1950 to take over the Philadelphia office of the Pennsylvania Association for the Blind. In 1961 a grant was made to him by the Vocational Rehabilitation Administration to develop special tools, and he produced a number of items before failing health made it impossible for him to continue in this work.

PETER J. SALMON (1895-   )
Partially seeing.
Agency executive.

His most notable contribution is a rational and practical program for all deaf-blind persons, including those with average and less than average capacity. Services to implement his ideas with respect to the deaf-blind were first worked out at local level in the Industrial Home for the Blind of Brooklyn, Salmon's base of operations since 1917. There he gradually had fostered action which was characterized by its understanding of the needs of blind people and their maximum participation in programs for their benefit. Salmon has acquired wide respect for the genuineness of his idealism and his ingenuity in implementing it. His program, which was to have excellent financial backing and handsome resources later in the century, was outlined in a fundamental blueprint published in the *Outlook for the Blind* in 1926. It looked forward to vocational placement, social service and a geriatric program. Salmon and his program became well known for generosity with methods. In an article entitled "Experimenting" published in the *Outlook for the Blind* during the depression, Salmon openly described seven specific and unusual markets his shop had unearthed, and which he might have been excused for monopolizing. His skill in management caused a number of his programs to become models for imitation by other agencies. One of these was the low vision clinic of Industrial Home for the Blind, another a speech and hearing clinic. Salmon was the chief proponent of the Hawes-Cooper Bill in 1928 which paved the way for the Wagner-O'Day Act. (See Senator Robert F. Wagner.) Subsequently, he was a part of virtually every constructive move for legislative action for many years as chairman of the AAWB Legislative Committee. His long-continued interest in the deaf-blind resulted in a program formalized in 1945. Later, under a grant from the Vocational Rehabilitation Administration, this program was carefully reviewed for its implications, which were published in a seven volume report entitled *Rehabilitation of Deaf-Blind Persons.* This and a subsequent seven-year pilot stndy had a profound influence on the amendment to the Vocational Rehabilitation Act of 1967 in which provision was made for the establishment of a National Center for Deaf-Blind.

SIR CLUTHA MACKENZIE (1897-1966)
Blinded in military service in 1915.
Sheep farmer, organizer, author, philologist.
He was the author of *World Braille Usage,* a study of the problem of international uniformity in braille systems, published in 1953 by UNESCO. This was a brilliant theoretical analysis, produced while MacKenzie was chairman of the World Braille Council. A New Zealander, he lost his sight at Gallipoli, was one of the leaders trained at St. Dunstan's. While at St. Dunstan's, he developed a flair for journalism and for organizing work for the blind. In London he began to edit *The Chronicles of the New Zealand Expeditionary Force.* Back in New Zealand, although he returned to sheep farming with profit, he also undertook to look after the welfare of St. Dunstaners there and later the civilian blind. This became an absorbing interest, and when World War II broke out he was asked to organize programs for the war-blinded of India, Burma and Malaya. It was at this time that he became internationally known in the field of work for the blind through his travels in behalf of the blind in the eastern half of the globe. Descriptions of his work were published in the *Outlook for the Blind.* At the same time he developed his interest in worldwide braille usage. His international viewpoint and dynamic personality gave him ubiquitous entree and in 1947 he was asked by the Chinese Government to "make a survey of blindness in China." He was keenly perceptive of the needs of blind people in relation to the various cultures in which they lived. These he had ample opportunity to observe at St. Dunstan's in Asia where a large number of races, religions and nationalities were fused. One of his most important contributions was encouraging farmers who had lost their sight to return to farming, for which he was able to offer practical contributions.

IAN FRASER, KT. (CREATED BARON OF LONSDALE 1958) (1897-)
Blinded in 1916 in military action.
Lawyer, legislator, organizer.
More than anyone else of his time, he projected in Britain the image

of the competent blind man of affairs and statecraft. Like Col. Baker of Canada and Sir Clutha MacKenzie of New Zealand, after losing his sight, he was trained under the guidance of Sir Arthur Pearson. He became chairman of the board of St. Dunstan's in 1921, and has continued in that office. However, he chiefly served blind people by making a career for himself in business and as a member of Parliament for many terms, beginning in 1924. He was national president of the British Legion and had a hand in legislation not only for disabled veterans, but also for British civilian blind people. He was also a governor of the British Broadcasting Company. His autobiography *Whereas I Was Blind* was published in 1942.

EVELYN C. MCKAY (1898-)

Sighted.

Research analyst, social worker, author, editor.

One of the professional staff which created the role of the American Foundation for the Blind in work for the blind. According to Robert Irwin, she was the associate with whom he "hammered out foundation policy." She drafted the recommendations for innumerable bills to be introduced both to the Congress and state legislatures. She was particularly interested in public assistance from the standpoint of legislative administration and research—most specifically, amendments to Title X of the Social Security Act. With Irwin, she recognized the tendency in work for the blind to neglect social work aspects in favor of education; she secured participation of work for the blind in the National Conference of Social Work in 1930. At her instigation a committee on statistics was established jointly between the National Society for the Prevention of Blindness and the American Foundation for the Blind, resulting in standard classification of cause of blindness, standard physician's eye reports and classification by amount of vision. This committee also paved the way for Ralph Hurlin's statistical analysis of the causes of blindness. She was the associate editor of the *Outlook for the Blind* from 1931 till 1943, the author of numerous articles implying the need for professionalization in the field and a redoubtable enemy of jerry-built programs. She promoted the training and certification of home teachers through the institution of summer courses which she organized first at Western Reserve and later at the University of Michigan. Her direct work with clients included administering a scholarship program for the American Foundation for the Blind and the placement of blind professionals a task for which she had an unusual flair. After retirement from the foundation she became a free-lance consultant to agencies for the blind and later became executive director of the Louis Braille Foundation for Blind Musicians. The author of this chronicle is indebted to her observation and memory for certain accuracies in its composition.

BERTHOLD LOWENFELD, PH.D. (1901-)
Sighted.
Psychologist, teacher, educator, author.
He focused the attention of psychology on the total effect of blindness in contrast, though not in opposition, to the work of Samuel Hayes. His diplomatic skill made acceptable not only his own interpretations, but also some of the apperceptions of Thomas Cutsforth, whose temperamental aggressiveness might well have caused him to be widely ignored but for the attention called to him by Lowenfeld. Like Cutsforth, he recognized the dangers of segregated education for blind children, but less heatedly. From Austria, where he received his doctor's degree at the University of Vienna in 1927, Lowenfeld visited the United States on a Rockefeller fellowship in 1930-31, at which time he was teaching at the Jewish School for the Blind in Vienna. He returned to the United States permanently in 1938, was on the staff of the American Foundation for the Blind from 1939 till 1949, and from 1949 until 1964 was superintendent of the California School for the Blind. He is the author of *Our Blind Children—Growing and Learning with Them* and of a detailed study of touch reading *Blind Children Learning to Read,* as well as numerous other articles published in journals. He wrote an extensive chapter dealing with psychological problems of visually impaired children, published in Cruikshank's *Psychology of Exceptional Children and Youth,* which is considered the most comprehensive presentation of this topic. In 1968 he made a study of the multihandicapped blind and deaf-blind children in the State of California, which was an important contribution to the data on which national legislation in behalf of the deaf-blind was based. As superintendent of a residential school for the blind, he encouraged widespread attendance of blind children in schools with the seeing. His stated opinion in this area was: "Institutions and services for blind individuals, unempeded by further handicaps, which separate the blind and keep them separated are regressive. Even though they may be temporarily beneficial to blind people, they are undesirable and inimical to the interest of the blind." He served on numerous committes including the Sensory Study Panel of the Research and Demonstration Service of the Vocational Rehabilitation Administration, as well as the National Advisory Council of that agency.

JENNINGS RANDOLPH (1902-)
Sighted.
Legislator.
He sponsored in the U. S. House of Representatives the Randolph-Sheppard Act, on which the vending stand program is based, and which is said to have put more money in blind people's pockets through gainful employment than any other program in work for the blind. The law was passed in 1936 and provided the opening wedge for the establishment of vending stands operated by the blind on federal property. The Commissioner of Education, later the Federal Security Administration and the Rehabilitation Services Administration were charged with the responsibility of administering the act by the designating licensing agencies, at state level. Two goals set forth were (1) to make surveys of concession stand opportunities for blind persons in federal and other buildings in the United States; (2) to make surveys throughout the United States of industries with a view to obtaining information that would assist blind persons in obtaining employment. A remarkable factor of this legislative phenomenon was that it succeeded without a special appropriation, though such an appropriation was authorized. Agencies responsible under successive reorganizations have carried the administrative costs, and the initial selling of the program was directed by the promotion skills of a group of blind men with exceptional missionary zeal, particularly Joseph Clunk as first chief of services for the blind in a federal agency and Leonard Robinson, whom Senator Randolph credits with having assisted him with forging the legislation.

MERLE E. FRAMPTON, PH.D. L.L.D. (1903-)
Sighted.
Educator.
His role was "constant dissenter." He led in counter-criticism of criticism of residential schools for the blind. Entering the field as principal of the New York Institute for the Blind in 1935, with academic credentials in sociology and theology, he very rapidly established a reputation for speaking out. Ultimately, this took the form of direct philosophical antithesis of the American Foundation for the Blind and Berthold Lowenfeld, with whom for many years he agreed on nothing, except perhaps Lowenfeld's statement that everything in the world should be opposed by something. In 1953 he coauthored a book, in the preface to which he said, "The residential school for the

blind has, from its inception up to the present, reflected the concrete expression of the people's will to realize the ideal of service to others. No temporary, no fancy flight of theories of nonsegregation, integration, institutionalization, no highly, publicized frills from the jargon of educational or social 'Don Quixotes' who tyrannize our present generation with baskets of words have detracted from the magnificent contributions of the residential school to blind people." His text contained a large number of quotations from educators of the blind, gathered from statements made by them from the time of Howe forward. The firmness of Frampton's opinions tended to isolate him from his colleagues, even in residential schools, but he continued redoubtable and apparently undismayed by this and was generally counted upon to take independent positions on questions receiving public review. In 1959 he served as executive secretary of a Congressional committee to study work for the blind in the United States. Proceeding both on a national and regional basis, this was remarkable for putting in print virtually every point of view which was current with respect to services for blind people.

LEONARD ROBINSON (1904-)
Lost sight at age of 11.
Lawyer, selective placement specialist.
He was the key lobbyist, independently and voluntarily, for the Randolph-Sheppard Act, and was acknowledged as such by Senator Randolph. While practicing law in Cleveland in 1931, Robinson attended the World Conference of Work for the Blind where he heard Joseph Clunk describe his placement activities in Canada. From then until 1936 when the act was passed, he pursued various leads which produced no result until he was able to get the interest of Congressman (now Senator) Jennings Randolph, who saw the possibilities of such a program, arranged for him to have his draft reworked by a staff member of the Senate Legislative Committee, and introduced the bill which eventually became the act. Robinson subsequently became one of its implementers with Clunk and continued in this work until his retirement in 1970.

As dawn breaks the spell of long night's study, the glare of currency breaks the spell of history. And streaks of currency have begun to show in some of the more recent careers enumerated in the above roster. We know that this is happening when names of the living come to mind thick and fast. And the glare of currency grows even brighter when their chronological enumeration, necessarily giving their right ages, might be just what someone is looking for to nudge them out of currency into history. These signs suggest that it is time to disclose what I have been able to distill philosophically from thinking about the people I have described. And if workers for the blind, for whom this material has been assembled, feel somewhat offended that such and such a one has not appeared in my listing, well and good. It is a sign that the principle of a personal approach to history has taken root. It is to be hoped that they will study and record their own deeds and those of their colleagues.

PHILOSOPHY

At this point you may well be thinking: What do all these people, so many of whom are dead, have to do with me? I can only say that I feel duty bound to inform you that when you encounter problems of blindness as a practitioner in a helping profession, you have a certain amount of tradition to deal with. Do not underestimate it. It is by no means a tradition of archaic magic, ancient superstition and modern ineptitude. If it were, you could merely write it off and approach the problems of blind people fresh, as a technician.

However, whenever a culture reaches a certain level of development, blindness begins to draw on the bank of general attention, and in the incorporation of altruism it is almost invariably an original stockholder. We find this in ancient Japan, in Italy, in France, in Britain—all of which developed durable institutions for the blind a very long time ago, though these institutions were not such as we would approve of today.

Scientific learning on the subject of blindness is sometimes called meager by 20th century social scientists of one sort or another. I think they are wrong to look for a science of blindness; rather, there is a very special aspect of humanism concerned with blindness, based on many sciences. And the historical literature of that humanism has had unique relationships with science and a sophistication which can hardly be challenged. The absence of eyesight seeps into every cranny of daily living, putting technology on the defensive in countless ways. The philosophy and common sense to master it cannot be puny.

Plato said, "The essence of equality lies in treating unequal things unequally."

Society's management of eye problems is one illustration of an unconscious effort to work out this formula; to understand the basic help and the attitudes toward giving and receiving help in a particular day and time inevitably will make a great difference in how problems of blindness are managed.

An episode in the life of Homer, attributed to Herodotus and undoubtedly more legend than fact, nevertheless raises the curtain on some rather advanced thinking about these things among the ancient Greeks. To understand the quotation, it is necessary to understand that Homer's original given name was Melesigenes.

> When Melesigenes arrived at Cumae, he frequented the assemblies of the elders, and there recited his verse. Admiring their beautiful structure, they fell into an ecstacy of delight. Joyful at the reception his poems had prepared for him among the Cumaens, and at the pleasure with which they had heard him, he one day proposed to them, that if the state would maintain him he would make the city of Cumae very celebrated. His hearers approved of the proposition, and engaged him to present himself before the council, where they would support him with all their interest. Melesigenes, encouraged by their approbation, presented himself at the House of Assembly on an audience day, and addressing the person who had the office of presenting those who had any request to prefer, he begged to be allowed to enter. This officer did not neglect to present him the first opportunity that offered. Melesigenes, as soon as that ceremony was over, addressed the assembly regarding the proposition he had formerly made. His speech ended, he retired, in order that the representatives might deliberate on the answer necessary to give him.
>
> He that presented him, and all those representatives be longing to the Elders' Assembly, where he had recited, voted for him. It is said that one only opposed the measure, giving for his reason, "that if they thought to feed *homers,* they would find themselves encumbered with useless folks." From this time the name of Homer, bestowed thus opprobriously on Melesigenes in consequence of his misfortune, was most generally used in speaking of him; for the Cumaens, in their dialet, called blind persons homers. Strangers always used this name in discoursing of the poet.
>
> The Archon concluded with saying, "that it was impolitic

to maintain the blind man." This caused the majority of the representatives to vote against the measure, the second time, and thus the Archon obtained more votes than opposers. The presenting officer communicated with Melesigenes on the subject, informing him of the progress of the debate, and of the decree. Deploring his ill fortune, he recited these verses:

"The illustrious daughters of Zeus, on their departure from these places, wished to immortalize this sacred town (Cumae) by my verses; but, deaf to my voice, the brutish herd disdained my harmonious lays. No, it shall not continue so! Whoever in blind folly heaped insults on my head shall not escape unscathed. I will courageously endure the ills dealt out to me by the Deity. Tis over, I will no longer rest in Cumae. My feet burn to depart hence, and my panting heart urges me to seek a foreign clime, and there to dwell, however insignificant the place may be."

On leaving Cumae, he pronounced a malediction against the Cumaeans, to the following effect: "That there never might be born in Cumae a poet who could render it celebrated, and give it glory."

Some indication of the treatment Homer thought due him is founded in the way he pictured the Phaeacian singer, Demodocus, in the following passage in the *Odyssey*.

Now came the herald along, leading the much revered singer,
The Muse's beloved to whom both evil and good had been granted,
For she took the sight from his eyes but gave him the gift of sweet music.
And Pantonous seats him in a chair bedizened with silver in the very midst of the guest near the base of a stately column:
Hanging there on a nail is his harp, the heavenly sounding,
Up over the singer's head, and he reaches his hand up to find it.
Before him the herald places a beautiful table with viands and
A full beaker of wine to drink when he wants it.

Certainly this instance of Greek democracy in action is not the worst example of a community's reaction to a blind individual's talents and problems. The Greeks have a bad name for exposing defective babies on hillsides and letting them die. But this story shows them at least giving the great epic poet a hearing and deciding against helping him on the basis followed by many communities today. "What we cannot do for all people of this kind, we must not do for one."

Ideals of a rehabilitation philosophy of work for the blind are more generous and daring. Dr. Richard Hoover has said its spirit is best captured in words ascribed to Aristotle defining equity: "Equity is justice that goes beyond the written law. It is equitable to pardon human weaknesses, and to look, not to the law but the moral purpose; not to the part, but the whole; not to what a man is now but to what he has been always or generally."

Anyone who feels a natural, unqualified approval of what the Cumaens decided about Homer will probably be uneasy with this statement of Aristotle's about equity, yet even to these it should give a tantalizing impression that he was closer to real justice than the civil law can be in a life where nature seems to abhor exact equality of human endowments. At any rate, the passage is curiously in harmony with rehabilitation philosophy as it has evolved. But the world had to wait a long time for our present day ideas of treating the individual needs of individuals individually, and in effect, "better than they deserve." Society's representatives keep coming back to Polonious's "each man as he deserves," and repeatedly need to be persuaded that they cannot be so exact as they think they can about what people "deserve."

Much early work for the blind cannot be considered rehabilitation at all. Henry J. Wagg, an Englishman, produced a very careful and thorough book entitled *A Chronological Survey of Work for the Blind,* starting in the 4th century when St. Basil established a hospital for the blind at Caesarea in Cappadocia and provided them with guides. In the 5th century, the Hermit of St. Lymnaeus established a Refuge for the Blind at Syr in Syria, special cottages being erected for their use. In 7th century France, St. Bertrand, Bishop of Le Mans, founded an institution for the blind, believed to be at Pontlier. Finally, there was St. Louis's extraordinary Quinze-Vingts. These early entries are records of custodial efforts, based on the asylum principle. Undoubtedly, such endeavors were far better than nothing in their day and time (which was often more rough and ready than our own), but they were not rehabilitation. Rehabilitation means participation by the blind individual in the doings of the world. Clear-cut programs to engineer this both in the Western World and also in the East were preceded by long periods of custodial treatment.

It is not a simple matter to give the essence of a philosophy strong enough to effect rehabilitation programs. The way ahead is by no means so clear as we wish it were. The best I can do at this juncture is to offer two exhibits which I have fashioned. Based on a certain amount of case study of workers for the blind, including those I have listed above, I have developed two rather informal job descriptions which attempt to capture in words the philosophy of successful workers for the blind by focusing on two roles. One role is the role of the counselor of state on blindness. When I say "state" I mean state in the political sense, i.e. any state: Texas, Lichtenstein, the United States, Roumania. The other level is the level of the hewer and hauler, fetcher and carrier—in fact, the "worker." This "grass roots" individual I will put first, signifying that he is the most important person in the life of the blind client and I call these practitioners masters of the art of teaching blind people.

Credo Ascribed to Certain Masters of the Art of Teaching Blind People

I hold the art of teaching blind people how to perform without sight among the highest callings which a human being may answer with his life. If at any time, through my own infirmity, or to fill a power vacuum, the day comes when I must become a mere executive, supervisor or administrator, I will remember that, no matter how it seems to the worldly, the true apex of work for the blind is personal service in direct contact with blind people, and that all organized work for the blind has no other end but this, as fully and well-performed as available knowledge permits.

During the years when it is my privilege to practice the art, I will do my uttermost, not only to extend my own effectiveness, and the effectiveness of others, but also to devise ways of imparting efficiency with all the tact and kindness of which I am capable, bearing in mind that the most cherished attribute a person has is his self-esteem, based on a sense of worth, the quintessence of which is independence.

I will keep in mind that a severe handicap, particularly in its early stages or if it goes for a long time untended, requires that an individual be a constant recipient of so much help that the burden recurrently seems intolerable, and that my actions and attitudes should never increase this burden by any kind of ostentation in my bearing toward my work or blind people. Without morbid self-effacement or subservience, I will avoid any form of encroachment upon the individuality of those I serve, especially subtle usurping of credit for their performance.

I will keep my emotions in such order that I will not seek exceptional satisfaction from relationships with those I help, and will steadily perform in such a way as to encourage them to rely on and be preoccupied with those persons it is most natural and desirable for them to know and to love.

To my working hours I will give the most complete attention of the most creative kind of which I am capable, dwelling constantly on every practicality which can render a human being without sight a person of value in his own eyes.

I will guard my tongue and my time, but give generously my knowledge and experience to others who are also devoted to this art which is my calling.

I will reserve my scorn for those who aspire to be my colleagues without true respect for the calling, who are cynical toward all these things in which I believe, and without diligence and care in performing their duties. These I will relentlessly harry out of the field by open and aboveboard strictures and sanctions without any regard for influence which such persons may muster to counterattack.

I will not spoil blind people, or encourage them to become mere charming enslavers of those around them. I will look to the long view in helping them, not to ease of the moment. But I will stop short of making myself a compulsive taskmaster over the people whom I serve.

No matter how my battles go, once a conflict is resolved, I will put it behind me and rest and recondition my heart, mind, and body for further action.

The counselor of state must be quite a different being, though this does not preclude his having once functioned at the grass roots, fulfilling the requirements sketched in the teacher's credo.

What Is Required in a Counselor of State on the Subject of Blindness

The list of requirements is as follows:

1. As much ease with blind people as with the sighted.

2. Real true familiarity with the things blind people can and cannot do.

3. Diplomacy in managing the embarrasing dictum "blind people can do anything."

4. Total absence of snobbishness toward the practitioner "down in the mud" with blind people.

5. Ability to deal with the national passion for the mechanical solution to blindness. (Also, the reverence for statistics and bigness.)

6. Ability to master the barricade "You will never know what it is to be blind" either by blindness itself or an intuitive quality which is an adequate substitute.

7. Willingness to keep up with a considerable number of areas, subjects, technicalities with which impaired eyesight involves the human being (finger reading, optics, statistics, small business, sociology, etc.). This is where the *narrow* subject of blindness becomes very *broad*.

8. Whereas all other counselors of state have many other worthy commitments, this counselor should have a judicious, but highly serious commitment to blind people in all *quid pro quos*. The able, ambitious fellow on his way somewhere has a disappointing tendency to sell out when the chips are down. However, there are exceptions when men on their way make fine contributions and manage their interests without conflict.

9. Ability to belong to the state of which he is counselor, and to blind people—not to agile folk who are champions at getting to such people as he.

10. Imagination and open-mindedness coupled with an uncanny ability to spot quacks, frauds and insane people.

11. A strong tendency to feel joy when other people flourish, to regard crisis and obstacles as worthy enemies and outcomes, resolutions and smooth motion as beloved friends.

12. Ability to keep his head when all about him are losing theirs and blaming it on him.

13. There must be no "13" for him (or her). He (or she) must fear no evil.

14. Whatever his education is, it should have given him some idea of what a state is, and how it has evolved.

15. Whatever his upbringing, it should have given him some idea of what a human being is, and how *it* has evolved.

EPILOGUE

It is lately the fashion to offer management improvement courses at which sample situations are offered to the class. I would like to illustrate my concept of the kind of task a counselor of state might encounter by the following imaginary situation with which he might be confronted as a representative of foreign aid in a country East of Suez. It is offered in parable form.

The Proper Way to Show a Blind Man an Elephant

Once upon a time there was an Asiatic prince, who granted an audience to a blind man, who had begged persistently to be heard for many days.

When the ceremonies of presentation were over (and at these the blind man acquitted himself very well), the prince bade the blind man say what his case was.

"My case is very hard," said the blind man. "I cannot see."

"My poor fellow!" said the prince, "but I knew this already. Indeed it was that which caused me to grant you this audience before many other petitioners who have been on our lists for a very long time. But what special thing is it that you have come to ask?"

"May it please Your Highness," said the blind man, "I am very tired of the old legend of the *Seven Blind Men and the Elephant.*"

"I know the tale well," said the prince, "and have always though it very much to the point."

"Highness," said the blind man, "I have no wish to contradict; only to seek your permission to demonstrate in the public square the proper way to show a blind man an elephant."

"What an idea!" said the prince. "What is the proper way to show a blind man an elephant?"

"First," said the blind man, "I would require an elephant. A beast with fine manners, a good disposition and natural compassion for humanity."

"My poor friend," said the prince. "I fear there are no such animals in my mews. Elephants are unpredictable at best. They have a certain aloofness from human affairs."

"I have heard," said the blind man, "that there is one elephant in your mews which possesses the traits I have in mind. Your Highness's white elephant."

"My white elephant!" said the prince. "But surely you know she is sacred. And though she is indeed sweet-tempered beyond belief, it is the sweetness of a royal princess, to whom no unkindness has been done in her whole life, and the last thing in which I can imagine her compliance would be a show in a public square. Put this out of your mind. Ask of us something else. Something reasonable. For example, I have learned one of my ministers has available an excellent begging corner for which our treasury would take only one fourth of the alms bestowed on you. Now that is something practical."

"This is more than kind of your Highness," said the blind man, "but I came to sue for an opportunity to demonstrate to the public the proper way to show a blind man an elephant."

"Again I ask," said the prince. "What is the proper way to show a blind man an elephant?"

The blind man was silent, and his face took on a respectful reserve which the prince could not help thinking had great, almost royal, dignity.

"Oh, well," said the prince. "It can't hurt at least to get into the subject somewhat. You know I went to Oxford, where they taught me to have an open mind. Be at the elephants' mews tomorrow at nine, and we will go into the matter a bit. The audience is over."

The blind man made a fitting obeisance, and the prince left the audience chamber hastily, because he was nervous at the thought of a blind man backing out of his presence.

The next day, when he met the blind man at the elephants' mews, he was feeling so foolish over having given in to the blind man's whim that he made short work of greetings and commanded that his white elephant be brought forth at once.

Then he felt somewhat embarrassed not to have been more friendly and, to make small talk, said, "We call her Eugénie, you know. Named for a French empress I knew years ago."

Hardly were the words spoken when Eugénie appeared through the doorway of the elephants' mews, looking not unlike an empress, glistening white in the sun, and with every mark of the excellent grooming she had at the hands of her elephant boy, who walked before her.

"Well," said the prince, "here she is."

To the prince's infinite surprise, Eugénie reached out with her trunk and began to explore the blind man by the touch system. He for his part began to caress her trunk. From there the prince saw the blind man begin to explore Eugénie inch by inch, leg by leg, tail, leg and leg, all over her sides, both ears and back to her trunk again. Then he asked her elephant boy to bring her to her knees, and climbing on her back he seemed to touch every fragment of her broad expanse, while she remained quite still, though occasionally reaching up to touch him gently with her trunk.

Finally he slid agilely to the ground and said, "May it please Your Highness, that is the proper way for a blind man to be shown an elephant."

"Well and good, well and good," said the prince.

"And I should like to demonstrate in the public square."

"I suppose it could do no harm," said the prince, "though it does seem to me you are making much ado. Do you want me to attend this demonstration?"

"I should be too much honored," said the blind man. "But why don't you give me the elephant?"

"Give you the elephant!" said the prince in great amazement.

"She is white," said the blind man. "She is no real good to you. Everyone knows you have privately become a Unitarian. You could give it out that I have a special dispensation to use her because of my blindness. We would then ask for gifts for her upkeep. That minister of yours who manages the begging corners could work out the financial details."

"How you do run on," said the prince. "You have no idea what it costs to feed Eugénie. My minister of finance tells me she is more expensive than my Rolls Royce."

"In that case," said the blind man, "whatever we were able to obtain from demonstrations could relieve your exchequer. It would be necessary for me to have my board and keep of course before anything were turned over to the state."

"Why don't you take the begging corner?" asked the prince.

"I have my dignity to think of," said the blind man. "If I demonstrate the proper way for a blind man to look at an elephant, I will be teaching the people something which they should know and improving your realm."

"Does it matter so much?" asked the prince.

"Yes, very much," said the blind man.

"Oh," said the prince. "How I hate modern politics!"

The examination question is, How, as consultant on blindness to this prince, would you go about sustaining his budding tenderness toward a rehabilitation philosophy?

For status figures, inventors, shining examples and stormy petrels I have as yet discovered no formula. It may well be that the teacher and counselor of state are the two basic roles in work for the blind, on whose affirmation all else depends, and which all the other actors must play, whatever else they do.

2

History of Federal Vocational Rehabilitation as It Affects the Blind

Louis H. Rives, Jr.

There is perhaps no better way to gain a grasp and perspective of a great nation's efforts to improve the lot of its people who are blind than through studying the development of each piece of federal legislation which affects them. By reading the legislative hearings, the Congressional debates, the statements made at the time by leaders in work for the blind who were for or against particular proposals, we can recapture the flavor and spirit of each movement forward in building a comprehensive national program to meet the needs of blind people.

For example, we can recapture the excitement among the members of the American Association of Instructors of the Blind when Samuel Gridley Howe realized that voluntary effort alone could not assure the provision of adequate books for blind children, and threw his influence into the fight for federal legislation to provide books for blind children. This resulted in the passage of the first piece of federal legislation specifically benefiting the blind, approved March 3, 1879.* Under this act entitled "An Act to Promote the Education of the Blind," an annual sum of $10,000 was made available to provide books and educational material to blind children throughout the country. From this beginning has come the ever-expanding program of books for the blind which we know today. Each of the amendments to this basic act tells a story of increasing need of blind people for educational

---

Note: Parts of this chapter appeared in *Blindness 1970* (A.A.W.B. Annual).

*Stat. 1879, Ch. 186.

material and of the willingness of our National Government to meet this need once it is made clear.

Just as interesting is the story of the passage of the Pratt-Smoot Act in 1931 which established in the Library of Congress the immeasurably important program through which blind people all over the United States can borrow, without cost, an ever-increasing number of braille and recorded books.

The stories of the Social Security Act of 1935, which for the first time committed the Federal Government to participate in the financial support of blind people, the Randolph-Sheppard Act of 1936 which recognized that blind persons could perform successefully as operators of vending stands in federal buildings, and the Wagner-O'Day Act of 1938 which gave a special preference to workshops employing blind persons in purchases made by the Federal Government are all interesting and are filled with differing philosophies, suspense, horse trading, controversy, and finally, accomplishment.

While all of these statutes have been milestones in the development of programs to serve blind people, none I think is of more significance and importance than the development of the vocational rehabilitation program through which scores of thousands of blind and visually handicapped Americans have been given the opportunity to lead full and productive lives in dignity and self-respect. The history of the federal-state vocational rehabilitation program began with the passage of the Smith-Fess Act which was signed by President Wilson on June 2, 1920. This act provided for an appropriation of $750,000 for fiscal year 1921 and $1 million for fiscal years 1922 to 1924, for payments to states cooperating in the vocational rehabilitation of persons disabled in industry or otherwise. Services under this first act were confined to counseling, job training, artificial limbs and other prosthetic appliances, and job placement. Federal funds were divided among the states on a population basis and each state was required to spend a dollar of its own funds in order to receive a dollar of federal funds. The Federal Board of Vocational Education was given responsibility for carrying out the act. In the states, the responsibility was vested in state Boards of Vocational Education. Authorization for the program was renewed in succeeding years.

With the Social Security Act in 1935 came the first permanent authorization for this program, providing for increased aid to vocational rehabilitation in recognition of such work in a permanent program for economic security.

During this period, from 1920 until 1943, the vocational rehabilitation program had meant little to blind people. Few if any, were accepted for services by state vocational rehabilitation agencies. Applicants who were blind were referred to state commissions for the blind (which received no federal financial assistance), or were rejected as poor risks for rehabilitation. In 1943, however, there was a great and pronounced change.

The comprehensive program for the rehabilitation of the disabled veterans of World War II gave impetus to a dramatic expansion in the vocational rehabilitation program for civilians. After deliberations and debates, a new law, the Barden-LaFollette Act, was signed by President Roosevelt on July 6, 1943 (P.L. 113-78).

Such persons as Robert Irwin, Francis Cummings, Barney Day, George Meyer, and Peter Salmon fought long and hard to liberalize the provisions of the new law and to make sure that they would be fully applicable in assisting blind people in preparing for and finding gainful occupations. One key provision of the new law made it possible for the portion of the state plan, under which vocational rehabilitation services were provided blind persons, to be administered by state commissions or other agencies serving the blind. This meant that commissions and other agencies for the blind, as well as rehabilitation programs for the blind located in state departments of welfare, for the first time could recieve federal funds to assist in their programs of vocational rchabilitation.

The statute required, however, that even in states where there was a separate program for the blind, the Board of Vocational Education would have to retain general responsibility for accounting to the Federal Government and for the approval of state plans. In practice, this requirement had little effect upon the operation and programs of the separate agencies for the blind. In addition to making it clear that blind people were eligible under the program and in opening up federal financing of agencies for the blind, the 1943 law vastly expanded both the concept and financing of rehabilitation.

The definition of "disability" was broadened to include mental illness and mental retardation as well as physical impairments. The scope of rehabilitation services was expanded to include hospitalization, medical treatment and surgery, to reduce or remove a handicapping condition, and economic maintenance to assist an individual to take advantage of other rehabilitation services in addition to those which had been authorized in previous acts, including diagnostic services, guidance, counseling, placement, prosthetic appliance, necessary training for the right job, training materials, occupational tools and equipment and suitable placement in gainful employment.

In the areas of financing, the 1943 law abandoned the old system which provided for the division of a specific federal appropriation among the states on the basis of population and required that each state spend a dollar of its own funds to earn a dollar in federal funds within the allotment, and substituted a so-called "open end" financing arrangement.

Under this new system, the Federal Government undertook, without limitation, to meet 100 percent of the costs of administration of the state programs, of guidance, counseling, placement, and rehabilitating war disabled civilians, and 50 percent of the costs of other rehabilitation services such as physical restoration, training and maintenance incurred by the state agencies in carrying out their programs.

The state agencies for the blind were quick to grasp the promise and potential of the new law. Staffs were increased manyfold, the range of rehabilitation services was expanded, vigorous programs to place blind persons in industry were launched and the basic pattern of the state vocational rehabilitation agency as we know it today was set. For the next 10 years, steady progress was made when thousands of blind people were rehabilitated into employment.

By the early 1950's, it became clear that changing times and changing needs were going to necessitate corresponding modifications in our basic vocational rehabilitation law. The "open end" financing provisions of the 1943 act were not in keeping with the times. Appropriations were not large enough to cover the expenditures which the states needed to make. This meant that each year the program would be mortgaged to pay last year's bills. There was an increasing awareness of the lack of qualified personnel and there was a ground swell for improved research to find better ways of serving disabled people.

As a result of studies and hearings in which there was full participation by organizations of and for the blind, a new law was drafted, passed by the Congress, and signed by President Eisenhower on August 3, 1954.

CHANGES IN THE 1954 ACT

The major changes in the 1954 act may be summarized as follows:

1. Financing provisions. The state's share under this act was determined by a formula which took into account the individual state's population and its per capita income. The object was to give greater financial support to states with relatively large populations and relatively small per capita income, calling for these states to pay smaller portions of the total cost of the state vocational rehabilitation program than other states with greater financial resources. The federal share varied from 50 to 70 percent, with the national average about three federal dollars to two state dollars invested in vocational rehabilitation.

2. Extension and improvement project grants to states. A new system of project grants to state agencies—extension and improvement grants—provided federal financial support at more favorable rates to induce states to develop new aspects of their programs and to extend their services to disability groups and geographical areas previously reached inadequately or not at all. Extension and improvement grants provided up to $3 of federal funds for each dollar invested by the state, up to a maximum of three years for each project.

3. Research and demonstration. Grants to encourage and support research into better rehabilitation methods and to conduct demonstrations across the country also were authorized for the first time. These grants are made to public and private non-

profit organizations, such as state rehabilitation agencies, voluntary groups, universities and rehabilitation facilities.

4. Training. Grants to support the training of more professional personnel for rehabilitation services included (1) long-term training grants to educational institutions and rehabilitation agencies for support of basic advanced professional training in the form of teaching grants, traineeship grants for students selected by the educational institution, or a combination of these two; (2) short-term grants for training less than a semester in duration, e.g. institutes, workshops, seminars and other training courses; (3) in-service training grants to state vocational rehabilitation agencies for staff development programs; and (4) rehabilitation research fellowships.

5. Rehabilitation facilities and workshops. The law also authorized for the first time the use of funds granted to the states for establishment (alteration, expansion, and equipping) of rehabilitation facilities and workshops and for the initial staffing of rehabilitation facilities for a period not to exceed one year.

6. Randolph-Sheppard vending stand program for the blind. The 1954 amendments included features to strengthen the provisions for giving preference to blind persons in the operation of vending stands on federal and other property.*

7. The provision of the law relating to the designation of the agency to administer the vocational rehabilitation program in each state was revised to include state Boards of Vocational Education, independent agencies whose primary responsibility was vocational rehabilitation, and, with respect to the part of the state plan relating to the blind, any agency authorized under state law to provide vocational rehabilitation services to the blind. As a result of this change, separate state agencies for the blind became directly responsible to the Federal Government without going through the state Boards of Vocational Education.

8. The act also contained a temporary authority for direct federal grants to public and other nonprofit organizations and agencies to bring about a substantial expansion in the vocational rehabilitation program.

---

*For full discussion, see article by Senator Randolph in *Blindness 1965*.

Progress under the 1954 act was swift and far-reaching. The improved financing provisions meant immediate increase in state and federal support. During the next 10 years, state and federal funds increased almost threefold to $150 million a year and about a million people were rehabilitated into gainful employment. Through the research program, new and better ways were found to serve severely disabled clients. Through the demonstration program, these new ideas were put into practice.

The training program opened up new avenues for recruiting qualified personnel and improved the skills of personnel already engaged in the rehabilitation profession. Tremendous impetus was given to the establishment, expansion and improvement of rehabilitation facilities which became an integral and essential part of the rehabilitation process. But even as the program moved vigorously ahead, it became apparent that the forces of change were again at work.

THE 1965 VOCATIONAL REHABILITATION ACT

By the early 1960's, the special needs of workshops and rehabilitation centers, the special needs of the severely disabled, the new emphases and financing arrangements in the bold programs in education, welfare, and employment placed demands upon the vocational rehabilitation program which were beyond the scope of the existing law.

Thus started the process of writing a new chapter in the story of federal rehabilitation legislation. The first step was the preparation by the Vocational Rehabilitation Administration of its suggestions for changes and improvements in the Vocational Rehabilitation Act. These recommendations were developed on the basis of experience gained in operating under the 1954 act. They took into account suggestions and consultation from all the major organizations and agencies engaged in the rehabilitation movement including the National Rehabilitation Association, the American Association of Workers for the Blind, the National Federation of the Blind, the National Association of Rehabilitation Centers, the National Association of Sheltered Workshops and Homebound Programs. Counsel was also sought from those who had been intimately involved in the training and research activities in vocational rehabilitation.

Based on the best advice available, the Vocational Rehabilitation Administration prepared a proposal for legislation which it felt would best meet the needs of the nation's disabled people. This proposal was then submitted to the Secretary of Health, Education, and Welfare who reviewed and modified it in the light of the objectives and requirements of other programs of the Department.

The revised proposal was then forwarded to the Bureau of the Budget where it was reviewed against the backdrop of our total national objectives and requirements. The resulting proposal was then forwarded to the Congress on March 12, 1965, with the recommendation that it be enacted as a part of the President's legislative program.

This legislative proposal contained several provisions designed to improve the vocational rehabilitation program. These were: (1) a new program with liberalized matching provisions to assist the states in determining the rehabilitation potential of severely handicapped persons; (2) a new program of direct grants for the construction of rehabilitation facilities and workshops; (3) a program of assistance to workshops, including workshop improvement grants, planning grants and technical assistance; (4) grants to assist in making long-range plans to meet the needs of disabled people; (5) changes in the requirements relating to the administrative location of the state rehabilitation agency so as to permit greater flexibility and to assure effective operation; (6) the establishment of the National Commission on Architectural Barriers to Rehabilitation of the Handicapped; (7) a program of grants to states and public and other nonprofit organizations in planning, preparing for and initiating special programs to expand vocational rehabilitation services; (8) the establishment of a National Research and Information Service on matters relating to rehabilitation; (9) the removal of the economic needs test in the provision of reader services to the blind and interpreter services to the deaf; (10) authorization of federal matching for management services provided by the state agency in the vending stand program or in other small business programs conducted under the supervision of the state agency; and (11) several other technical and clarifying amendments to the existing law.

Bills embodying these legislative proposals were introduced by Senator Lister Hill on March 15 as S. 1525 and Mrs. Edith Green of Oregon on March 18 as H.R. 6476. Hearings were held in the House and in the Senate at which time interested individuals and organizations had an opportunity to give their views about needed changes in rehabilitation legislation. After deliberation by the House Committee on Education and Labor, a modified bill was prepared which was introduced by Congressman Dominick V. Daniels of New Jersey on May 20, 1965 as H.R. 8310.

This bill was passed by the House of Representatives on July 29. While there were relatively minor differences between H.R. 8310 as passed by the House and the Administration bill, there were two points of variance. One was the fact that the bill as passed by the House permitted the states to remove all services from a consideration of economic need. The other and far more important one was in the method of financing proposed. H.R. 8310 provided for the same matching rate in all states (i.e. 75% federal by FY 1967) for expenditures made for vocational rehabilitation services under the basic support program.

Under the administration proposal, the matching rate for grants for the support of rehabilitation services would have continued the variance according to the state's per capita income from 50 percent in the richer states to 70 percent in the poorer states. Also, in the area of financing, the allotment system proposed in the House bill would have allotted funds among the states from an annual authorization giving equal weight to population and per capita income, where the Administration proposal on the other hand would have allotted the sums appropriated each year on the basis of a formula which gave much greater weight to per capita income than to population, which means relatively larger allotments to the poorer states.

On the Senate side, the press of other important legislation prevented action on rehabilitation legislation until October 1, when S. 1525, which was the Administration proposal, was passed.

The differences between the bills passed by the House and Senate would have to be resolved and agreement reached if there were to be new vocational rehabilitation legislation. It was clear that the basic bar to agreement would be the financing upon which there were deep and sincere philosophical differences. Negotiations and discussions to find financing provisions which would be acceptable to both Houses were carried on tirelessly by the conferees appointed by the House and Senate as the day of adjournment drew nearer and nearer.

Finally, when it seemed almost sure that time would run out, a compromise was reached which provided for the allotment of funds on the basis favored by the Senate and for the matching of expenditures in accordance with the methods favored by the House. As soon as this basic compromise was reached, the other differences were quickly resolved and almost in the closing hours of the session, the Vocational Rehabilitation Act Amendments of 1965 were passed by the Senate and the House and sent to President Johnson who signed it into law on November 8, 1965.

In the rush for adjournment and the necessity for compromise, some areas requiring change were omitted and the authorizations for appropriations were limited in duration. These gaps were largely filled and the appropriations authorizations were extended and increased by the Rehabilitation Amendments of 1967 and 1968. The 1965 act established the basic framework and provided the federal financial support for the vocational rehabilitation program as it will continue for at least a decade. It is important, therefore, to study it in detail.

The 1965 amendments changed the federal financing provisions in the basic federal-state vocational rehabilitation program. It specified dollar limits or maximum authorization for allotment among the states—$300 million for fiscal year 1966, $350 million for fiscal year 1967, and $400 million for fiscal year 1968. The matching rate was set at 75 percent federal funds and 25 percent state funds.

Appropriations were authorized only for these three years. For subsequent years, it was necessary to ask Congress for further legislation to extend or revise this new financing system. These funds continued to be allotted among the states on a formula which reflected a state's population and its per capita income squared (in relation to national population and income).

To assure that the increased federal funds did not replace state funds but were used to increase the total finances available, the law provided that the state funds in any state must be no less than they were in fiscal 1965 and further, that should state funds be less, federal funds will be reduced.

The state rehabilitation agencies were authorized to provide vocational rehabilitation services to handicapped individuals to determine whether they could reasonably be expected to become able to engage in gainful employment.

Under previous law, state rehabilitation agencies were expected to determine—after diagnosis but before any rehabilitation services were rendered—whether or not a handicapped person could become employable after rehabilitation services. For large numbers of handicapped persons, with severe disabilities or complicated problems or both, this was virtually impossible. As a result, many of these handicapped individuals did not receive services. This modification enabled a handicapped person to receive services up to a maximum of six months to evaluate his employment potential. Within this period, the state agency could observe his response to services and determine whether further services could be expected to result in employment. In the case of mentally retarded individuals and any other designated by the Secretary of Health, Education, and Welfare, such services would be rendered to a maximum of 18 months.

The former program of "extension and improvement" grants to states was replaced by grants to states for two general purposes: (1) the development of methods or techniques which were new in the state for providing services, or (2) projects to serve those who have catastrophic or particularly severe disabilities. Federal funds for these grants were allotted on the basis of population.

For each state, the federal share for the first three years of such a project was set at 90 percent for all states; for the remaining two years, it was set at 75 percent. The act authorizes appropriations for these innovation grants of $5 million for fiscal 1966; $7 million for fiscal 1967; and $9 million for fiscal 1968.

Each state was encouraged to conduct statewide planning for rehabilitation during the fiscal years 1966 and 1967. Federal grants covering 100 percent of the cost of such statewide planning were authorized, with the amount for any state not to exceed $100,000 annually.

The planning activities were designed to accomplish three general objectives: (1) to bring into being a well-defined picture of state resources for rehabilitating the disabled and a clear picture of foreseeable needs, (2) to help assure orderly growth and development and a minimum of duplication, and (3) to arrive at an organized statewide plan by which all disabled persons needing rehabilitation services could receive them by the year 1975. It was expected that this plan would be meshed with the facilities planning.

Because the Administration and the Congress strongly wished to do everything possible to rehabilitate more disabled people without delay, provisions were included in the new act for project grants to expand vocational rehabilitation services.

These grants were available to both state agencies and voluntary nonprofit agencies. However, the objective must be the rehabilitation and return to gainful employment of larger numbers of disabled individuals. Federal grants are available for paying part of these projects, the federal share to vary according to the individual project.

Under the previous law, a state vocational rehabilitation agency had to be located either under the state Board of Vocational Education or organized as a separate agency or commission of state government.

Under the new act, the agency could be a separate commission or agency. It could be located within the state unit administering or supervising the administration of educational or vocational education, or it could be part of a larger state organizational unit which includes two or more of the following state functions: education, health, welfare, or labor. The 1965 law continued the authority for the administration of vocational rehabilitation programs for the blind by any agency of state government which was authorized by state law to carry out this function.

There was, however, a basic change relating to the organizational structure of the rehabilitation unit which is applicable to state agencies for the blind. Under this provision, the state vocational rehabilitation agency must include a vocational rehabilitation bureau, division, or other organizational unit which (1) is primarily concerned with vocational rehabilitation, or vocational rehabilitation and other rehabilitation of disabled individuals, and is responsible for the vocational rehabilitation program of such a state agency; (2) has a full-time director; (3) has a staff employed on rehabilitation work on a substantially full-time basis; and (4) is located at an organizational level and has an organizational status within such state agency comparable to that of other major organizational units of such agency.

Prior to the 1965 amendments, the federal law provided that certain services of the vocational rehabilitation program could be provided without cost only if the handicapped person was financially unable to pay the cost himself, within the state's requirements regarding the individual's economic need. The law eliminated economic need as a prerequisite for vocational rehabilitation services as far as the Federal Government is concerned. Each state, however, is at liberty to apply such economic need tests as it wishes or as may be required by state law. However, the state agency still has to take into account any similar benefits the individual may have by way of compensation, pension or insurance.

For the first time, the act authorized federal funds to help construct new rehabilitation facilities and workshops.

This new grant program also assisted in the acquisition of existing buildings and the expansion, remodeling, alteration and renovation of rehabilitation facilities and workshops. Such projects may also include assistance with the costs of initial equipment and the acquisition of land. The object here was to aid in expanding the number of rehabilitation centers, workshops and special rehabilitation facilities needed in the U. S. as a part of the total effort to develop adequate rehabilitation programs and services.

The amendments authorized federal appropriations of $1.5 million for fiscal year 1966; $7 million for fiscal year 1967; and $9 million for fiscal year 1968. Since funds are granted on a project basis in that section of the law, there is no statutory allotment system. The federal share of such a project varies according to a formula, with a minimum of 33 1/3 percent and a maximum of 66 2/3 percent.

In connection with this construction effort, the act authorized federal grant assistance in the costs of initial staffing of rehabilitation facilities and workshops, including not only those constructed through this grant program but other facilities and workshops constructed with other financing after the date of enactment of the law. Federal assistance with initial staffing was authorized at a maximum of 75 percent of staffing costs in the first year, 60 percent in the second year, 45 percent in the third year, and 30 percent in the fourth and final year.

A special provision of the act authorized assistance in the construction of residential accommodations in connection with workshops for mentally retarded individuals and such other categories of handicapped individuals as the Secretary of Health, Education, and Welfare may designate.

To provide an orderly method of determining state needs and priorities in developing centers and workshops, the act authorized grants to pay part of the cost of continuing statewide planning. This was expected to provide a pattern of review within each state which would minimize any overlapping in the developing of community and state resources, and would aid in reaching decisions on the best use of federal, state and voluntary funds.

In further support of sound projects, the act authorized planning grants, where needed, to aid project sponsors in developing well-conceived plans for construction of centers or workshops.

The 1965 amendments authorized appropriations for two grant programs for workshop improvement (training services projects, and improvement grants) as follows: For fiscal 1966—$1,500,000; for 1967—$9,000,000; and for 1968—$14,000,000. The act also provided that grants under the workshop improvement section be made only if the workshop concerned met the safety standards established by the Secretary of Labor.

The following provisions completed a plan to achieve a comprehensive program for workshop improvement in this country:

1. Training services projects. The act authorized a five-year program (beginning July 1, 1966) of grants for projects to provide more and better job training for handicapped persons in workshops and rehabilitation facilities. Grants were authorized to states or to voluntary agencies.

This program authorized grants for the following: (a) provision of training in job skills, work evaluation, work testing, tools, equipment, job tryout and related services; and (b) the payment of a training allowance to the handicapped trainee, at a rate up to $25 per week plus $10 for each dependent (but not exceeding $65 per week per trainee). These training allowances for the handicapped in training in workshops or rehabilitation centers were limited to two years for each individual.

It is the responsibility of the state vocational rehabilitation agency to determine the suitability of the handicapped individual for such training and to determine that the training to be provided will meet the individual's needs. For these training services projects, the federal share was set at 90 percent. To be eligible to participate in such a project, a workshop must meet the criteria adopted by the Secretary on the advice of the National Policy and Performance Council.

2. Workshop improvement grants. The act recognized the desire of many workshops to make improvements in their methods of operations, so they can provide the most modern and effective services to handicapped persons. The introduction of criteria as a result of the work of the National Policy and Performance Council undoubtedly stimulated many other workshops to seek improvements in their services and their general operating methods. Therefore, the new law authorized workshop improvement grants during a five-year period beginning July 1, 1965. Improvement grants were designed to help workshops analyze, improve, and increase their professional services, to similarly elevate their business operations, and to generally make more efficient and effective the total operations of the workshop.

The act authorized federal funds to pay part of the cost; thus, the federal share of any project will vary from one situation to another.

3. Technical assistance. One of the recurrent requests stated by workshop operators in many places was for the help of experts in business management, shop layout, professional services, sales management and the many other facets of a total workshop operation. The act made specific provision for this need. The Rehabilitation Services Administration can meet these requests through

panels of experts in the various fields who can be placed on duty for short periods of time to advise and help the workshop in overcoming its specific problems. In some instances this has been done through contracts with the state rehabilitation agency. This technical assistance is furnished without charge to the workshop.

4. National Policy and Performance Council. In making grant funds available to state agencies and workshops for training services projects, it is necessary to have available certain criteria which reflect the general capacity of a workshop to provide the training services needed. Therefore, the act called for the establishment of a National Policy and Performance Council, composed of 12 members selected from the fields of vocational rehabilitation, workshops, state or local government, business, the professions, labor and the general public.

The Secretary of Health, Education, and Welfare appoints the members and chooses a chairman from among the membership. Each member serves a term of four years (except that initial appointments will be made for lesser periods, to begin a system of automatic rotation of council membership). The council is responsible for advising the Secretary on the policies and criteria to be used in making grants for training services projects, for making recommendations on workshops improvement generally, for assessing the effectiveness of the workshop improvement section of the act, and for providing such other advice and services as the Secretary may request.

The 1965 law encouraged local jurisdictions (counties and cities) to make local funds available for increasing vocational rehabilitation services to their disabled citizens. Such local funds can be matched with federal funds at the same rate that other state funds are matched. For the purpose of this matching procedure, the "statewideness" requirements of the federal law and state plan may be waived. This provision of the act established in the Department of Health, Education, and Welfare a National Commission on Architectural Barriers to Rehabilitation of the Handicapped, consisting of the Secretary or his designee as chairman, and not more than 15 members. These members were chosen from among the general public and from private and professional groups working with and having knowledge of architectural problems and their solution.

This commission functioned in an effort to capitalize on the extensive and successful work done in recent years by many public and voluntary groups, aimed at making buildings more accessible to, and more usable by, seriously handicapped people. It was aimed to overcome the barriers faced by disabled people in wheelchairs, those on crutches and braces, the blind, those with severe cardiac conditions, and others who were prevented from working and leading a normal community life by these obstacles. The commission functioned for three years with an annual appropriation of $250,000 for its expenses. A final report was furnished in December 1967.

To further complement the 11-year-old research grant program of the Rehabilitation Services Administration, a new program of intramural research activities was authorized. This permitted the Rehabilitation Services Administration to undertake certain research and developmental activities which can be carried out more expeditiously through direct activity than by grants.

The 1965 act authorized a maximum period of four years of federal financial assistance to any individual pursuing a course of professional study in rehabilitation.

Federal Matching for Management Services in Vending Stands and Other Small Businesses

The 1965 act authorized (effective July 1, 1966) federal matching for management services provided by state vocational rehabilitation agencies to vending stands and other small businesses established under the supervision of the state agency.

Reader Services for the Blind and Interpreter Services for the Deaf

The act authorized federal matching in expenditures made for providing reader services for the blind and interpreter services for the deaf without regard to the client's economic need or his eligibility for similar benefits from other sources.

Vocational Rehabilitation Amendments of 1967 and 1968

On October 3, 1967, Public Law 90-99 was signed into law as the Vocational Rehabilitation Amendments of that year. These amendments provided for an allotment base of $500 million for fiscal year 1969, and $600 million for fiscal year 1970, thus extending the federal authorization to the end of that year. The amendments also provided for an additional year for comprehensive statewide planning, establishment and operation of the National Center for Deaf-Blind Youths and Adults, a program of projects with states for providing vocational rehabilitation services to handicapped migratory agricultural workers and members of their families, and removed resident requirements from the federal Vocational Rehabilitation Act. The new law also provided for a fixed allotment to the District of Columbia to enable that jurisdiction to receive an increased share of federal vocational rehabilitation funds.

On July 8, 1968, President Nixon signed Public Law 90-391 which was known as the 1968 Vocational Rehabilitation Amendments. The following provisions are covered in that legislation:

1. Extends the authorization of appropriations for grants to the states for vocational rehabilitation for an additional year with authorization of $700 million for fiscal 1971 and increases the federal share from 75 percent to 80 percent effective July 1, 1969.

2. Extends and increases the authorization of appropriations for innovation grants (formerly extension and improvements) to $3.2 million for fiscal 1969, $5 million for fiscal 1970, and $10 million for fiscal 1971, and authorizes reallocation of unused allotments.

3. Extends and increases the authorization of appropriations for research, demonstration and training to $80 million for fiscal 1969, $115 million for fiscal 1970, and $140 million for fiscal 1971.

4. Authorizes a minimum allotment of $1 million to each state.

5. Authorizes the expenditure of up to 10 percent of a state's allotment for vocational rehabilitation services under Section 2 of the act for construction of new rehabilitation facilities.

6. Establishes a grant program to public and other nonprofit agencies for recruitment and training of manpower to serve in programs for the handicapped and for the recruitment and train-

ing of handicapped persons to serve in various public service occupations.

7. Authorizes the Secretary of Health, Education, and Welfare to approve sharing of state agency finances and administration with other state agencies involved in programs for handicapped individuals.

8. Broadens state plan requirements to include evaluation of rehabilitation potential, personal and vocational adjustment, and follow-up services.

9. Authorizes the Secretary of Health, Education, and Welfare to spend up to $1 million to evaluate the effectiveness of the various programs under the act.

10. Authorizes services to families of handicapped persons.

11. Redefines "rehabilitation facility" to include sheltered workshops and eliminates the term "workshop" from the act.

12. Authorizes initial staffing for up to four years and three months for all types of rehabilitation facilities constructed under the act.

13. Extends and increases the authorization of appropriations for construction of rehabilitation facilities under Section 12 of the act to $10 million for fiscal 1969, $20 million for fiscal 1970, and $30 million for fiscal 1971.

14. Extends and increases the authorization of appropriations for improvement of rehabilitation facilities under Section 13 (formerly workshop improvement) to $10 million for fiscal 1969, $20 million for fiscal 1970, and $30 million for fiscal 1971.

15. Establishes a new program for comprehensive evaluation of rehabilitation potential of the disadvantaged with authorization of appropriations of $50 million for fiscal 1969, $75 million for fiscal 1970, and $100 million for fiscal 1971.

16. Increases the ceiling on the authorization of appropriations for the President's Committee on Employment of the Handicapped to $1 million annually and removes the terminology limiting the Committee's program to the physically handicapped.

17. Authorizes the service of an optometrist as a rehabilitation service.

The purpose of this chapter has been to describe the history of rehabilitation as it has been influenced by federal legislation.

3

International and National Projects on Blindness

Douglas C. Mac Farland

I should like to begin by setting limits for the topic assigned. A discussion of all the federally financed research projects on blindness would itself provide enough material for a book. Government research in the area of blindness is supported by the Veterans Administration, the Office of Education, several branches of the National Institutes of Health, as well as the Social and Rehabilitation Service. I am, of course, most familiar with the research conducted by the latter agency and should like to confine most of my remarks to projects that have been funded by it and its predecessors, VRA and OVR, since 1954 when the Vocational Rehabilitation Act was amended to include funds for research, demonstration, and training activities. If you are interested in obtaining information regarding a wide variety of research, let me suggest that you get in touch with the American Association of Workers for the Blind for their publication on this subject (AAWB, 1970).

DEMONSTRATION GRANTS

Our agency has spent more than $10,000,000 on a wide variety of research projects designed to improve the lives of blind persons. As alluded to previously, funding supports both research and demonstration projects. The blind population of the United States constitutes such a small minority and is so widely scattered geographically that it is essential to support demonstrations of the special techniques that have been developed in order to have them gain acceptance throughout the country. A simple example of a "demonstration" is the constellation of services usually provided to a newly blinded person in order to help him adjust to the disability and to learn useful methods of performing tasks without the use of sight. Through experimentation some years ago, it was determined that these services could best be provided as part of a total curriculum taught in a special center over a period of four to six months. Rehabilitation adjustment facilities for the blind today are commonly accepted in this country as well as in many other parts of the world. It was necessary, however, for our agency to fund a number of centers and to support special staff in others in order to demonstrate what should be included in the course, average time to gain proficiency, the ratio of instructors to students, and most important, the results that could be obtained under optimum conditions.

For many years since the inception of our research and demonstration program, selected demonstrations were supported. The sole purpose of these projects was to introduce new techniques and to make it possible for public and private agencies alike to obtain personnel and equipment in order to experiment with these new techniques. The idea was to support the program with 90 percent federal money for a period of three to five years, at which time the program would be well enough established so that it would be carried on by the local agencies. Perhaps the best example of a "selected demonstration" was the establishment of more than 30 optical aid clinics (Brinkley, 1970) throughout the country. These clinics introduced advanced technology in the field of optics, financing salaries for ophthalmologists and other necessary technical personnel as well as providing special microscopic and telescopic lenses that were prescribed for persons with small amounts of residual sight. The clinics have long since proven their worth for thousands of legally blind persons who, properly fitted and trained in the use of these special lenses, are now able to read normal print and to do some of the tasks which heretofore were impossible for them.

I am describing selected demonstration projects as background for our research program even though they are no longer supported through this funding mechanism. Selected demonstrations are now financed through a special section (P.L. 89-333, Section 3) of the Vocational Rehabilitation Act, which means that far more can be replicated and the research and demonstration money is freed for purposes more in line with the original intent of Public Law 565, (P.L. 83-565, Section 4) which expanded the VR Act. Demonstrations are still very much a part of our research program, but they must be unique in character and have a built-in research component. Except for very unusual circumstances, demonstration projects now founded by our office are not duplicated in several areas of the country. They are chosen for support because they provide an opportunity to test an especially promising hypothesis as well as applying both new and old techniques to the solution of significant problems in our field.

Perhaps the best way to illustrate how a demonstrative effort can be of practical value is to give a brief description of a few programs that have been completed. I administer a small division within the Rehabilitation Services Administration that carries among other responsibilities the continuous development and expansion of new employment opportunities for the blind. We must constantly be alert to new work horizons and survey the components of each of the new vocational opportunities to determine whether they are practical for blind persons. In the best interests of those we serve we should not become concerned with short-range jobs or fail to explore all requirements of the job.

Successful rehabilitation of a blind person or any severely disabled individual usually involves the work of many professional persons, and temporary failure must be expected occasionally. This makes the ultimate solution that much more difficult. Therefore, when we were approached about seven years ago to support the training of blind computer programmers and to help develop the techniques necessary for these individuals to become successful, we were more than a little skeptical. While a few blind persons had become successful mathematicians, this was the rare exception. We felt these same difficulties would be encountered in higher proportion in work with complex computers. Nevertheless we funded a project at the University of Cincinnati Medical School under the direction of Dr. Theodore D. Sterling (RD-2689). He was able, with the help of his students and colleagues, to devise successful techniques for dealing with card readout and other problems inherent in computer programming. In fact, the study, which was a combined research and demonstration project, was extremely successful. At the end of a three-year period only a very few of the more than 30 persons trained did not find rewarding employment as computer programmers.

Since that time, the students have moved to progressively more difficult jobs, and some of them are now highly respected systems analysts. What is more important is that the techniques developed by Dr. Sterling and his colleagues have made it possible to open a new avenue of employment. At the beginning of the program, a blind computer programmer was virtually nonexistent. Today, there are more than 450 blind persons successfully employed in the field and seven schools that have adopted Dr. Sterling's methods of instructions; in some instances they have improved upon them to the extent that they now operate continuous training courses for blind students.

Over the past several years, typing directly from dictation equipment has proven highly satisfactory for blind persons with the appropriate training and interest. Recently, with the introduction of more sophisticated equipment, the demand for medical transcribers was greatly expanded. It is now a common practice for doctors to dictate in their homes and offices, from remote parts of the hospital, and even while driving in a car. Obviously, increased demand meant the possibility of many hundreds of additional jobs for blind persons if they could be properly trained in the spelling and use of medical terminology. At the same time there were no satisfactory training materials available (Hathaway, 1967).

In conjunction with the Hadley School, our office sponsored several meetings of experts to consider how this difficult and expensive problem could be solved. Eventually it was determined that in order to provide efficient training, *Dorland's Medical Dictionary* along with the medical speller should be put into braille and made available to a number of schools training medical transcriptionists who had the necessary personnel and were willing to train blind students. To indicate the magnitude of this problem I need only say that *Dorland's Medical Dictionary* transcribed into braille constitutes 48 volumes, plus supplementary material (the medical speller and glossary of pharmaceutical terms taken from the *Physicians' Desk Reference* which will involve approximately 10 additional braille volumes). The expense for developing the plates and producing a few additional copies came to approximately $50,000, an expense that no single agency or training facility could afford. If the Federal Government had not been willing to underwrite the research and subsequent book production, a substantial work opportunity for blind persons would have been lost.

There are numerous examples of similar demonstration projects that have paid rich dividends for the blind funded by the Social and Rehabilitation Service. Though they may be of great interest and worthy of further study by professional persons working in the field, these should suffice to exemplify the demonstration aspects of our research and demonstration program; expanding employment opportunities will be discussed in detail in a later chapter.

BLINDNESS RESEARCH GRANTS

I should now like to turn to several areas of research that have yielded valuable information since the inception of the program and have contributed directly or indirectly to helping blind persons live happier and more productive lives. Research has made it possible for us to expand the number of testing instruments used for determining intelligence, aptitude, and personality. Although there is still need for more work in this area, we have given the psychologist and educator additional refined tools to help them better understand the potential of blind persons with whom they work. One example of research that filled a very apparent need was the development of a nonverbal intelligence test by Harriet and Philip Shurrager (1964) from the Illinois Institute of Technology. The test is undergoing standardization. It has, however, a very high correlation with the Wechsler-Bellevue Verbal Scale, an intelligence test that has heretofore been used rather extensively with blind persons. The value of a nonverbal instrument needs no further elaboration.

In sociological research we have been afforded the opportunity to conduct attitudinal studies in an attempt to understand the effect that certain attitudes of the sighted public have on how a blind person reacts to society and some of the reasons for certain behavioral patterns. Conversely, it is also very important to study the attitudes of blind persons toward the sighted community to determine what differences exist, if any, and how such differences can be minimized. Additional information is being obtained through the conduct of longitudinal studies to determine success and failure characteristics of certain groups and underlying reasons for these, where they are discernible. A third broad area of investigation is in the field of medicine. In spite of the vast amount of knowledge we now have concerning ophthalmology it is still painfully true that a large percentage of blindness even in an advanced country such as the United States is classified as "cause unknown." While such conditions continue to exist, there will be a tremendous need for the development of new methods and techniques for diagnosis, treatment, and surgery of the eye.

In order to concentrate on ophthalmological problems, a few years ago Congress authorized the creation of the National Eye Institute, part of the National Institutes of Health, formerly covered under the activities of the National Institute for Neurological Diseases and Blindness. It is expected that most of the eye medical research sponsored by the Federal Government will be supported or initiated by this new organization. Eye medical research is a vast and complex subject that should not be included for extensive discussion in such a short period of time, nor should it be attempted by one who is not trained in the field.

I think it important, however, even in this brief discussion of research, to indicate the importance of ophthalmological research and at least pinpoint one area of study and the impact that this will have on our field of work. It is a well-known fact that diabetes is fast becoming the major cause of blindness in this country. Physicians tell us that unless something is done to combat this disease it will in time cause more blindness than cataracts and glaucoma, the only two conditions that are now responsible for more blindness in this country. To put the problem in its proper perspective from a standpoint of rehabilitation, one third of all persons now referred to rehabilitation adjustment facilities are suffering from diabetes. At present our medical researchers are expanding a great deal of effort attempting to develop treatment to counteract the severity of the problem. Medical researchers have discovered that some of the damage caused in the eye by this disease can be eradicated by a burn technique using laser beams, the product of newly developed technology. There are some research projects currently underway to study the relative effectiveness of several methods of photocoagulation incorporating the ruby, argon and xenon lasers and other techniques in order to determine to what extent they can be effective in arresting damage done to the eye by the disease and also to compare results with those achieved by other surgical techniques.

A fourth and final area of research which I should like to touch upon is the development of hardware useful to the blind person in dealing with some aspect of his disability. Research in the development of various pieces of apparatus ranges from work on a simple folding cane to the interface of computers and braille embossing equipment in order to develop a high-speed technique for the production of braille, which hitherto has been a relatively slow process. Again I shall not attempt to catalogue the new pieces of equipment that have been developed to aid blind persons in the home and on the job. As indicated previously, descriptions of these can be obtained from the American Association of Workers for the Blind (AAWB, 1970). I certainly do not wish to leave the impression, however, that during the past 16 years we have done more than merely scratch the surface. We have not yet come to a point where we can take advantage of our tremendous advances in technology in solving the problems of the blind.

Let me give one illustration of the difficulties encountered and the great frustrations that can ensue from dealing with what on the surface would appear to be a very simple problem: a cane that could be folded into a number of pieces or telescoped so that it would fit comfortably into the user's pocket. The cane must, however, when extended be comparatively light in weight, well balanced, and rigid enough to provide immediate feedback from the tip of the cane to the user's hand. It must also be sturdy enough to withstand the rigors of normal use, without bending or breaking under daily stress conditions. To many who were given the requirements, this seemed a very simple problem and one that could be solved in a few weeks. However, it is significant to note that 25 years elapsed before we finally achieved a cane model that met the specifications set forth above (Brazil, 1969). MIT and others now have developed a practical folding cane but not without considerable expense and frustrating failures along the way.

Many other hardware items have been adapted or developed during the past 15 years—electronic meters, mechanical measuring devices, special tools, compasses, and many other devices that have made both work and recreation more available to blind persons. I deliberately chose to discuss a simple illustration rather than describe some of the more complex reading devices that are now under consideration (Bliss, 1967).

Stanford Research Institute (Drs. Linville and Bliss) has developed a print-to-tactile reading device that makes it possible for a blind person to scan ordinary print and to read it one letter at a time from a cell of vibrating reeds. Maximum speed achieved on this machine is 50 words per minute. I am sure the researchers themselves would be the first to agree that the reading device is far from ideal; however, it does indicate that solutions are being sought to the vital problem of making print directly available to the blind.

Another major breakthrough is being sought in the development of "sight substitutes." These are more in what might be termed the exotic range. The first (1969) is a device developed by Dr. Paul Bach-y-Rita, San Francisco and his associates at the Institute of Medical Science. It is Dr. Bach-y-Rita's hope to miniaturize the device and to increase the number of contact points. It operates with the use of a video camera attached directly to the head of the subject. The camera is movable and therefore the subject is able to scan the room, viewing a number of objects. Impressions picked up by the camera are transmitted to the surface of the back. The device emits a pattern of stimuli from mechanical points, roughly corresponding to what the video camera is scanning. After a short period of time, the subject is able to interpret these patterns and recognize the objects being viewed. Dr. Bach-y-Rita and his associates believe that ultimately, the device attached to the back can be incorporated in a flexible pad and when miniaturized it will not only be useful in recognizing objects but can be used as a means of travel.

Other researchers (Vaughan and Schimmel, 1966) have been working on a different type of visual prosthesis. Instead of using mechanical stimuli on the skin's surface, it is the intent of the researchers to make a direct implant on the visual cortex of the brain. There are, of course, many problems involved before such an experiment will be totally successful. We are perhaps many years away from the implant of a vision substitute, but I am firmly convinced that success is possible within the next few decades. Whether the device when completed will be universally feasible, reasonably economical, or even widely accepted is a question yet to be answered. We do know, however, that at least one brain implant was conducted in England a few years ago. The light point resolution was only 39 contact points as opposed to a projected 10,000. It nevertheless did prove that implants can be achieved and that a person can receive and recognize crude light patterns. For detailed description of the research and related experiments, we would recommend the report on the conference (RD-2064) of visual prostheses held in Chicago, June 1969.

As indicated at the outset there are literally hundreds of research projects which have interest for anyone working in our field. I hope that I have accomplished my purpose by citing a few in order to describe the research program and to pique your interest.

INTERNATIONAL RESEARCH GRANTS

Now I would like to outline what we are currently doing in our international program. We are presently working with a number of foreign countries, supporting research and demonstration projects with excess currency available through Public Law 480 funds (Agricultural Trade, 1954). The program is restricted to research projects, usually of five years' duration, the philosophy being that we encourage research, or, in many instances in the developing countries, demonstrations that when proved practical will be continued by the local government or private organizations. The program has several excellent advantages. It permits us to work with the local people in developing much needed rehabilitative services, incorporating either training or medical components. The research is generally beneficial to the United States because it provides valuable information to us which might not otherwise be available. For example, in discussing medical research earlier, I alluded to the great need for study and experimentation in the use of photocoagulation and other techniques needed to alleviate the destruction caused by hemorrhaging and other ill effects on the eye resulting from diabetes.. It is possible by conducting research projects in developing countries to obtain a great deal more data because of the much larger number of subjects who can participate in the research. There are approximately 450,000 persons who meet the definition of legal blindness in the United States as opposed to 15 million throughout the world. India, alone, estimates more than 4.5 million blind in its total population. With this in mind, then, one can readily understand that our international program is indeed a two-way street.

Let me cite one additional example in the field of medical research. In most of the underdeveloped areas of the world, eye hosptials are rare and in the outlying areas almost non-existent. Therefore, a technique must be employed whereby mobile units are used to move eye doctors, ancillary personnel, and equipment to the hinterlands, performing thousands of operations under very crude conditions. It is possible for a young doctor working in one of the eye camps to obtain more surgical experience in six months than might be available to him in many years in the United States. Because of the nature of our law governing expenditures of excess currency under Public Law 480, we are not permitted to support ongoing service projects. We have, however, initiated a number of mobile eye clinics, as local demonstrations to work on unique problems. For example, there is one area in Southeast Asia known to us that is reported to have more ophthalmological difficulties resulting from allergies than any other population of its size in the world. It is readily understandable that it would be to everyone's advantage for us to establish mobile eye care in that area. The allergies result from a profusion of flowers that seem to thrive in that climate. It is obvious that much could be learned from working with patients seen in that section of the world. We believe that this would be extremely valuable in solving some of the difficult allergy problems we encounter here in the United States.

There are, of course, many relatively mundane demonstration projects that are proving successful overseas but do have a certain amount of spin-off for us. Let me conclude by citing one located in New Delhi, India (Deshmukh, 1967). This project has been designed to train blind persons from New Delhi and outlying areas in what is termed light engineering work (semiskilled factory work) in the industrial areas of India. The course, including travel instruction, assembling, packaging, and machine operation, is generally concluded in about a four-month period. So far, the program has finished four classes. In every instance, more than 90 percent of the students have been successfully placed in employment. This may not seem like a remarkable record until one realizes that it has been accomplished in a country where there are 80 million persons underemployed, 30 million unemployed, and where thousands of trained engineers are forced to take laboring jobs because opportunities in their own profession do not exist at present. One would think that under such conditions training blind persons would be a futile endeavor. This, however, is obviously not the case. The lesson to be learned by all of us who are engaged in training and placement of disabled workers is that appropriate training is the key to success—surveying the employment field regardless of how overcrowded it may be and then providing the best training available. Perhaps this project does not have a direct relationship to our own vocational rehabilitation program here in the United States, but if nothing else, it provides an inspiration for any of our counselors who feel that their job in assisting disabled persons to find employment is a difficult one.

I hope that the foregoing sampling of research will prove enough to whet your appetites and that you will delve deeper in our field of endeavor whether your interest is as a professional worker or a volunteer who wishes to do something constructive with a few hours of extra time.

REFERENCES

Agricultural Trade, Development and Assistance Act of 1954, as amended (P. L. 480). Program is financed with U. S.-owned foreign currencies accumulated from the sale of agricultural commodities in developing nations.

REFERENCES

Bach-y-Rita, Paul: Tactile television system. San Francisco, Institute of Medical Sciences, RD-3109, 1969.

Bazell, Seymour: Design and development of a collapsible folding cane. Chicago, ITT Research Institute, RC 38, 1969.

Bliss, James C.: Optical-to-tactile conversion aids for the blind. Stanford, California, Stanford University, RD-2475, 1967.

Brinkley, Sterling B.: Optometry and the vocational rehabilitation program. *AAWB Blindness Annual,* 1970.

Deshmukh, Durgabai: To establish a technical training center and sub-contract workshop for the blind. New Delhi, India, The Blind Relief Association, Project No. 19-P-58132-F-01, 6/67 - 2/72.

Hathaway, Donald W.: Development of a braille medical dictionary. Winnetka, Illinois, Hadley School for the Blind, RD-2603, 1967.

Shurrager, Harriett C.: *Manual for the Haptic Intelligence Scale for Adult Blind.* Chicago, Illinois Institute of Technology, RD-1412, 1964.

Sterling, Theodore D.: Investigation into optimum employment procedures in computing. New York, Association for Computing Machinery, DR-2689, 1968.

U. S. Government Sponsored Research to Study Blindness—1970 Supplement. American Association of Workers for the Blind, Inc.

Vaughan, H. G. and Schimmel, Herbert: Preliminary study of feasibility of electrocortical prosthesis. New York, Albert Einstein College of Medicine, RD-2064, 1966.

4

The Private Agency

Allan L. Ward

It seems highly appropriate in describing the private agency and its services to give an in depth description of an outstanding agency. The efforts of the private agency will then be described by discussing the work which is done in one particular center—the Arkansas Enterprises for the Blind. The reader should keep in mind that agencies have many common characteristics as well as individual differences.

Arkansas Enterprises for the Blind is a volunteer, nonprofit organization incorporated under the statutes of Arkansas as a rehabilitation center for the blind and visually handicapped. The program was begun in 1939; the center was opened in 1947, and is governed by a board of directors elected by the Lions Clubs of Arkansas. It provides evaluation, comprehensive personal adjustment, prevocational training, and selected vocational training all of which are used to assist people with visual limitations to function as independent individuals with potential for self-support.

The center of the complex of buildings making up the agency occupies a full city block and includes five modern two-story, specially designed buildings surrounding an open quadrangle. Other home-size units stand on adjoining property which equals two more city blocks. Its staff consists of approximately 90 persons, with a training capacity of approximately 100. The process through which the trainee passes can be described by discussing sequentially the activities he encounters.

Initially, formal application is made for admission to Arkansas Enterprises for the Blind. Usually this formal application is made by the appropriate representative of a state agency, often the home counselor. In other instances family members or other sponsoring agencies may submit this application. The formal application is reviewed by the admissions committee of Arkansas Enterprises for the Blind. A letter of acceptance from the center sets the date for the person to arrive.

ACTIVITIES AT THE CENTER

Monday of each week throughout the year is used to begin the process of introducing new trainees to AEB activities. When a trainee arrives at a public conveyance point such as an airport or bus station, he is met by a representative of the center. He is taken to his dormitory, introduced to his dormitory supervisor who takes him to his room and helps him unpack and orient himself to the room. Following this, the dormitory supervisor takes him to the office of the administrative assistant. The administrative assistant interviews him, reviews with him the processes of center operation and certain fundamental policies, advising him of the aspects that most immediately involve him. On the day of the trainee's arrival at the center, the administrative assistant sends a letter to the home counselor advising him of his clients arrival at the center.

The new trainee then goes for an interview with the director of training or the coordinator of trainee services. The center policies are reviewed with him and his training program discussed. They talk with him regularly throughout his stay at the center. Following this, he is given an extensive orientation tour of the entire facility by one of the professional staff members. A conference is scheduled for each trainee with the executive director of Arkansas Enterprises for the Blind during his first month at the center. The new trainee is immediately assigned to his center counselor with whom he has a conference within the first few days. The counselor provides him with a ready source of information, and the trainee knows that he may call on his counselor at any time for aid and assistance.

After arriving on Monday, the trainee is examined on Tuesday by the staff physician to verify previous medical examinations, identify the possibility of any communicable disease, and to identify any new condition that would influence the person's training.

Based on the examination and in conjunction with the previous report supplied to the center, whenever necessary, a special diet is recommended. Any necessary medication is prescribed and the dosage indicated. Where necessary, the physician refers the trainee to a specialist, such as a dentist, dermatologist, etc., for any further examination. Diabetics, for example, receive an automatic foot inspection and are taken to a podiatrist if necessary. They are weighed each week and any gain or loss is noted. When any other condition, such as obesity, necessitates weight records, this may be checked daily.

It is expected that persons on special diets will bring their dietary listings with them. These are reviewed by the nurse and kitchen staff and discussed wtih each trainee. Food is specially prepared for each meal that will meet with the needs and restrictions of each particular diet.

Prior to the arrival of the trainee, the scheduling committee has analyzed the background information concerning him, and has prepared a schedule for his first month of evaluation. This schedule takes into account his past medical record—especially in areas such as physical conditioning and mobility where physical exertion might be contraindicated by various physical problems, until his tolerance for activity can be determined by observation and tests.

The new trainee then begins his work in a variety of the training areas. The staff evaluates his performance level in each area and keeps careful daily records of his level and progress. These records form the basis of progress reports which will be prepared at the end of the month for evaluating the trainee's performance and progress in all areas and the steps he needs to take toward his vocational goal. These areas of training are divided into five major categories including orientation and mobility, personal management, work evaluation and prevocational training, educational services, and social and recreational activities. Educational services include the area of alpha communicative techniques, braille, abacus, typing, academic instruction and oral communication. Recreation and social skills include physical conditioning, social skills and recreation. Personal management includes techniques of daily living, home management and grooming. Orientation and mobility includes the detailed training sequences and classes in concept development. Work evaluation and prevocational training is divided into the two major areas of shop and crafts.

The trainee is advised that he can see any staff member on the same day that his request is made by notifying the information center. The staff member will be informed immediately and will schedule the trainee at his earliest convenience no matter what the trainee's concern may be, whether it is housing, schedule, finance, a personal problem or some other consideration. On Thursday of each week the supervisors from each area meet with the records of their departments and review the overall schedule of all persons.

Once a month the trainee's schedule is reviewed and discussed by the supervisors after discussion with the personnel in their area. Requests for changes in the schedule can be made by the trainee, the center counselor, an instructor, or a supervisor. One month before termination, a full staffing is held with written reports being submitted the day prior to the oral discussion.

Reports are sent to the home counselor monthly. The first month's report is an evaluation of all the areas in which he has been observed along with recommendations for necessary training. Following that, there is a progress report each month. At the completion of training, a terminal report is written. This is prepared three days prior to the trainee's termination so that it can be sent by mail to arrive in the counselor's office by the time the trainee returns home.

During the first week, the center chaplain confers with each new trainee. For any who wish to attend a place of worship of their choice, he will assist in making contact with the appropriate group and arranging transportation. He is available during the afternoon and also at night in his counseling role.

The trainee is expected to remain on the campus during his first two weeks of evaluation in order to become acquainted with the center and also for his own safety until he can be fully evaluated by the mobility department. At the end of two weeks the mobility department issues him a safety approval slip indicating how, with whom, and under what circumstances he is qualified to travel safely. At some time during the first two weeks the staff social worker interviews the trainee for approximately two one-hour sessions in order to secure a comprehensive social history.

By the third week, a series of tests are administered to the trainee. These generally include the Wechsler Adult Intelligence Scale (WAIS; Wechsler, 1955), the Pennsylvania Bi-Manual Work Sample (Roberts, 1945), The Rotter Incomplete Sentences Blank (Rotter and Rafferty, 1950), and any others felt necessary after observation and study of the trainee or his records. If the trainee is under undue tension during this initial period, the testing may be postponed until a later date. When the records indicate that these tests have been given prior to the person's coming to the center, they may be waived, and/or additional tests may be given.

During the first month the trainee is screened by the optical aids area to see if he has any degree of usable vision that may be benefited by the use of such aids. When the screening affirms such a potential benefit, he is given a thorough optical aids examination as quickly as possible.

The orientation and mobility department administers a hearing screening test during the first month; if there is any indication of reduced hearing ability, a full examination is scheduled by a professional audiologist. At some time during the first two months after his arrival, the trainee is interviewed by the staff psychiatrist. Those whose records indicate some type of problem are dealt with first. Those necessitating additional time are scheduled accordingly.

In addition to his regular training schedule, the trainee attends a large group discussion three times a week. This is held in the auditorium and consists of a variety of presentations on policies and procedures, visiting lecturers speaking on a variety of topics and presentations on subjects requested by the trainees themselves. Twice a week the trainee meets for a small group discussion. Each small group consists of approximately 10 persons usually supervised by one of the professional staff members with at least a master's degree. These discussions offer the trainee an opportunity to express himself concerning the ideas and emotions that he experiences in connection with his visual problem and related areas of life.

During the evening hours and weekend periods, various instructional rooms are open for study and practice, such as the typing room, the braille-writing rooms, etc. In addition to the study activities, a comprehensive recreational program provides activities each evening and weekend. These consist of formal visits to places of historical or artistic interest, to performances of classical and contemporary variety on stage and on film as well as an array of informal game nights, outdoor barbeques and talent shows.

The specific time of termination is determined on the recommendations of the staff, in consultation with the trainee and the home counselor. On the day of departure, the staff member takes the trainee to the transportation terminal and sees him safely on his way.

STAFFING PATTERN

The organization of the center includes the executive director who is directly responsible to the board of directors. His immediate aids include an administrative assistant and an assistant executive director. Directly responsible to the executive director are the director of training, the director of public relations, the director of research and staff development and the chaplain-field representative. Assisting the director of training is the coordinator of training services. The aforementioned positions constitute a cabinet that meets weekly with the exctuive director.

Six supervisors of training activities are responsible to the director of training. The six supervisors of training activities include the chief of psycho-social services and the supervisors of personal management, work evaluation and prevocational training, orientation and mobility, educational services and social and recreational activities. Responsible to the supervisors are instructors and instructor's aids who teach in the various areas already outlined in the training sequence. The staff meets twice weekly to discuss trainee problems.

The office of public relations offers a continual series of articles and materials to the public through the media such as newspapers, radio and television, on stores of interest and education so that the public may become more fully cognizant of the potential and achievements of blind persons.

In order to keep the staff up-to-date on new developments and training techniques and to provide an active interchange of ideas, the staff development office plans and supervises in-service training through regular monthly meetings, quarterly meetings, and a special annual meeting. To these are invited professional workers in various fields related to the work and services of the center. A staff development library provides background reading materials in the various aspects of work with the blind.

Another important aspect of the center's services involving work with blindness is the growing internship training program. Persons hired by various state agencies or private agencies necessitating varying degrees of intensive training are sent to Arkansas Enterprises for the Blind for comprehensive preparation in orientation and mobility, counseling and rehabilitation teaching which may stress any of the particular sub-areas involved. The internship program is coordinated through the office of staff development and provides daily seminars to integrate the materials being observed in the daily classes, schedules periods of observation, instruction and practice teaching, and develops an individual program geared specifically to the needs of each intern.

Another adjunct of the overall AEB program is the research area. This concentrates on finding new and better ways to offer training services. During the last several years, for example, the center has received training grants through the Social and Rehabilitation Services Administration of the Department of Health, Education and Welfare for developing the optical aids clinic, for demonstrating the effectiveness of orientation and mobility training for persons outside the rehabilitation center, for preparing blind students for college work, for training blind persons as taxpayer service representatives, for developing a major communications syllabus, and for testing the effectiveness and use of newly developed ultrasonic binaural sensors. Additional proposals under consideration include new methods of training blind computer programmers, of serving the elderly blind in their home communities, of meeting the needs of the preschool child, of training vending stand operators, of training phone answering service personnel for various government or private agencies among them.

The source of financial incomes and categories of expenditures of the private agency are various. Of its 100 percent input, AEB receives 76 percent from tuition paid by rehabilitation agencies; 9 percent by sponsoring Lions Clubs; 5 percent from memberships, memorials and miscellaneous gifts; 7 percent from federal research grants; and 3 percent from sales of such items as light bulbs. The expenditures of AEB can be catalogued in four main categories; 58 percent of the expenditures are for professional services; 28 percent for operations and maintenance; 9 percent for administration and office; and 5 percent for public education.

In looking at a specific private rehabilitation agency, we have reviewed the training program of Arkansas Enterprises for the Blind and its structure, as it assists people with visual limitations toward the goal of leading active and productive lives.

REFERENCES

Roberts, J. R.: *Manual for the Pennsylvania Bi-Manual Work Sample.* Minneapolis, Education Test Bureau, 1945.

Rotter, J. B. and Rafferty, Janet E.: *Manual for the Rotter Incomplete Sentences Blank.* New York, Psychological Corperation, 1950.

Wechsler, D.: *Manual for the Wechsler Adult Intelligence Scale.* New York, Psychological Corperation, 1955.

5

Developing Special Programs for Subprofessionals and Volunteers

Robert L. Pogorelc

The critical shortage of professionally trained personnel in the fields of health, recreation, education, and social welfare, coupled with the increasing public demand for these types of community services, has led to the development of government legislation and voluntary agency programs involving the expanded utilization of volunteers. "Volunteerism" (or "voluntaryism," as it has been termed on occasion) is not only fundamental to work for the blind,* but this field of social endeavor has pioneered in the use of volunteers in many unique ways. The purpose of this paper is to discuss present volunteer utilization in agencies which provide service to blind individuals, to identify some of the current problems affecting the use of volunteers in this field, and to consider ways in which community agencies serving the blind might utilize volunteers more effectively.

BLIND AGENCIES USING VOLUNTEERS

At the present time, more than 400 voluntary agencies and organizations provide direct services to blind persons, through the use of professionally trained and qualified mobility instructors, braille and typing teachers, home economists, occupational therapists, psychologists, social workers, counselors, work evaluators, etc. In addition, many of these agencies also utilize volunteers for reading, friendly visiting, shopping trips, social, cultural, and

*It is intended that references to the "blind" throughout this paper also include the "severely visually disabled."

recreational trips, and so forth on behalf of blind persons. Volunteers also serve on boards of directors, advisory committees, and as administrators and supervisors in these agencies and organizations.

Notable examples of volunteer utilization within agencies for the blind, 1968, can be found in every part of the country. At the Braille Institute of America in Los Angeles, 1445 volunteers have given over 104,000 hours of service in 11 different service categories. The New York Jewish Guild for the Blind has over 300 volunteer workers serving in every area in which professional staff are engaged, in accordance with their individual skills and interests.

The Phoenix (Arizona) Center for the Blind is heavily dependent on its 350 volunteers, who donated 25,000 hours of their time on over 8,500 separate assignments. At the bare minimum wage, this represents a value of $35,000, which would double their present budget.

The Hadley School for the Blind in Winnetka, Illinois, utilizes over 150 volunteers, without whom their program would be severely handicapped since the contribution of manpower which volunteers represent is considered beyond estimate. The four locations of the Massachusetts Association for the Blind received the services of over 500 volunteers who assisted clients with tasks for which there is no substitute for sight to an extent not possible by existing staff.

In addition, national organizations utilize the services of volunteers across the country for specific programs. The National Society for the Prevention of Blindness has over 17,000 volunteers, mostly young mothers providing preschool visual screening, as well as those serving as officers and directors of its state affiliates and national organization.

The National Braille Association has more than 2100 members who are, for the most part, dedicated volunteer braillists from all parts of the United States. A unique group of volunteers is the "Telephone Pioneers," who, as veteran employees of the Bell Telephone System throughout the country, volunteer to repair talking-book machines in their respective localities. This group numbers in excess of 3600.

These are just a few examples of volunteer utilization, gleaned from comments and reports submitted to the Office for the Blind and Visually Handicapped, Rehabilitation Services Administration, U. S. Department of Health, Education and Welfare, in response to a recent survey.

PROBLEM IN USING VOLUNTEERS

The problems involved in the use of volunteers are, in many respects, similar to those generally found in personnel management. Personnel policies in the areas of recruitment, selection, training, motivation, assignment, supervision, and recognition of volunteers vary from outstanding to grossly inadequate in agencies serving the blind, as they do with respect to paid staff members, and as they do in all types of public and private organizations, both profit and nonprofit. To the extent that the personnel policies and practices concerning volunteers pose problems which are common to those encountered with other staff members, the implementation of the modern principles and practices of personnel administration can resolve or reduce these difficulties. However, certain personnel problems which are peculiar to the area of volunteer utilization have been identified, and have particular implications for agencies for the blind.

The most critical of these is the recruitment problem, which of course, threatens the very lifeblood of voluntary activity. In the past, voluntary agencies serving the blind had, with some exceptions, relatively little serious competition for the services of volunteers. Several factors, however, have developed rather recently which alter this situation considerably. First, the enactment of federal legislation promoting the use of volunteers in various health, education, and social service fields has both stimulated volunteer activity and increased the competition for their services. Many of these programs, in addition, are highly challenging and exciting to young people, who often forsake or postpone promising business careers for the opportunity to serve. Examples of these federal programs include VISTA, the Peace Corps, Operation Headstart, community action groups, civil rights activities, projects devleoped under the Higher Education Act of 1965, and so forth. Secondly, the effects of the low birth rate of the depression years are being felt, with a resultant decrease in the availability of volunteers in the middle-age range who have enough experience, knowledge, skill, time, energy, and dedication to inherit and carry on the leadership function in our community agencies. Thirdly, the outbreak of riots and other forms of violence which beset almost all of our large metropolitan areas has caused many individuals to be wary of venturing (especially at night) into the downtown sections where many of our agencies, and often the blind clients, are located. Fourth, the increased number of working women tends to suggest that the capable woman of middle years whose children are grown, or almost so, is less likely to be found among volunteer ranks. In many cases she has returned to teaching or to business. Fifth, many young volunteers are subject to the mobility of our times; because of transfers and promotions and job changes, there are likely to be short terms of service among volunteers, or they may never return to the volunteer ranks in a new, unfamiliar community. Sixth, as the various professions become more complex and demanding, both in training and experince, it becomes difficult for some professional staff members to accept a lay person in any significant role. If volunteers are utilized at all, they are assigned to menial tasks, regardless of their abilities, training or experience, or they are treated in such a manner as to make them feel incompetent, unneeded, and/or a burden to the professional staff. Needless to say, any volunteers who might remain with the agency under these circumstances will function at a level which will "justify" the professionals' attitude toward them.

The problems indicated above should not be considered to be a complete listing of those affecting volunteer recruitment, nor should it be assumed that all agencies have these difficulties. However, the problems discussed above may provide a basis for investigation regarding the factors involved for those agencies which do have volunteer recruitment problems.

Although a deficiency in any one area of personnel management can and does affect one or more other areas, either directly or indirectly, the aspect of volunteer recognition is probably the next most critical area to be considered in the utilization of volunteers. It is not intended that the importance of other areas, especially training and supervision, be minimized, but the fact that volunteers contribute their time and energies without recompense should emphasize the need for appropriate recognition of their efforts. Unless the individual volunteer perceives his voluntary experience as personally satisfying and worthwhile in terms of his expenditure of time and effort, he will not continue to serve. If he leaves, the best programs of recruitment, selection, training, assignment and supervision will have been for naught. Obviously, every potential volunteer in work with the blind does not have the appropirate personality and temperament to serve successfully, but it is the agency's responsibility to maximize the opportunity for satisfaction among those who do. The concept of recognition is inherent in the idea of satisfaction, since it is a rare individual who will continue to perceive his efforts as satisfying without adequate recognition. Various mehtods of recognition have been adopted by agencies for the blind, including outings, picnics, recognition luncheons and dinners, certificates, awards, etc. It would appear that this area is sufficiently important to justify intensive study concerning the development of new and innovative way of accomplishing the desired objectives.

It is beyond the scope of this chapter to discuss the various methods and techniques involved in the selection, training and development, assignment, and supervision of volunteers. However, it is imperative that agencies serving the blind become aware of and implement the principles and practices which have been successfully utilized by organizations with highly developed volunteer programs, particularly the American Red Cross, the Boy and Girl Scouts of America, and similar organizations.

EFFECTIVE USE OF VOLUNTEERS

In an attempt to stimulate increased effectiveness in the utilizations of volunteers among agencies serving the blind, a few proposals are offered for consideration in addition to those mentioned above. First, it may be desirable, and perhaps, necessary, to reimburse volunteers for expenses incurred in the course of their volunteer activities. There are, undobutedly, a number of individuals who would be willing and eager to volunteer their services; but because they live on a small, fixed income they are unable to afford the expense of transportation to and from the voluntary agency, or the expense of eating meals in a restaurant while on volunteer duty. It would appear that many retired persons have the available time and the inclination to serve, but fall into the limited income category, and, rather than place themselves in the embarrassing position of asking for expense reimbursement, either avoid becoming involved or drop out after becoming aware of the cost. The amount of money involved might be considered nominal to the agency or to salaried individuals, but not to those who must account for every dollar. This concept has been termed "paid volunteers" which, at first blush, appears to be a contradiction in terms. However, this terminology is being increasingly used to describe volunteers for whom expenses are reimbursed. Secondly, it is suggested that the agencies for the blind carefully review their activities in order to identify those tasks, presently being performed by paid staff members, which might lend themselves to assumption by volunteers, either in their entirety, or at least in part. This would free the paid staff for activities which cannot properly be delegated to volunteers, or permit the assignment of volunteers to tasks which do not justify the use of paid staff in relation to other, more appropriately professional, activities.

A secondary benefit of this task review might be to provide a basis for recruiting volunteers with specific training and/or experience, as required by the task itself. Identification of the task and of personal requirements necessary for its completion might suggest a specific resource for the recruiting of volunteers. Thirdly, administrators of agencies for the blind in a particular geographic area might consider the establishment of central volunteer bureaus, either exclusively for their agencies or in conjunction with other types of voluntary organizations. Another possibility might involve the identification of volunteers with particular skills and/or experiences, and the sharing of these individuals among the area agencies on an "as needed" basis, since some activities are of a short-term nature, and some volunteers will accept assignments involving only one specific task, e.g. teaching English or performing magic tricks, because of their particular expertise in that field. Fourth, a concerted effort should be made among national, state, and local blind organizations to establish training programs for agency administrators and staff regarding the problems and principles of volunteer utilization and to prepare manuals and guidelines for the subject which can be utilized on an on-going basis.

SUMMARY

In summary, the need for increased services to blind individuals far surpasses the supply of trained professional staff. In order to reduce the impact of this problem, both professional workers for the blind and the public in general must be made aware of and accept the fact that volunteers are making and can make significant contributions to this field. In addition, the application of sound personnel policies and practices, plus the development of innovative ways to recruit and utilize these volunteers, can lead to the provision of more and better services to the blind, within the limits of present financial and manpower resources.

Part Two
Blindness and Its Impact

6

Eyes and Vision

William D. Rusher

This chapter represents an effort to present some aspects of ophthalmology to those who work with handicapped people. This material is not intended to be a scientific text for the medical student, general physician or ophthalmologist. It is intended as a source of information for nonmedically trained personnel who are interested in helping those who have visual limitations. It is also an attempt to dispel some popular, but false, myths and old wives' tales regarding vision, eyes and their use.

Because ophthalmology is a broad field of medicine, intimately connected with many other medical specialties, it is difficult to abstract and condense the subject into a relatively short, readable chapter which can serve as a reference for those not medically trained. Yet this is the assigned task and the direction in which the effort has been made.

Of necessity, much will be omitted. Some purposefully as being of minimal value to the intended reader and some through inadvertence on the part of the writer.

The eyes are living, precisely engineered optical instruments which are unbelievably delicate in structure and function, yet are able to stand years of abuse, injury, neglect, and indifference and still perform.

Compared to the finest camera, the eye can automatically aim and focus itself in less than half a second, adjust its aperture size, record the picture on three-dimensional color film which has an instantaneous development time, and is self-renewing after each exposure.

ANATOMY

The eyes are forward outpouchings of the brain to which they are connected by nerve trunks. About thirty percent of the entire brain is concerned with vision. This area of the brain is as far removed from the eyes as it can be and still be in the head. The visual cortex, as it is called, is located posteriorly, behind and above the ears. Visual impulses must travel from the front of the brain to the back where seeing actually occurs. One may have a visual handicap because that part of the brain does not work, even though the eyes may be "normal." Therefore, visual limitation is not limited to affectations of the eyes alone. An individual with a 20/400 brain cannot see 20/20. Since the visual mechanism is a long and diverse one, sight can be affected by innumerable conditions interrupting the visual tracts at any point in their course. An infection, inflammation, tumor, hemorrhage, or clot can obstruct the visual pathway somewhere between the eye and the visual center in the posterior brain and not directly involve either the eye or the visual cortex.

The eye is formed as a combination of two spheres of different sizes. The anterior (or front) one-sixth portion is smaller than the posterior portion and has a radius of about 7.5 mm. The posterior five-sixths portion has a radius of about 12 mm. Therefore, the diameter of the larger section of the eye is about 24 mm or just a little less than one inch (25 mm = 1 inch). The eye weighs about 7 grams and its volume is about 6.5 cubic centimeters.

The eye is made up of three separate layers. These layers are continuous in both anterior and posterior portions. The outer layer is tough, fibrous, protective, and relatively inelastic. The anterior part of this layer is called the cornea. It is analogous to a watch crystal. It is virtually a transparent disc, consisting of five distinct layers and it has strong optical properties. The cornea is exquisitely sensitive and can be very painful when injured—for example, by a scratch, a foreign body, or by burning from ultraviolet light from the sun or a sunlamp. It is subject to a number of diseases and can cause blindness if sufficiently damaged. An enormous amount of study has been and is being carried out regarding the cornea. As a result, corneal transplants now enjoy about a 75 percent success rate and are becoming a leading surgical means of sight restoration.

Posterior to the cornea and continuous with it is the sclera, or the white part of the eye. Although the material making up the cornea and sclera are practically the same, their architecture is different, rendering the sclera opaque. This results partially from the random deposition of the scleral fibers similar to the effect obtained when a box of toothpicks is emptied all at once on a table. The tissue fibers of the cornea, on the other hand, are laid down in regular rows, in laminated layers, resembling the structure of plywood. This arrangement offers very little resistance to passage of light, rendering the cornea practically transparent. The sclera is less susceptible to disease or injury since the major portion of it is deep in the bony orbit, surrounded by a protective fat pad; however, it does not escape entirely.

The visible anterior portion of the sclera, between the eyelids, is covered by a thin, moisture-producing membrane called the conjunctiva. The conjunctiva also lines the inner surfaces of the eyelids and folds on itself when blinking occurs. Inflammation of this layer is known as conjunctivitis. This can result from many noxious agents and is commonly called "pink eye."

The middle layer of the eye is made up of blood vessels and structures derived from blood vessels. Posteriorly, this vascular layer is called the choroid. Its primary function is one of nourishment for the internal parts of the eye, particularly the retina. The anterior part of this layer undergoes remarkable change and becomes an annular or ring-shaped organ known as the ciliary body. (This is a muscular ring with about 70 radial folds extending posteriorly. It has several functions, one of which is associated with accommodation, to be discussed later.)

The most anterior segment of this layer is known as the iris. Thus the iris is made up of blood vessels. Architecturally, the blood vessels are arranged in arcades or loops of vessels larger at the periphery and becoming smaller toward the center of the eye where there is a round mobile opening called the pupil. These vessels do not normally carry blood, but they may when disease occurs.

Collectively, the choroid, ciliary body, and iris are known as the uvea. When the uvea becomes diseased, it is called uveitis. This can be acute or chronic, localized or widespread, and can produce minimal to severe visual damage, even total blindness. Sympathetic ophthalmia is a form of uveitis.

The posterior layers of the iris and the ciliary body contain a very large quantity of pigment-bearing tissue cells. One of the functions of this material is to act as a screen to control the amount of light entering the eye through the pupil. The pupil, which is actually a hole in the center of the iris, is controlled by a set of constrictor and dilator muscles which automatically decrease the pupillary diameter in bright light and increase its size in dim light or darkness. This operates similarly to the iris diaphragm in the camera. When the pupillary opening is small, distant objects are clearer and the depth of focus is greater than when the pupil is dilated or widely opened.

The innermost layer of this three-layered organ is the retina. The retina is the thin nerve layer lining the inside of the globe. It extends anteriorly to just behind the ciliary body. The same layer extends forward to cover the ciliary body with a film of fluid-producing cells known as the ciliary epithelium. This layer produces the fluid called aqueous humor which fills the anterior chamber or the space behind the cornea and in front of the crystalline lens. The crystalline lens is located immediately posterior to the iris.

The retina is the nerve center of the eye. It is made up of 10 layers of tissue, yet is less than one mm thick. There are about 135 million separate nerve elements in the retina of each eye. Remember that the whole eye is less than one inch in diameter. The nerve elements sensitive to light are called rods and cones. They are located in the posterior layer of the retina, next to the middle layer of the eye, the choroid. The cones are concerned with day and color vision, the rods with night vision and motion. The cones are most numerous in the central posterior part of the retina, along the visual axis, in a small depression called the macula. The cones are packed very closely together in the macula and each cone located there has a separate nerve fiber connecting it to the visual cortex in the posterior brain. This is the area in the retina which permits acute discreet, sharp vision. This is the only part of the retina capable of seeing 20/20.

The rods are located primarily in the periphery of the retina where the cones are very thinly distributed. The rods contain a pigment called visual purple which is bleached when light stimulates the retina. The rods provide for peripheral or side vision. The stimuli from four to eight rods are collectively gathered by one nerve fiber and carried to the brain. In subdued light, insufficient to stimulate the cones, the rods provide form vision, appreciation of motion, and spatial relationships necessary to function adequately at night. This helps explain why one can see an object better in the dark if he looks slightly to one side, above, or below it. Rods are also important in persons who have a disease known as retinitis pigmentosa, in which the rods are damaged early in life and cause night blindness, which is one of the earliest symptoms of this disease.

The retina is subject to and reacts to disease and injury just like the brain. If a portion of the retina is damaged by disease or injury and its function is lost, it is not recoverable. The damaged retinal elements may heal but a nonvisually functioning scar replaces the damaged part and the eye loses a corresponding segment of sight. Disease or injury can produce such an event. The retina is subject to several infectious agents. It is very susceptible to damage from pressure as occurs in glaucoma. It is easily damaged by trauma, such as sudden hard blows on the eye. The retina may be damaged by diseases which cause bleeding into or around it, and it is subject to breakdown with formation of holes which in turn causes retinal separation or detachment.

The eyes rest in roughly cone-shaped bony orbits. The orbits are oriented horizontally in the skull with the innermost sides of the cones being parallel and the apices of the cones deep inside the head. The eyes are moved by six muscles attached to each eye. These extraocular muscles are paired. There are two horizontally opposed muscles, two vertically opposed, and two which are set at an oblique angle, above and below each eye. When one turns his eyes to the right, the horizontal muscle on the outside of the right eye (on the ear side) contracts but the horizontal muscle on the inside (nearest the nose) of the left eye must contract to turn the left eye to the right in concert with the right eye. The extraocular muscles therefore function as paired yoke muscles.

Three different nerves control the function of these muscles. The lateral rectus muscle (the horizontal muscle on the ear side of the eye) is supplied by the sixth cranial nerve, the abducens nerve, so named because it abducts the eye (i.e. it turns it outward).

The superior oblique muscle (an obliquely placed muscle running across the top of the eye, which rotates the eye in a clockwise fashion) is supplied by the fourth cranial nerve, the trochlear nerve, so named because it operates through a pulley.

The remaining four muscles, the superior, medial, and inferior recti muscles and the inferior oblique muscle, are all innervated by the third cranial nerve, called the oculomotor nerve.

The horizontal muscles turn the eyes from side to side, the vertical muscles turn the eyes up or down, and the oblique muscles rotate the eyes clockwise and counterclockwise.

The muscles can move the eyes 30 degrees in 0.1 second using only 1/50 of their available muscle power. The extraocular muscles are extremely richly supplied with blood vessels and nerves. Because of this they are, per unit area, the strongest muscles in the body.

EMBRYOLOGY

Two weeks after conception, ocular structures are identifiable in the embryo, which at this stage is 2.5 mm long. At four weeks the eye is shaped like an eye. At four months all ocular structures are present and identifiable. Following this, development consists of differentiation and maturation of component parts. Yet at birth, the eye is not fully developed. Visual stimulus (light) is needed for the full maturation of the macula. The eye attains its adult size at about eight years of age.

Eighty percent of children are born farsighted (hyperopic). Five percent are born nearsighted (myopic). Fifteen percent are born with "normal" eyes.

Hyperopia (farsightedness) increases to age eight, then gradually decreases until maturity is reached. Myopia (nearsightedness) increases after age seven up to about age twenty-five, after which little change occurs.

GROWTH AND DEVELOPMENT

At birth, the eye is relatively larger in relation to the rest of the body than is true in an adult. Hence, most infants appear to have "such big eyes."

The crystalline lens at birth is nearly spherical and is very pliable like soft plastic. The lens continues to grow throughout life and its consistency changes with aging. As one gets older the lens becomes larger and harder (more glasslike), and is unable to change its shape as readily as in youth. This causes presbyopia (old sight) which becomes noticeable around the age of forty years. This is usually the time when an individual begins to experience trouble reading small print at near distances. As this change takes place, some of the inherent magnifying power of the eye is lost and near objects look blurred. To compensate for this, one may push an object farther away, rear the head back, or both, in an effort to see more clearly. This is when people say, "I see fine at a distance, but my arms are getting too short." This is a universal condition and is a function of time. It is not usually related to disease. At this time in life, reading glasses becomes necessary to provide the needed but insufficient natural magnification.

The iris at birth contains very little pigment on its anterior surface. Hence, most infants' eyes are some shade of blue. As time passes, more pigment is deposited on the anterior iris and the eyes become green, hazel or brown. An irregular deposition of pigment in the iris may produce freckles.

As aging proceeds, the skin of the eyelids, which is the thinnest skin of the body, loses some of its elasticity and in extreme cases may droop and wrinkle markedly, producing a cosmetic blemish known as blepharochalasis.

Alterations in the depostion of fat in the skin of the eyelids may produce irregularly outlined yellow plaques in the lids, frequently nearest the nose, which are another cosmetic blemish known as xanthelasma.

The same type of alteration of fat metabolism occurs in the

periphery of the cornea, where a whitish ring is often seen in old eyes. This is called arcus senilus.

The aforementioned conditions are usually harmless. Xanthelasma and arcus senilus, when occurring in young people, may signal abnormally high blood cholesterol levels.

The vitreous, which is the mass of jellylike tissue filling the posterior eye cavity, undergoes aging changes which include liquefaction and condensations of fibrin material causing suspended masses known as vitreous floaters.

Aging also produces regular changes in the choroid and retina. Since the choroid is made up of blood vessels, "hardening of the arteries" (arteriosclerosis) causes choroidal sclerosis. This may affect blood supply to the retina which when diminished reduces retinal function and can adversely affect vision.

BINOCULAR VISION

Binocular vision is variously designated as fusion, stereopsis, or depth perception. It is the ability to see with both eyes as if they were one while providing an individual with an appreciation of depth. Without this ability, one is unable to tell with accuracy how far objects are away from him.

Binocular control is a learned process and is not well developed before age six months. Before this, one's eyes may move independently. Hence a newborn infant may look at the ceiling with one eye and the floor with the other.

Stereopsis is a variable phenomenon and can be weak or strong. It continues to develop during the first six or seven years of life. However, if it fails to develop before the ninth birthday there is little chance for its development thereafter.

Conditions which interfere with the normal binocular control are varied. There are two conditions which are frequently encountered which are not the result of disease or injury.

The first is strabismus. This is also known as squint or crossed or walleyes. A child may be born with this condition or it may develop early, usually in the first year. The visual axes are not properly aligned. One eye may turn in or out, up or down. If this happens and vision is equal in each eye, diplopia, or double vision results. This is intolerable, and one eye, usually the weaker, is suppressed. The one being used then develops better vision. If uncorrected and allowed to progress, the squinting, suppressed eye fails to develop good vision and the child grows up with a healthy eye which does not see well.

Another condition affecting development of binocular vision is anisometropia. This is a condition where there is a marked difference between the refractive errors. For example, one eye may be nearsighted, the other farsighted. Since an infant is mostly concerned with immediate surroundings, he may use the nearsighted eye and ignore the farsighted one, although the eyes may be perfectly straight with the visual axes well-aligned. Again, the unused eye does not develop properly. Anisometropia can be diagnosed very early in life.

The condition produced by either of these events is known as amblyopia, which literally means dim vision due to any cause. Where there is no physical abnormality or disease the term amblyopia exanopsia applies.

These two conditions, strabismus and anisometropia, can and must be recognized very early in life in order to prevent amblyopia. The diagnosis of these conditions is not difficult and most all can be treated and often corrected. It is tragic to see an adult with an amblyopic eye which could have been corrected in childhood, yet two and one-half million Americans have, to some degree, a crossed eye causing reduced vision.

It is vital to recognize these conditions early. It is never too early to examine one's eyes. It is recommended that all children have a complete ocular examination before going to school. If there is any suspicion of visual difficulty, the eyes should be examined, regardless of the tender age.

Since visual acuity is a function of age, attention, intelligence, experience, and the ability to communicate, it is obvious that one is unable to say precisely what a one- or two-year-old can see. By the time a child is three or four years of age, visual acuity testing meets with greater success. By age five acuity can usually be measured very accurately.

DISEASES

There are scores of diseases affecting vision. It is beyond the scope of this chapter to name or describe them all. What follows is an outline of some of the more common causes of visual impairment.

A. Hereditary Conditions

1. Myopia (nearsightedness) is a common condition in which the eyeball is relatively too large or has too much magnifying power, or both. In myopia, parallel incident light rays are brought to focus in front of the retina causing images of distant objects to be blurred. Myopic individuals see clearly at near distances. The range of clear near vision depends upon the refractive error. Myopia generally is first noticeable after age seven or eight years. It increases through the teen years to about age twenty-five years regardless of external factors such as close work, lighting, rest, vitamins, etc. Eye exercises have no effect since eye size and refractive power cannot be altered this way. Long-standing myopia of high degree may produce retinal degenerative changes or detachment. Visual deficiencies of myopia are correctible with concave lenses (minus lenses).

2. Glaucoma is an internal eye disease, in which the intraocular hydrostatic pressure is abnormally high, causes damage to the retina and optic nerve. The incidence of glaucoma is 2 percent in persons over the age of forty. There are two general types:

a. Chronic glaucoma accounts for more than 90 percent of all glaucomas. It causes insidious visual field loss and rarely produces physical symptoms until very late in the course of the disease.

b. Acute glaucoma, occurring in less than 10 percent of cases, is dramatic. It causes halos around lights, agonizing aching eye pain and rapid visual loss. Acute glaucoma can produce blindness in less than twenty-four hours. It is an ophthalmological emergency requiring prompt, definitive treatment (usually medical and frequently surgical).

The diagnosis of glaucoma is made by physical examination of the eyes. One of the instruments utilized is called a tonometer, with which the intraocular hydrostatic pressure can be measured. Untreated glaucoma produces blindness. One of every eight blind people is a victim of glaucoma.

3. Retinitis pigmentosa, a genetically determined degenera-

tive retinal disease affects retinal rod function early in life (six to twelve years of age), causing varying degrees of night blindness. It affects both eyes and is more prevalent in men than women. Progressive visual field loss is characteristic of this disease. There is no known effective treatment.

4. Albinism, a disease affecting the metabolism of melanin, (body pigment which regulates color of eyes, hair, skin, etc.) has a sex-linked inheritance factor. It causes poor retinal development and nystagmus (shaking eyes). There is marked reduction in retinal and uveal pigment rendering the eyes very light-sensitive. Albinos characteristically have pink eyes with poor vision, white eyebrows and eyelashes, white hair, and pale, often freckled, skin.

5. Macula degeneration is a term used to denote a group of conditions involving loss of central or reading vision. This can occur in an infant, juvenile or adult. It primarily affects central vision, leaving peripheral or side vision intact.

B. Congenital Conditions

1. Ptosis (drooping eyelid), a condition in which one or both upper eyelids hang down like a curtain, is due to a derangement in muscle or nerve function necessary to raise the lids. This may cause backward head-tilting in order to peer under the lids or may so obstruct vision in an eye as to cause poor visual development.

2. Syphillis (the great disease imitator) can cause inflammatory changes in any or all coats of the eye, separately or collectively. The effects of this infection may be present at birth or may not become evident until years later, perhaps even until adulthood. Associated diseases include mental deficiencies, deafness, bone, skin, hair, and teeth affectations. The most common congenital syphilitic eye lesion is interstitial keratitis which is inflammation of the cornea. This often produces corneal opacities which reduce visual acuity.

3. Cataracts at birth are often the result of German measles (rubella) in the mother during the first three months of pregnancy. The virus causing rubella has an affinity for the developing lens tissue, which it affects in the embryonic eye, causing lens opacities.

C. Trauma

Injury constitutes the leading cause of blindness between the ages of five and fifteen years. A myriad of physical agents damage the eye. Lacerations or puncture wounds are common. Industrial chemicals (acids and alkalis), foreign bodies (B.B.'s and cartridge casings), vegetable matter (thorns and briars), minerals (rocks and abrasives), toys with sharp corners, and countless other agents have been known to destroy sight. The use of industrial safety glasses has markedly reduced ocular injury in recent years.

D. Infections

Almost any infectious agent, bacterial, viral or fungal, can affect the eye. There are some agents which have a particular predilection for the eye, such as the large trachoma virus.

1. Trachoma is the world's leading cause of blindness. It affects one-sixth of the world's population. It causes scarring on the front of the eye. Peoples in lands bordering on the Mediterranean Sea and in Far East Asia are particularly prone to contract this disease. Trachoma is rare in the United States, except in Indians, Eskimos, and Mexicans.

2. A small virus, known as herpes simplex, causes corneal ulceration. This is the same organism which causes "cold sores" at the corners of the mouth and around the nose. It is difficult to eradicate and is very painful.

3. Ophthalmia neonatorum is an infection in a newborn's eyes contracted by passage through the birth canal. Protection against this is provided by the Credé procedure, which is applying silver nitrate drops to the eyes shortly after birth.

E. Metabolic Conditions (affecting the body's use of nutrients)

1. Diabetes mellitus is a disease caused by disturbances in carbohydrate and fat metabolism. The typical ocular disease is in the retina where hemorrhages and exudates occur. The uvea, optic nerve, lens, and extraocular muscles can also be affected. Diabetes can cause refractive changes, e.g. false myopia. It is currently believed that the duration of the disease is more important in ocular changes than is the severity of diabetes.

2. Hypertension (high blood pressure), causes blood vessel spasm, retinal edema (swelling), hemorrhages and exudates (fluid portion of blood escaping from blood vessels). These changes are often reversible early in the disease.

3. Arteriosclerosis (hardening of the arteries), causing hard-

ening of blood vessel walls (arteries and veins) eventually leading to occlusions (vessel blockages) which cause death of tissue served by the occluded vessel. These changes are irreversible.

4. Tumors (autonomous new growth)

a. Retinoblastoma (a tumor of developing retinal elements) is the typical tumor of childhood. Seventy percent occur before the age of four years, 30 percent are bilateral. The incidence is higher in whites than blacks. The children of an individual cured of retinoblastoma will have a 50 percent chance of developing the disease since it is determined by an autosomal dominant gene.

b. Malignant melanoma (a tumor of adults). The average age at discovery is fifty years. It occurs in 0.02 to 0.06 percent of eyes. It is usually unilateral and about 85 percent arise in the choroid. It is rare in Negroes.

5. Retrolental fibroplasia (RLF) is a bilateral retinal disease of premature infants. It is characterized by disorganized growth of immature retinal tissue. It is caused by excessive oxygen given premature infants during the first few weeks of life. The retina is replaced by fibrous tissue which ultimately becomes detached. Once blindness occurs, there is no hope for sight restoration.

F. Degenerative Conditions (retrogressive tissue process)

1. Cataract, an opacity in the crystalline lens, may vary in size, location, and density. There are many causes but cataracts are most frequently due to aging and are most commonly found in elderly persons (senile cataract). Most cataracts are bilateral but they seldom progress at the same rate. There is no medical treatment for cataract. Surgical extraction is indicated when the cataract decreases visual acuity sufficiently to prevent the person from leading a normal life.

2. Retinal detachment occurs when the retina peels off the back of the inside of the eye. This is actually a separation of the nine inner layers of the retina from the outer tenth layer. When this occurs, the individual may see "soot," "lighting flashes," or "a curtain coming down (or up)" before the eye. These individuals should be examined very carefully, particularly if they are very nearsighted, have had previous ocular surgery, or have sustained ocular trauma.

OCULAR EMERGENCIES

There are several true ocular emergencies which demand immediate ophthalmological evaluation. Some of the most frequent ones are listed below (not in order of importance):

1. Trauma.
2. Corneal ulcer.
3. Severe conjunctivitis.
4. Orbital cellulitis.
5. Chemical burns.
6. Acute iritis (uveitis).
7. Acute glaucoma.
8. Central retinal artery occlusion.
9. Retinal detachment.

DEFINITION AND CAUSES

A person is considered legally blind if (1) vision in the better eye as measured at a distance of twenty feet using the Snellen chart is no better than 20/200 with correcting glasses or if (2) the widest diameter of the visual field in the better eye subtends an angle of twenty degrees or less.

The commonest causes of blindness are as follows: in infants, congenital defects; in children, injury; in adults, cataracts, vascular diseases, glaucoma, trachoma, trauma, and degenerative conditions.

VISUAL ACUITY

Visual acuity is measurable by many means. Pictures of different objects, circles and dots of different sizes, letters, and numerals may be used. Herman Snellen (1834-1908) is credited with developing a system by which acuity can be expressed as a fractional number. His test chart consists of letters or numerals, each stroke of which subtends an angle of one minute, with the whole character occupying five minutes of arc at the stated distance.

The numerator of the fraction denotes distance, the denominator denotes the size of character seen (20/20=10/10=1/1=1). The term "20/20" may be considered as unit vision.

Many expressions have been devised to denote visual acuity

as a fraction. Those which enjoy most widespread use compare patient's acuity with the average normal acuity for a given distance. A reading of 20/20 indicates the line on a visual testing chart seen by average normal eyes at twenty feet.

Tests for near vision are made on the same principles as for distance. One which is used frequently is the Jaeger type.

A ray of light entering the eye passes through several refracting (light-bending) media: first the cornea, then the aqueous humor, the pupil which controls the amount of light passage, then the crystalline lens, and then the vitreous (or jelly body) finally reaching the central retina (the fovea centralis in the macula). The cornea is a strong refracting instrument but it has no power of accommodation. The optical function of the cornea is to refract light through the pupil and it needs to be clear and uniformly curved.

The variable refractive part of the eye is the crystalline lens. The lens is an elastic organ located behind the iris. It is biconvex (like a magnifying glass). In young persons, the lens is capable of infinitely precise instantaneous adjustments in shape which produce images on the retina of objects in space at varying distances from the eye within a range of twenty feet. This is called accommodation. Accommodation is the result of contraction and relaxation of the ciliary muscles from which the lens is suspended by radial supporting fibers known as zonules. Contraction and relaxation of the ciliary muscles cause the lens to change its shape. As the lens becomes more convex, or oval, nearer objects are perceived best. Light rays entering the eye from distances greater than twenty feet are considered to be parallel and no accommodation is necessary. In this state the eye is unaccommodated or at rest. No ocular work is required to see objects twenty feet or farther from the normal eye.

When the eye is healthy and of normal size, the unaccommodated eye may receive and focus parallel incident light rays from a source twenty feet or farther away into a sharp image on the retina. This is known as emmetropia (sight in proper measure). Emmetropia is ideal but not common since most people have some degree of refractive error.

Variations from emmetropia are collectively called ametropia (sight not in proper measure). Some of these variants are as follows:

1. Hyperopia (far sight).
2. Myopia (near sight).
3. Astigmatism (not at a point).
4. Presbyopia (old sight).
5. Anisometropia (different refractive errors in the two eyes).
6. Aniseikonia (different image size in the two eyes).

These conditions may exist alone as in simple myopia or in combination (hyperopic or myopic astigmatism) to which would be added presbyopia in people over forty years of age. The two eyes in the same person may vary. One eye may be nearsighted, the other farsighted and one or both may be astimgatic and/or presbyopic.

Astigmatism refers to varying degrees of refraction in different meridians of the eye. For example, the vertical meridian may be a stronger refracting medium than the horizontal or vice versa. This would produce two different focal planes neither of which might fall on the retina. Blurred vision would result. Most astigmatism is related to the shape of the cornea.

Various symptoms in addition to visual problems may be produced by refractive errors. Children may frown, blink frequently, or be unusually clumsy. Adults may complain of "eyestrain," headache, or dizziness.

VISUAL FIELDS

The field of vision is all that is seen above, below, and to the sides, when the eye is fixed on any object in space. The visual field changes each time the eye moves. Normal visual fields extend almost ninety degrees to the temporal side, about sixty degrees nasally, forty-five degrees up and sixty-five degrees down.

Because of the separation of the eyes, one can see slightly farther around to the right of an object with the right eye and to the left with the left eye. The images thus presented to the brain are not exactly alike. By fusing these two slightly different images into one, the brain provides us with depth perception. We can then tell which object is closest or farthest away. This ability is variously known as fusion, binocular vision, or stereopsis. If the eyes do not work together in this fashion, one may be unable to accurately estimate distances to objects in space. This is particularly noticeable in strange surroundings and can easily be demonstrated by covering one eye and attempting to judge distances. There are other clues which may help in this instance, such as size (things look bigger when they are close, smaller when far away), shadows, knowledge of size, shape, and distance from experience.

Because light crosses the center of the eye before it strikes the retina, one sees objects above with the lower part of the retina, below with the upper part of the retina, to the right with the left part of the retina, and the left with the right part of the retina.

Since the retina is nerve tissue, quite similar to brain tissue, its function is irrevocably lost when it is damaged by disease or injury, and the portion of the visual field mediated by the damaged retina is also lost.

If the central retina (the macula) is diseased, discreet reading vision is lost. If a part of the peripheral retina is damaged, the corresponding portion of the visual field is lost. If the entire retina is destroyed, total blindness results in that eye.

Many conditions can produce loss of visual field. A common one is glaucoma. The normal hydrostatic eye pressure is maintained by an elaborate system of fluid production and drainage within the eye which is controlled within very narrow limits.

Most glaucomas are caused by a defect in the mechanism which drains the fluid from the eye. This filtering mechanism (or drain) ceases to function normally or becomes stopped up. The water pressure then builds up to the point where normal retinal health cannot be maintained.

The retina is very sensitive to pressure, particularly the anterior peripheral part which is the last to develop and is generally the weakest part.

If the pressure within the eye rises to high levels rapidly and remains elevated, the retina is literally squeezed to death and permanent loss of visual field results. This is the case in acute angle closure glucoma where functional vision can be lost in a matter of a few hours.

If the pressure rises very slowly, as is the case in most glaucomas, there may be no physical or ocular symptoms; but, if untreated, it can produce very gradual retinal death and visual field loss. This may occur so slowly over such a prolonged interval that the individual is not aware of the problem until significant visual field loss has occurred. It may take years for this type of glaucoma to cause blindness and the victim may never have a pain. That is one reason this type of glaucoma is like a thief in the night. It can rob one's vision and never be noticed until late in the disease.

As peripheral retinal function is lost from such conditions, the peripheral visual fields become smaller. That is, one loses the ability to see normally to the sides, above, or below. As this condition continues unabated, the visual fields get smaller and smaller (contracted) until only a small central area of visual field remains. In long-standing simple glaucoma, the remaining visual fields may be quite small (as if one were looking out through the breech of a double-barreled shotgun) with all the side vision gone.

According to the definition of legal blindness, if the widest diameter of the remaining visual field in the better eye is no more than 20 degrees, this person is blind, regardless of the visual acuity. Thus one can have 20/20 vision in both eyes and be legally blind. Legal blindness does not imply total loss of sight.

The following statistics should prove thought-provoking:

10,000,000 people in the world are blind
350,000 people in the United States are legally blind
35,000 Americans go blind each year
2,500,000 Americans have, to some degree, a crossed eye—causing reduced vision in one eye of one half that number
10,000,000 children in the United States need eye care

If this chapter will help expand the understanding of ophthalmology for persons outside the medical field, the intentions of the author will be fulfilled.

GLOSSARY

Accommodation—Adjustment of the eye for seeing at different distances. This is done by the change in the shape of the crystalline lens by the action of the ciliary muscle.

Amblyopia—Dimness of vision from any cause.

Amblyopia ex anopsia—Dim vision due to disuse, without organic disease.

Ametropia—Refractive error in which image is not focused on retina when eye is at rest. Includes myopia, hyperopia, and astigmatism.

Anisometropia—Differences in size and shape of images seen by the two eyes.

Aphakia—Absence of the crystalline lens.

Aqueous—Watery fluid filling the space between the cornea and crystalline lens.

Asthenopia—Uncomfortable vision, eye fatigue.

Astigmatism—Refractive error in which light rays do not come to a single focus in the eye. Caused by different degrees of refractive error in the various meridians of the eye.

Binocular vision—Stereopsis, fusion. The ability to see the same object at the same time with two eyes and fuse them into one visual image.

Cataract—Opacity in the crystalline lens.

Chalazion—Cystic, inflammatory enlargement of a meibomian gland in the eyelid.

Choroid—The vascular intermediate posterior nourishing coat of the eyeball.

Ciliary body—Part of intermediate coat of eyeball between iris and choroid, consisting of ciliary processes and ciliary muscle.

Concave lens—Lens which diverges light. Known as diverging, reducing, negative, myopic, or minus lens, denoted by (—) sign.

Cones—Retinal nerve elements concerned with visual acuity and color in lighted surroundings (day vision).

Conjunctiva—Mucous membrane lining posterior portions of eyelids and anterior, exposed sclera.

Contact lens—Small, thin, usually plastic lens fitting directly on cornea.

Convergence—Bringing the visual axes of the two eyes to focus at a near point, causing the eyes to turn toward one another.

Convex lens—Lens which converges light. Known as converging, magnifying, hyperopic, or plus lens, denoted by (+) sign.

Cornea—Transparent, watch crystallike anterior outer coat forming anterior wall of aqueous chamber.

Corneal graft—Surgical procedure in which a section of diseased, opacified cornea is replaced with clear cornea from donor eye of recently deceased person.

Crystalline lens—Transparent, colorless, pliable, continually growing body suspended in eye between aqueous and vitreous, functioning in accommodation.

Cycloplegic—Drug which temporarily puts ciliary body at rest, paralyzes accommodation, and dilates the pupil.

Cylindrical lens—Segment of a cylinder, the refractive power of which varies in different meridians.

Diopter—Unit of measurement of lens power, or refractive strength.

Diplopia—Seeing one object as two.

Emmetropia—Refractive condition of eye at rest in which image of distant object is focused directly on retina.

Epiphora—Excessive production of tears.

Esophoria—Tendency of an eye to turn inward.

Esotropia—Manifest inward deviation of one eye.

Exophoria—Tendency of an eye to turn outward.

Exophthalmos—Abnormal protrusion of eyeball.

Exotropia—Manifest outward deviation of one eye.

Field of vision—Entire visual area seen while fixing on one object in space. Visual field changes each time eye moves.

Floaters—Particles of cells or fibrin which move in the vitreous.

Fovea—Part of the posterior retina adapted for most acute vision; located in the center of the macula.

Fundus—Posterior layers of eye visible with ophthalmoscope.

Fusion—See text on binocular vision.

Glaucoma—Increased intraocular pressure with resultant retinal and optic nerve damage.

Hemianopsia—Blindness of one half the field of vision, one or both eyes.

Heterotropia—Strabismus. Manifest deviation of visual axis of one eye, out of alignment with fellow eye.

Hyperopia—Farsightedness. Refractive error in which point of focus of parallel incident light rays is behind the retina.

Iris—Circular, colored membrane, suspended in anterior chamber in front of crystalline lens.

Lens—A refractive medium with one or both surfaces curved.

Macula lutea—Small indented area of posterior retina, surrounding fovea, comprising most visually sensitive part of retina.

Miotic—Drug which causes constriction of pupil.

Mydriatic—Drug which causes dilatation of pupil without affecting accommodation.

Myopia—Nearsightedness. Refractive error in which point of focus of parallel incident light rays is in front of retina.

Nystagmus—An involuntary rapid movement of the eyeball, which may be horizontal, vertical, rotatory, or mixed of two varieties.

Oculist or Ophthalmologist—Interchangeable terms for physician who is a specialist in diseases of the eye.

Oculus dexter (O. D.)—Right eye.

Oculus sinister (O. S.)—Left eye.

Oculus uterque (O. U.)—Both eyes.

Ophthalmoscope—Lighted optical instrument used to view inner ocular structures, particularly the fundus.

Optician—One who makes or deals in eyeglasses and/or optical instruments and fills prescriptions for glasses.

Optometrist—Nonmedical person trained in measurement of refraction of eye for prescribing glasses. Not licensed to use or prescribe drugs or perform surgery.

Peripheral vision—Ability to see motion, form, and color of objects outside direct line of vision.

Presbyopia—Old sight. Gradual lessening of accommodative power, due to physiologic changes, causing blurred near vision after age 40.

Ptosis—Drooping eyelid.

Pupil—Round hole in center of iris, analagous to iris diaphragm in a camera.

Refraction—Bending of light, change in course of light rays passing from one medium into another of different density. Also, the act of determining the refractive error of the eye and correcting with glasses.

Refractive error—Defect in focusing mechanism which prevents light from focusing directly on retina.

Refractive media—All transparent parts of the eye which have refractive power.

Retina—Inner layer of eye composed of light-sensitive nerve elements.

Rods—Retinal nerve elements concerned with motion and vision at low levels of illumination (night vision).

Scotoma—Blind spot in visual field.

Snellen chart—Chart used to test visual acuity. Consists of lines of letters, numbers, and symbols drawn to Snellen measurements.

Strabismus—(see Heterotropia) A manifest deviation of an eye.

Sty—Acute infection of glands of Zeis or Moll in eyelid.

Tonometer—Instrument for measuring intraocular pressure.

Trachoma—A viral disease of the conjunctiva and cornea, producing photophobia, pain, and lacrimation characterized by redness and inflammation.

Uvea—Entire vascular intermediate coat of eyeball, comprised of iris, ciliary body, and choroid.

Uveitis—Inflammation of uvea.

Visual acuity—Measurement of detailed central vision.

Xanthelasma—A form of xanthoma affecting the eyelids and characterized by soft, yellowish spots, or plaques.

Zonules—Fine strands of tissue stretching from ciliary body to entire lens equator (360 degrees), holding the lens in place and functioning in accommodation.

7

Attitudes and Blindness

John H. Wallace

One of the most often used words in contemporary times is the term "attitude." This seemingly simple term is indeed a very complex construct which permeates virtually every aspect of our behavior. How many workers lose promotions or even their jobs because supervisors deem them to have poor attitudes toward their work? How many graduates students do not earn their degrees because professors believe they have poor attitudes? Before a recent championship game in professional football involving literally thousands of dollars for each player, the television analyst emphatically stated that the game hinged not on which team had the strongest offense or strongest defense, nor on any individuals, but that it would be won by the team which had the winning attitude. Perhaps we can say that Helen Keller had a winning attitude.

WHAT IS AN ATTITUDE?

Attitudes cannot be observed; like intelligence, they must be inferred from behavior. The scientific study of attitudes as a controlled variable was pioneered by Thomas and Zaniecki (1918). At that time, they defined an attitude as an internalized counterpart of an external object representing the individual's subjective tendency to act toward the object. There have been many subsequent definitions of the term. One of more recent vintage and perhaps more parsimonious has been given to us by Sherif (1965) who defined an attitude as follows: Attitudes refer to the stands the individual upholds and cherishes about objects, issues, persons, groups, or institutions. Perhaps the key to Sherif's definition is the word "stands." When an individual takes a stand on an issue, he usually commits himself. Cinema fans probably remember a rather common scene in the old cowboy horse operas when the cattleman, threatened with the possibility of sheep herders moving in on his grazing territory, gruffly exclaimed to the dashing hero, "You are either with me or against me." Perhaps the term attitude is analogous to the term pregnancy or obesity in that all three terms are clearly dichotomous. Either one is pregnant or not pregnant, either one is obese or not obese, either one has an attitude or does not have an attitude toward some object or event, usually called a referent. In other words, if an individual has an attitude he is no longer neutral toward the referents of the attitude. He is for or against, positively inclined or negatively disposed in some degree toward them, not just momentarily but in a lasting way as long as the attitude in question is operative.

Two fundamental points on which most definitions of the term "attitude" agree are that attitudes are socially formed and that attitudes are selective. Attitudes are selective in that they provide a basis for discriminating between alternative courses of action. For example, if an individual has a very positive attitude toward one movie star and a negative one toward another and there are two movies starring each of these actors in town, his attitude would most likely determine which movie he would see. Attitudes also introduce consistency of response in social situations of an otherwise diverse nature. When an avid football fan has a favorite team, one certainly can predict his behavior if "his" team wins. Most assuredly the team's victory will leave him with a warm glow and a pleasant disposition; however, one can predict that a loss will leave him troubled and disappointed. Any individual's behavior becomes highly predictable when his attitudes are understood.

SOURCES OF ATTITUDES

As previously mentioned, attitudes are socially formed. They are based on cultural experience and training and are therefore revealed in cultural products. According to Sartan (1962), an individual usually learns his attitude from one of the following sources or combinations of these sources: specific experiences, communication from others, imitation of models, and institutional factors.

One way we learn our attitudes and beliefs is through specific experience with the referent of the attitudes. For example, after several pleasant experiences in dealing with a person, we usually come to like him. By contrast, a series of frustrating, negative experiences will usually engender an unfavorable attitude. Sometimes even a single experience produces a strongly favorable or unfavorable attitude. For example, a man who has suffered unpleasantries with a policeman may learn in one isolated experience to have an unfavorable attitude toward all policemen. He is, of course, generalizing his unfavorable reaction in a specific situation to policemen in general.

Many of our attitudes are formed as a result of communication with other people. Of particular interest is the informal instruction which children are given in the family. Like many other aspects of behavior, attitudes and beliefs acquired in childhood tend to be the most stable. A child does not enter the world with ready-made beliefs and attitudes about it. Order and meaning to his phenomenal field are first learned from his observing the views of others and especially from his family. These attitudes constitute a frame of reference helping to shape his experiences. Although they may be modified in particular details in the light of new indoctrination and personal experience, they will rarely be supplanted by an entirely new set of attitudes and beliefs.

Of course, all indoctrination is not successful. For it to be effective, the individual who is being influenced must have a favorable and respectful attitude toward whoever is trying to influence him. As mentioned above, in the home situation, a child is very likely to feel positively inclined toward his mother and father. In the school situation his teachers may carry a lot of prestige in his eyes.

Another way in which our attitudes are developed is through the imitation of models. In a particular situation, we observe another person's behavior. We interpret his behavior in terms of the attitudes and beliefs his action implies. If we identify with him and respect his judgement, we are likely to accept this (inferred) way of perceiving and feeling about the situation.

For example, suppose that Billy Joe and his mother are walking down the sidewalk and see a blind man standing on the corner. On seeing this man wearing dark glasses and carrying a long, white cane, Billy Joe's mother suddenly grabs his arm and rushes across the street to the opposite sidewalk. She shudders and almost pulls Billy Joe down because of the suddenness of her quick movements. This behavior on his mother's part defined this blind person as one to be avoided. Remember that Billy Joe believes that his mother is far more powerful than he is and that her way of interpreting things is most often correct. By being led to see the situation as unpleasant, Billy Joe will probably acquire an attitude of fear toward blind persons as has his mother.

Children and adolescents often are quite vigilant in observing how their parents react to different people. They learn attitudes by observing whom their parents respect, whom they regard as friends, and whom they dislike. It is important to note that such evaluations may be acquired without the child's direct interacting with such people.

Many institutional factors function as sources and supports of our attitudes and beliefs. For example, consider the description of a well-known organization. Members of this organization wear the same types of uniforms. They greet each other with formal salutes and language. There is a definite structured hierarchy of power. All activities fit into an organized schedule. One might guess this to be a brief description of a military organization or even a highly ritualized religious order. From this description, some rather good guesses can be made as to the general character of the attitudes and beliefs of this organization. There is an implicit division and differentiation of power. There is an attitude of respect for one's superiors. Discipline and teamwork are stressed in behavior. The different parts of the institution—the uniforms, the physical plant, the behavior—have a meaning which fits in with certain beliefs and attitudes.

PREJUDICE

Of particular interest to social scientists are attitudes which are unfavorable toward one group or another. Such attitudes are commonly known as prejudices. Prejudice has been defined as an attitude emotionally resistant to change. Unlike a simple misconception, a prejudice is actively resistant to all evidence that would unseat it. A concrete example of this phenomenon can be illustrated by utilizing an earlier example of the formation of an attitude toward police officers. Suppose that an individual is hostile and resentful toward policemen. He perceives them as rude, unethical bullies who take great delight in stepping on others. When a policeman moves next door to person with an unfavorable stereotype of policemen and turns out to be a very friendly, sociable person who is helpful and a good neighbor, the person with the unfavorable stereotype can simply explain this case as an exception. On the other hand, even a few examples of police behavior consistent with the stereotype will tend to further reinforce his prejudicial attitude.

Prejudices are learned in the same manner as other attitudes. They are acquired by means of specific experiences, communications from others, imitation of models, and institutional factors. One may ask then why these particular attitudes are so emotionally resistant to change. Several factors have been identified which support prejudice.

Socioeconomic status seems to be a factor related to prejudice. It is understandable that the poor people in the ghetto who feel they are being discriminated against will have strong negative feelings toward those whom they regard as responsible for their frustrations. Certainly the Black Panther movement is an illustration of this phenomenon. On the other end of the continuum, individuals from a higher socioeconomic class may feel threatened by lower socioeconomic groups. They may perceive this lower socioeconomic group as a threat to their security and cherished ideals. This is certainly exemplified in the current crisis concerning the busing of children from suburban areas to the inner city and vice versa.

Another factor related to prejudice is an individual's personality. The findings of Adorno (1950) with regard to the authoritarian personality suggest that prejudice in some people may be due to unconscious anxieties and hostilities. Frequently, prejudicial attitudes against groups are projections.

Prejudices usually come in clusters. Being prejudiced against one group tends to go along with being prejudiced against other groups. For example, if an employer has negative feelings toward hiring blind persons, he most likely would feel much the same way about employing other disabled persons. Research findings have clearly indicated significant correlations between negative attitudes toward blindness and antiminority, antiNegro, and pro-authoritarian attitudes.

ATTITUDES TOWARD THE DISABLED

The sources of our attitudes toward the disabled are the same as the sources of any attitudes. This is readily evident when one reviews the unfolding development of attitudes toward the disabled from ancient times to the present. Current attitudes toward handicapped persons have incorporated a variety of historical attitudes.

The ancient Greeks believed that the physically impaired were inferior. The sick could expect consideration from society only as long as their condition was capable of improvement. Even harsher were the Spartans who systematically killed all deformed and disabled children in order to upgrade their race.

Oberman (1965) reviewed the ancient Hebraic attitudes toward the disabled as found in Old Testament references toward disability and came up with these conclusions: "Disability and disease were interpreted as being expressions of displeasures of the Lord and His punishment upon the afflicted. Illness and physical defect marked the person as a sinner and they were considered both a punishment and a means of atonement." This attitude is quite apparent in the following Biblical verses:

> The Lord shall smite thee with a consumption, and with a fever, and with an inflammation, and with an extreme burning. . . . (Deuteronomy 28:22)
>
> The Lord shall smite thee with madness, and blindness, and astonishment of heart. (Deuteronomy 28:28)

In the selection of priests, the disabled were automatically eliminated as candidates. This dictum has been followed even in modern times.

Kanner (1964) reported that the Romans made special use of many of their disabled population. It was not unusual for the wealthy to keep a "fool" or "jester" for the amusement of the household and guests.

The following story was reported by Seneca in one of his epistles to Lucilius:

> You know that Herpaste, my wife's fool, was left on my hands as a hereditary charge, for I have a natural aversion to these monsters; and if I have a mind to laugh at a fool, I need not seek him far. This fool has suddenly lost her sight. I am telling you a strange but true story. She is not aware that she is blind and constantly urges her keeper to take her out because she says my house is dark.

At a later time the fools became the playthings of princes and the courts. The jesters were recruited from persons with misshapen bodies and from mental defectives. The kept fools, of course, occupied an exceptional position among the mental defectives or otherwise handicapped. The vast majority of the more severely retarded did not fare as well. However, in many "uncivilized" areas, they were regarded superstitiously as blessed "infants of the good God" and were allowed to roam unmolested.

It was during the period of "enlightenment" and "reform" that the mental defectives and other disabled individuals were at their worst. It was then that many of them became victims of the prevailing demonism. Even Martin Luther referred to the feebleminded as godless. Thus the disadvantaged individual not only felt the frustrations resulting from lack of capability, but he suffered social ostracism and personal feelings of unworthiness as well.

We like to believe that in the twentieth century our civilization has progressed to such a level that we are no longer confronted with the negative attitudes of the past, and that these attitudes have been replaced by more positive ones of acceptance of the disabled. Without question, we have made great strides in eliminating prejudices. This is readily evident in the huge numbers of our disabled population who are functioning and productive members of our society. McGowan and Porter's (1967) contention that widespread prejudice toward the disabled still exists seems to be well-founded when one reviews the current research in this area. Take the epileptic for example. The major problem for the person with epilepsy is no longer in the area of medical knowledge but rather in the realm of public understanding and acceptance. The social image of the epileptic is lagging far behind the present availability of scientific fact, with the result that these people still face frustratingly unjust written and tacit restrictions which were devised in an era when all people with epilepsy were considered to be hopeless, untreatable, and unsafe.

In a survey of state laws early in 1962, Olender found that in many states, by law or by administrative policy, people with epilepsy were not permitted to drive, marry, and to have children. Surveys have also revealed the resistance adults with epilepsy face in finding employment. Although a concern for safety is usually given as a reason, their opinion was that emotional bias was the real cause for this. Further surveys indicate that there are no significant differences for accident rates with properly placed epileptics than with others. Nevertheless, workmen's compensation laws often fail to give relief for injuries suffered by employees who have epilepsy. Similar difficulty is experienced in the epileptic's effort to obtain life insurance.

Caveness (1960) reported on a public attitude study conducted over a ten-year period. The sampling technique included representative members of all groups throughout the country. Some of his findings indicate that 90 percent of the population have an awarneness of epilepsy; that 18 percent would object to their child playing with a child who has epilepsy; 4 percent believe that epilepsy is another form of insanity; and 11 percent firmly believe that people with epilepsy should not be employed. On the positive side, his last survey, completed at the end of the ten-year period, detected a distinct improvement in social attitudes in contrast with the findings of ten years before.

Barker (1953) made a survey of the frequency of jokes about physically defective persons. In five collections, including 6,909 jokes, 4.1 percent of the jokes were concerned with such persons. Disabled persons were clearly deprecated in 80 percent of the jokes. Only a single joke in this series placed a disabled person in a superior position. In the remainder the attitude expressed toward disabled persons was neutral or the significance was not clear. Although the jokes in these collections frequently deprecated the persons to whom they referred, this tendency was stronger with jokes about the disabled than with jokes about some other classes of persons. For example, jokes about farmers, salesmen, judges, and dentists deprecated the subject of the joke in 49 percent of the cases.

Whiteman and Lukoff (1962) presented high school subjects with six photographs of college boys to be placed in rank order according to a number of behavior and personality characteristics. One of the college boys was photographed sitting in a wheel chair and this picture was presented with the wheel chair blocked out. Ray found that being represented as "crippled" influences the ranking of the stimulus subject to a statistically significant degree—when identified as "crippled" he was judged to be more conscientious, to feel more inferior, to be a better friend, to get better grades, to be more even-tempered, to be a better class president, to be more religious, to like parties less, and to be more unhappy than when depicted as "noncrippled."

Examples of negative attitudes toward the disabled are also evident from the changing terminology in rehabilitation. When a term or description becomes so emotion-laden that its use is prejudicial to a group, the term is changed. During the past 50 years, the number of changes indicate the depth and diversity of prejudice. Crippled has been changed to handicapped; idiot, imbecile, and moron, once good clinical terms, are no longer acceptable professional terms; leprosy has become Hanson's disease; the blind are becoming visually impaired; the poor are now the disadvantaged; the epileptic now has a convulsive disorder; and a few years ago the severely disabled became the catastrophically—involved by act of Congress.

Thus far some of the public attitudes toward the disabled have been reviewed. What about those of us who are professionally employed in the field of rehabilitation?

Gellman (1965) and Bell (1962), in studies concerned with the attitudes of rehabilitation workers toward the handicapped, found evidences of negative attitudes. It seems that many rehabilitation workers tend to categorize handicapped individuals and view them as "cases" rather than as unique individuals. Even rehabilitation workers are not exempt from having unfavorable attitudes toward the disabled, whether they be conscious or unconscious.

IMPORTANCE OF HAVING POSITIVE ATTITUDES TOWARD THE DISABLED

Why should we even be concerned about positive attitudes of acceptance of the disabled? A review of the literature indicated that many professional practitioners ascribe a good deal of the individual maladjustment of blind persons to devaluating societal stereotypes.

The findings of Sommers (1944) in an attitudinal study using questionnaries supported this contention. The questionnaries revealed a wide variety of attitudes and feelings among the visually handicapped. They indicated that emotional disturbances and maladjustments result more frequently from the conditions and social attitudes of the blind person's environment than from the sensory handicap itself.

Harold Yuker (1965), an authority in the field of attitudinal measurement, made the following commentary with regard to the importance of public attitudes toward the handicapped:

> If the attitudes of the nondisabled person are negative and rejecting, he will avoid the disabled individual and try to minimize the interaction between them. He will not want the disabled person as an associate or friend, possibly not even as a neighbor. If the person with the negative attitude is an employer or personnel manager, he will not want to hire disabled persons. If, on the other hand, the attitudes of the nondisabled persons are positive and accepting, he will tend to be friendly and warm toward the disabled.

Perhaps the most damaging aspect of negative attitudes toward the blind by the public is that all too often these negative attitudes are adopted by the blind and become attitudes of the blind. Too often the blind accept the limitations the public think they have and thus do as much to make the imagined limitations real. Some blind persons are ashamed to carry a white cane and they try to bluff sight because they perceive the public attitude that somehow faulty sight is not "altogether respectable."

ATTITUDE CHANGE

How can a prejudiced attitude be changed? A review of the literature indicates that the compendium of findings is inconclusive and many times contradictory. Urban and Ford (1967) reported the following factors which affect attitude change:

> (a) The more *extreme* the attitude, the less susceptible to change. (b) Similarly, the more *intense* the attitude, the more immune to modification it is presumed to be. (c) Also, the more *complex* the attitude, the harder it will be to effect change in the attitude system. (d) The degree of *consistency* within an attitude system is important. A consistent attitude system tends to be a stable one, with the elements mutually supporting one another. (e) The *centrality* of an attitude, reflecting the degree to which it is intimately related to the person's fundamental goals and objectives in life, is thus an additional factor.

As previously stated, an attitude is usually determined by a whole set of influences, some of which are unfavorable to the object. For example, consider the following possible attitudes and beliefs of an employer toward hiring handicapped workers.

1. A belief in the rights of all citizens to have equality of opportunity.

2. A belief in judgment of a person's ability to do the job instead of his disability in another area.

Among the factors that might cause an unfavorable attitude to the employment of the handicapped are the following:

1. A belief that hiring the handicapped would cause increased insurance rates.

2. A belief that hiring the handicapped would cause a higher accident rate.

3. A belief that hiring the handicapped would lower production.

4. A belief that turnover would be higher.

One way for an attitude change to occur is to get new information relevant to the attitude. For example, new information to the effect that hiring the handicapped is good business, or information stating that insurance and accident rates are not higher where handicapped individuals are employed might change the attitude of an employer mildly opposed to hiring the handicapped.

A second reason an attitude may change is because of a change in perception. For example, a politician who is unfavorable toward a bill which is somewhat detrimental to his constituency might not have thought of this bill in relation to its importance to the United States as a whole. Perceiving this bill in relation to its value to the country as a whole might alter his attitude toward the bill in a favorable direction. Most attitude change is not so much the matter of changing values but rather a matter of changing our perception of the situation in relation to values already held.

A third way in which an attitude may be modified is through a change in motivation. Actually, either of the two previously mentioned factors can foster a change in motivation. In turn, a change of motivation can cause one to perceive a situation in a new way or evaluate new information differently. For example, an employer who has been indifferent or hostile toward employing handicapped persons may change his whole attitude toward employing the handicapped when a close friend or relative becomes disabled.

Another factor related to attitude change is group affiliation or the influence toward conformity which a group exerts on its members by virtue of an individual's identification with the group and group objectives. The penalties for nonconformity many times are unpopularity, ostracism, or loss of prestige. A good example of an organization which utilizes this concept is the President's Committee on Employment of the Handicapped. Also, community organizations emphasize the need to help particular minority groups, such as the handicapped, and influence their ability to find jobs by pressuring members of the industrial community.

Many of our attitudes change because of the influence of prestigious persons. These individuals may be close friends, experts, or persons we admire such as actors or professional athletes.

When we see someone like Jerry Lewis or Henry Fonda sponsoring a particular fund drive for a charitable organization, we may be influenced to contribute to this fund drive if we are admirers of these men. We may feel that their affiliation with a particular charity automatically legitimizes the fund drive and makes it a worthy cause.

Two additional factors are significantly related to attitude change. First, a person must be aware that he has a prejudicial attitude in order for effective change to occur. Secondly, when attitudes become more liberal toward other minority groups, then the attitudes toward specific disability groups, such as the blind, also become more liberal. In other words, as the environment changes, individuals within the environment also change.

SUMMARY

Attitudes refer to the stands an individual upholds and cherishes about objects, issues, persons, groups, or institutions. Most authorities agree that attitudes are socially formed. According to Sartan, attitudes are learned from one of the following sources or combinations of these sources: specific experiences, communication from others, imitation of models, and institutional factors.

Prejudice has been defined as an attitude emotionally resistant to change. A historical review of the treatment of handicapped and disabled segments of our population has indicated much prejudice and many unfavorable attitudes.

Most authorities agree that the public's attitude toward the blind and other disability groups play an important role in their rehabilitation. When negative attitudes are present, rehabilitation is retarded.

Numerous factors are related to attitude change. An individual may alter his attitude because he receives new information relevant to the attitude, because of a change in motivation or perception, because of a change in group affiliation, or because of the influence of a prestigious person.

REFERENCES

Adorno, T. W. and others: *The Authoritarian Personality.* New York, Harper, 1950.

Barker, Robert G.: *Adjustment to Physical Handicap and Illness.* New York, Soc. Sci. Res., 1953.

Bell, A. H.: Attitudes of selected rehabilitation workers toward the physically disabled. *Psychological Reports, 10*:183-186, 1962.

Caveness, William F.: Trend in public attitudes toward epilepsy over the past decade. *Epilepsia, 1*:385-393, 1960.

Gellman, William: Roots of prejudice against the handicapped. *J. Rehabil., 25*:329-341, 1965.

Kanner, Leo: *A History of the Care and Study of the Mentally Retarded.* Springfield, Thomas, 1964.

McGowan, John F., and Porter, Thomas L.: *An Introduction to the Vocational Rehabilitation Process.* Washington, D. C., Vocational Rehabilitation Administration, HEW, 1967.

Oberman, C. Esco: *A History of Vocational Rehabilitation in America.* Minneapolis, Denison, 1965.

Olender, Jack H.: *The Legal Rights of Persons with Epilepsy.* Washington, D. C., The Epilepsy Foundation, 1962.

Ray, M. H.: The Effect of Crippled Appearance on Personality Judgment. Unpublished master's thesis, Stanford University, Stanford, California, 1964.

Sartan, Aaron Q. and others: *Psychology: Understanding Human Behavior.* New York, McGraw-Hill, 1962.

Sherif, Muzafer and others: *Attitudes and Attitude Change: The Social Judgment—Involvement Approach.* Philadelphia, Saunders, 1965.

Sommers, V. S.: *The Influence of Parental Attitudes and Social Environment on the Personality Development of the Adolescent Blind.* New York, The American Foundation for the Blind, 1944.

Thomas, W. I. and Zaniecki, F.: *The Polish Peasant In Europe and America.* Boston, Badges, 1918.

Urban and Ford: In *Attitudes and Blindness.* Pennsylvania Department of Public Welfare, Office for the Blind. A workshop conducted for the staff of the Office for the Blind. Harrisburg, Pennsylvania, 1967.

Whiteman, Martin and Irving F. Lukoff: Public attitudes toward blindness. *The New Outlook for the Blind, 56*:153-158, 1962.

Yuker, Harold E.: Attitudes as determinants of behavior. *J. Rehabil., 31*:15-16, 1965.

8

Research on Psychological Factors Associated with Blindness

Mary K. Bauman

It sounds so simple to talk about the psychological impact of blindness and yet it is not at all a simple question. First we can ask, impact on whom? Although blindness happens physically to an individual, psychologically it happens not only to him, but to a family, to a community, to a school, to an employer, and in fact, to a whole culture.

This, of course, is also true of other disabilities or handicaps. Much of what we have as a reaction to blindness is also found in the reactions to other kinds of disabilities. Yet there is a good bit of evidence that blindness is regarded as different, and wc must cope, as we talk about the psychological impact, with the fact that throughout history blindness has often been regarded as a "different" thing. The blind person was rejected more in some cultures; he was protected more in other cultures. Even our own culture, in terms of the amount of legal action that has been taken, shows a significant difference. I do not know what the count today is, but a few years ago something like 10 times more legal action had been taken with regard to blind people than with regard to any other single disability. This legal action included income tax exemptions, postage adjustments, the possibility of having a companion travel without charge, etc. This makes it pretty clear that even today blindness appears to be different from a lot of other disabilities in our culture. In fact, as far as I know, there is no agency or commission for the deaf in any state, no commission for the cerebral-palsied, certainly no commission for the person with heart problems. But the number of commissions for the blind established by the legislatures of a number of states seems to say that those legislatures see blindness as a different problem which requires a different solution.

A certain amount of research supports this. In research in which nonhandicapped persons rated the various handicaps, blindness has stood out as the one that looked worst or in some way significantly different from the others.

Yet, there are some ways in which blindness has not stood out. It is interesting that we have in many places developed quite a good integration of blind children into regular classes. I would also like to point out that we do not have a college for the blind although we do have a college for the deaf. Moreover, I remember with interest an occasion when someone asked about having a college for the blind in a group of rehabilitation workers and they were all horrified at the thought. We are not horrified at the thought of residential schools for blind children, but we all turn on anyone who suggests we need a college for blind people.

EFFECTS OF BLINDNESS

We live in a very competitive culture. We are not really very honest about it, because we insist that all men are created equal and then we work like mad to be better than the next fellow, are ashamed when our children do not get the best records in school, win the highest scholarships, and so on. So we really are constantly living in a kind of psychological conflict in which any disability is a real handicap. All men are not created equal; the blind infant is not equal; the blind adult does not have a chance to be equal in a lot of ways. But rehabilitation tries to make it as equal as it can. Those involved in rehabilitation are in the business of making men equal even if they were not created that way.

The psychological impact of blindness is affected by a great many factors including the age at which vision is lost and the cause of the loss. One of the arguments that blind people get into is whether it is better to lose your vision suddenly, completely, forever, or to lose it gradually, bit by bit. If you have lost it suddenly, you are likely to think that is the best thing; if you lose it gradually you cannot help feeling that there was some advantage to this in that the adjustment could come slowly and gradually. My own experience is that when it comes slowly there is always the hope that maybe not much more will go—and the fear that it all will. The tension created by that situation is, I think (speaking as a psychologist on the outside) a different kind of impact of blindness than the impact of sudden loss.

The psychological impact is much affected by the nature of the individual's family, whether he be a congenitally blind child or an adult.

Let's talk about congenital blindness and the impact of this on a family. Anytime that a family knows there is going to be a baby added to it, there is a period of mental readjustment along with months of change in which the center of activity of that family is changed. Everyone knows that this must be experienced, but they expect to get something great from it—another member of the family! The family also anticipates that by and by mother will be back to taking care of the two-year-old and the four-year-old, to cooking good meals for father, and so on. But when the child is born blind, that hope, that attitude of readjustment, is changed. Except in a family where blindness is hereditary and everybody is pretty used to it, a whole new set of information has to be gained. How does one bring up a blind child? It may be a blow to their feeling of status as a family. In many cases this birth is the beginning of a lifelong sense of guilt on the part of one or both of the parents; so very many parents say "Why did this happen to us," and are searching for what they did wrong. I think this was more true a generation ago than it is now. Some of the causes of blindness in recent years, particularly retrolental fibroplasia, which was associated with the medical profession's learning how to preserve premature children, was quite clearly not the fault of the parent. I feel that the attitude of guilt in families has changed somewhat as a result of this, as well as the attitude of communities.

PARENTAL REACTION TO BLINDNESS

Nevertheless, there is no doubt that the blind child's coming into the family changes that family's feelings about the new addition to the family; in some cases we know that the psychological reaction of that family is a very extreme one. I know of no residential school that does not have a few students who have no families. They were abandoned and nobody knows who their family was. I have examined psychologically more than one adult who had been discovered only weeks or months before I saw him or her. That person's family had hidden the individual successfully for years in the back room of some house somewhere because they were unwilling to let anyone know that there was a blind child in the family.

Much more frequent is rejection which is hidden or sugar-coated in what one might call overprotection. In all too many cases, families do too many things for the child in order to hide deep rejection feelings. Many times the reaction of the family is to try to compensate or overcompensate. Sometimes they say, in effect, "My child is blind but he is a great musician," or "He is a great mathematician," etc. Very frequently, the family's behavior in this connection is unrelated to the talents of the child and pushes the child to try to be something that he really cannot be. I have seen some completely ridiculous examples of this kind of thing in which the parent has informed me, for example, that the child has great musical talent although teachers of the child say he is not very good. The family's own psychological needs compel them to try to find compensating superiority, while a lack of appreciation of the child's true talents can create very great problems for the youngster himself. There are also a great many sensible families who, fortunately, have had some good advice early in the blind child's life and who are trying to be reasonable about his upbringing. In many cases though, they have genuine confusion. They do not know whether they should expect as much of the blind child as they do of the seeing siblings. They do not know whether they should discipline with the same firmness. They do not know how to supplement the experience of the blind child although they have sense enough to realize that there are some things the blind child cannot readily learn. What kinds of toys should he have; what kinds of games can be played; how can they develop friendships for the child who cannot readily run down the street and develop his own friendships? What about wheeled vehicles—what about a bicycle, what about a tricycle?

They have a reasonable concern about their child's being in a dangerous situation. How often should they say, "Don't cross the street, don't go off our play area"? These are real problems of real people and in many cases the rehabilitation worker will be asked to help solve them.

There is no easy answer. Just to say, "Expect as much of this child as you expect of the sighted brother or sister," is not enough of an answer. We sometimes take refuge in saying, "just love him," but more is needed. One also must teach a child and discipline him. There *are* standards, and the family must manage these standards so that it is possible to live with this blind child.

CONCERNS OF THE BLIND

Now, let us imagine, as we talk about psychological impact, an ideal situation for a congenitally blind child. We can define an ideal situation as a family that understands, loves, gives as much supplementary experience as possible, and does not make a great issue of it. What does the blind child who grows up in such a family feel about being blind? Louis Rives says that at first the child does not know he is blind. He may hear the word (in a sensible family, the word is used), but other words are also applied to a child, and what does "blind" mean anyway? As a very small child, Rives did not perceive himself as different from other children; in fact, he says, "Normal is what *you* are." He assumed no one saw anything he did not see. Then he remembers realizing there were things his friends could do that he did not seem to be able to do. They would say there is a bird in the tree; he did not hear any bird so how did they know there was a bird in the tree? Very gradually, he recognized there were some things his friends could do that he could not do, and that was what "blind" meant—that he could not see the bird in the tree, he could not see that it looked as if it were going to rain, and so on.

What happens from there on depends very much upon the blind child's own ability and upon this environment that we are talking about. Lowenfeld, who is one of the authorities in the field, said that blindness has only two effects in and of itself: (1) It affects certain cognitive functions. There are certain kinds of things that cannot be explained to a person who has been totally blind from birth. One cannot explain the difference between red and green, for example, to someone who has never seen color at all. (2) Lowenfeld feels that the other inherent limitation growing out of blindness is the problem of mobility. He emphasizes the mobility issue more than I would perhaps because I have great faith in being able to overcome the mobility problem. But I do appreciate the fact that without useful vision there are hazards in travel that the rest of us do not have. I had a very good friend who reached my office one day breathless, and with a look of anguish on his face. He said, "You didn't tell me they changed the direction of travel on your street." He had almost been knocked down because he was accustomed to traffic coming from the right on that street and the city had, since his last visit, changed to the opposite. That kind of thing is part of what Lowenfeld was referring to. Another example is the fact that, for most of us, going up or down a curb requires no thought at all; it must always require a certain amount of concentration when one cannot see that curb. With the best of cane technique, one must locate the curb and react to that cane. There is a far more complex process involved even for a good traveler. That dependence which limits a person to going when a friend is willing to go, and sometimes where a friend is willing to go; that dependence which makes the individual ask for help when he would so like to be independent —this certainly has a psychological impact upon what would like to be a very free and independent spirit.

Teenagers also worry about other things, particularly teenagers in a public school setting. A boy in such a setting is likely to feel concern about athletic competition. In many schools swimming is not available so games that involve a ball are likely to be the way in which athletes demonstrate how good they are. The impossibility of a totally blind boy's being a football hero or a baseball pitcher or a home run hitter makes a difference in this area called "impact of blindness." When the boy is a little older, the fact that he cannot drive also seems to make a big difference. In some of my research with adults, I have asked, "In what way does blindness most handicap you." A very large percentage of the men said that not being able to drive most troubled them. It was not just the inconvenience of dependence upon others; there seems to be an association with driving a car that seems different from just the convenience. There is an element of power in being able to control a car and make it go where one wants it to go. When it is impossible to do this, there is a psychological impact in that fact.

Another area of impact is the adjustment to sex relationships for both boys and girls. Here blindness can create some very real psychological problems in the inability to observe sex differences; how a girl behaves in relation to a boy, and how a boy behaves in relation to a girl. Again, on the basis of years of work with teenagers, I see the adolescent period as one of many psychological problems related to social skills and to the whole intersex relationship. These problems have often been blamed on residential schools, but I think it is inherent in the situation itself.

If the individual had normal vision until age 20 or 30, and then lost his vision, we have a completely different kind of psychological impact. What blindness means to that person is complicated by what it meant to him when he could see.

Here we go back to what blindness means in our culture. Is blindness indicative of a beggar? Is blindness indicative of a completely dependent person? If a person were always sorry for blind people and now suddenly became one of them, how could he help being sorry for himself? If, as is true in many cases, the blind person was not presented in a very favorable light in his early experience, he essentially is in the position of rejecting himself.

THE ADJUSTMENT PROCESS

The concept of adjustment to blindness which occurs to an adult has been given a lot of attention by a lot of people. A psychiatrist named Cholden pretty much popularized the concept of mourning for the lost sighted self, and Father Carroll has carried it one step farther by indicating that one is indeed mourning for a dead individual. The sighted self is dead and until one has mourned and buried the sighted self, one cannot get started as a blind person. I do not believe that this necessarily happens to everybody, but there almost always is a period of seeking to adjust. This can be a period of emotional tension, instability, and unreality in thinking about oneself. Further, there is a period of very real learning about how to get along without vision. A great deal of the adjustment problem of a newly blinded person is real; it is not emotional only: What do you have in your hands—it doesn't feel like anything you can remember; how do you shave, how do you feed yourself without spilling the food, how do you cut your meat? These are very real, practical problems. One can call it mourning for an old self that was capable of cutting meat, but the therapy that is really effective is teaching the person here to cut the meat without seeing it, not psycho-analyzing him and talking him out of problems that are real. Perhaps I am not a good person to talk about the psychological impact of blindness, because I seek a practical way of dealing with it. I feel that the best therapy usually is learning how to deal with the problem. The individual can then develop a different concept of himself and will be very much more comfortable with not being able to see. If the person can live in an environment where people know it is not easy, are sympathetic with the fact that it is not easy, and help him make it easier, that's the best possible therapy.

Now, unfortunately, not everyone lives in such an environment. The first impulse of most families, and of many nurses, ophthalmologists, and so forth, is "I'll do it for you." It is a nice gesture but nobody learns anything when somebody does it for him. To a certain extent a family also has to adjust; they also have a period of mourning. The psychological impact of blindness is not just on the person but also on the family. The first thing they want to do is make up for blindness by doing as much as they can for the individual.

Rehabilitation counselors have to understand that and yet fight it. They must learn to do this gracefully—not hurt their feelings but help them to realize that nobody is getting anywhere this way, that only by learning to do gracefully as many things as he can will the newly blinded person ever "adjust."

Sometimes blindness happens to an individual in a family where there is at least one person who is really looking for somebody to take care of. Usually it is a woman whose children are grown and no longer need her, and who was just at the point of feeling pretty useless when a son or a husband loses his vision;

here is someone to whom she can devote the rest of her life. Rehabilitation counselors have to deal with this and it is not easy. They must sense that person's need: the fact is that she does need something to do with her life, but what she is trying to do will all too often be a boomerang. For the first six months, doing everything for a newly blinded person may yield a great sense of reward. By and by however, it is likely to result in a feeling, not so much of being needed as of being exploited. All too often the gentleness gets a little rougher, the sweetness a little more bitter, and the whole family is much less happy than if the individual had learned to do what he could for himself early, easily, and comfortably without anybody's making a great fuss about it.

Sometimes blindness happens to someone whose life as a sighted person was not very successful by his standards, or perhaps by anyone's standards. The individual who has been struggling as a sighted person may find in blindness a socially acceptable solution to all those struggles. Consequently, in some cases, the psychological effect of blindness is very comforting. Here is a good excuse for not being a great success, for not making a lot of money, for any of the kinds of things that competition and/or failure has represented for that individual. Now everyone can understand why he is not going to be a great success. This is a completely different kind of psychological reaction and a tough one for the rehabilitation counselor, because as soon as this person tries to succeed, he fears that he may again fail. It is thus pretty hard to motivate this kind of individual. I think that when a counselor has a motivation problem with an individual it would be well to understand the kind of person he was before he lost his vision, because maybe that is where rehabilitation really has to start—with an understanding of the effect of competition and threat of failure upon the person before visual loss.

To some extent the impact of visual loss is a very practical one. People do lose their jobs when they lose their vision. That is a practical problem, that is a question of income. While the individual may be in a state that has a "blind pension," it is really not much money to try to live on. A father who suddenly cannot earn the money to take care of his family may find that the family is no longer looking upon him with quite the respect that he was accustomed to. It may be difficult to get the children to do what he wants them to and may be difficult to get his wife to recognize him as the head of the house if she is going out to earn the money now. These are practical psychological problems that people who lose their vision have to face. A fair number of men who lose their vision are abandoned; their wives simply pack up and go, usually taking the children with them. That does not help one to accept himself as a blind person.

Some people deny their visual loss. This most frequently occurs when loss is not total. Some clients do not admit how little they can see and as a result do things that are really quite foolish. They have accidents because they refuse to carry a cane—they are not going to advertise the fact that they are blind. They keep trying to do a job where there is some danger because they will not admit that they cannot do it. They may manage because they know the job well and because they get some fellow worker to do part of it (which hides from the supervisor the fact that they really can no longer do this job). These are kinds of psychological impact which quite definitely end in efforts to deny the visual loss, and quite frequently as a result to deny the help of a rehabilitation counselor. They do not want to talk to someone from an agency for the blind because "I'm not blind."

One kind of psychological impact is to use blindness as a weapon, a way to control the environment. The attitude is one of "You've got to take care of me." The individual may take this attitude toward the state, ie. the state owes him a living. Still more personally, he may control a family by insisting upon having things done for him. He insists on being taken somewhere because this is proof of the devotion of his family. This, too, is a psychological problem which counselors will face inevitably in a certain number of cases. Very frequently, the newly blinded person narrows his world to the point where he thinks he has eliminated most of the ways in which he may look foolish, or in which he may get hurt. Consciously or unconsciously, he drops these activities from his daily life. The placement man is thus a threat to him. The counselor urges mobility training and he is scared to death. He has reason to be scared, and it requires patience and understanding to accept his fears. There has to be communication in which the counselor understands what he is saying without any words, and he can understand what the counselor is trying to say with lots of words. The only common ground is feeling. One must try to appreciate what is going on inside this personality, and to recognize that because failure is not a pleasant thing, many people do not try because they are afraid of failure. To them, it may be preferable deliberately not to try and to defend their right not to try with everything they can. The counselor must sense the fear, sense the anxiety, sense the need to move slowly with sure ground under each step along the way.

RESEARCH ON PSYCHOLOGICAL IMPACT OF BLINDNESS

This paper will omit discussion of most research related to "hardware" and try to give a quick overview of some of the research which might be called psychologically oriented. The research falls mainly into three groups, somwehat related to passage of time: What is blindness made of, what are blind men made of and what is the environment in which they live made of?

The first research was "What is blindness made of." Psychologists were curious about how blind people learned without being able to see, the kinds of concepts they had, and how they compensated for not being able to see. When I first came into this field there was a very real belief in the ability of other senses to compensate. The phrase that was used by many psychologists was the vicarüsm of senses. Within the vicarüsm of senses, if blindness eliminated one source of information all the others were supposed to improve automatically so that the blind person was able to get the same information in some other way. However, studies that were made with reasonable care soon showed that a blind person might develop better attention to other sources of information, such as anditory information, but he heard no better than sighted people did. He might develop attention to tactual information and thus be able to make discriminations that the sighted person would not ordinarily make, but sighted persons could be taught without too much time and effort to make that same level of discrimination. The senses did not improve with loss of sight, but the use of information from the senses was improved.

When I came into this field there was a very real acceptance of something that was called facial vision, by which it was meant that a blind person could feel when he was approaching something, such as a wall. It was supposed that there were sense receptors in the blind person's face that were not in anyone else's face. Some people had good facial vision and they could tell when they were coming to a tree or a pole; other people had medium facial vision and they could tell when they were coming to a wall or could distinguish a doorway through a wall; and of course some people had very little facial vision and could not depend upon it.

Then some really good work on this was done, chiefly led by Dallenbach, Worchel, and that group, and it became quite clear that the blind person was using hearing. He heard when he was coming to a wall, and when his hearing was stopped off, he had no more facial vision than anyone else. It was also quite clear that blindfolded sighted people, within a rather small amount of time, could learn to respond to this sound. It thus had nothing to do with blindness as such. In fact, in one of Worchel's studies, the person who unquestionably had the best facial vision was a sighted girl who was blindfolded.

So we got rid of some of the misconceptions, and I do emphasize how recent they are. Within the last 20 to 25 years we have come to grips with the fact that blindness is made of a loss of sight and that is all it is made of. It is not made of any compensating ability to hear or to feel things with the face or anything of that sort.

This fact has pretty much stopped that kind of research, but the new question is how far can the senses be pushed. There is work being done on this. For example, Emerson Folke in Louisville has been experimenting with speeding up material which is read. Sighted people who are good readers can read faster than anyone who can read aloud. The blind student, particularly at the college level, who must get his information by listening to tape recordings, or by someone reading face to face, has to put in a great many more hours of study in order to cover his college courses than the sighted student. I suspect that Emerson Folke, a very competent young man, was greatly irked by this, and probably his own need motivated him to try to develop equipment that would speed up this reading. He has been studying just how fast he can move up a recording and still understand it. Of course, there are some people who do not understand it very well as soon as it is speeded up while other people can use varying speeds with reasonable comprehension. This work is progressing and perhaps some day it will provide solutions to the long hours of listening that are required for most totally blind persons who try to go to college.

Carson Nolan, of the American Printing House for the Blind, has worked on differentiation tactually and its relationship to learning braille. He has been concerned with being able to predict the ability of a young child to learn braille and he has developed a test of tactual discrimination chiefly based on different kinds of sandpaper from very fine to very coarse. He found some relationship between the young child's ability to discriminate his samples and to learn braille at that age. This is the kind of research that one might say is now concerned with the physical compensations for blindness.

Now, what are blind men made of? Again, some early concepts seem weird at this point. For example, there was an early opinion that blind people had more speech defects than sighted people, and several studies seemed to prove it. As nearly as I can tell blind children have no more speech defects than sighted children have; they respond to the same kind of speech training that sighted children respond to, this is therefore a completely exploded concept.

Then there was a concept that blind men were made of a great deal of verbal ability. Cutsforth was one of those who thought that blind people were extremely verbal, by which it was meant that they can say a lot of things but they do not know what they mean by it. We must admit that certain concepts are weak or missing. A person can not tell red from green if he never saw red or green. The blind person may use the words and one might call this verbalism, but on the whole I am inclined to feel that is not an important component in blindness.

One of the aspects of blindness that has not had a great deal of research attention is that related to the combination of blindness and the effects of aging. New studies are being planned in this direction. New Jersey, for example, has a committee specifically studying its aged blind and their needs.

In the late 1940's and the early 1950's, I was involved in something called the "adjustment study" which was the first big description of blind people and what they are made of. In a way we were describing not just the blind people but the opportunities they had. For example, we found that people with pretty high IQ's were often doing factory work; that was the only work anyone could get for them. It was not that the man with the IQ of 126 wanted to do factory work, but he would rather be independent doing factory work than be on welfare. So he willingly did it. MacFarland, in his study in New Jersey, compared a blind person doing a job with a sighted person next to him doing the same job and consistently found higher IQ's in the blind persons. It would be possible to argue that the blind person had to be brighter in order to do this job, but I am inclined to think that the blind person just could not get any other job and settled for some job rather than no job.

There was a time when people said publically that a blind person had to have about 10 more IQ points to do a job. Today, I think we can prove that is not true—a blind person does not have to have 10 more IQ points to do the same job.

The adjustment study did show that certain psychological measurements make fair predictions of what an individual will do within a defined cultural opportunity. The structure of the study was simply that the rehabilitation counselors in five different states chose three defined groups of clients or ex-clients: (1) Those whom they regarded as eminently successful. These were independent people, living pretty normal lives, who were employed and had been employed consistently over a defined period of time. (2) Those who were the opposite of that. They were not successful. They were maladjusted, dependent individuals who had not been employed for a long time or had never been employed. (3) A middle group which seemed to be employable and had promise, but were not at that moment employed and had not been for six months; we might call these the promising but unemployed group.

We tested them, we interviewed them, we studied the case history folders, some of them two inches thick, and all these facts were inter-related in careful studies. We found out that we could, by a combination of ability, interest, dexterity, and personality, define those who were likely to be successful and those who were not very successful; we could also make some predictions about the middle group as to which way they would be likely to go.

Then, about 15 years after that, I was curious about whether we had been right, so we went back and tried to find those people. We found roughly 80 percent, and studied what had happened to them in the intervening years to see whether the counselors had been right in their selections and whether we had been right in our tests. We found that the counselors were pretty much right; about 85 percent of the cases who had been successful still were successful. However, only around half of the unsuccessful were still unsuccessful. A succession of rehabilitation counselors had worked with them and tried to train and place them. Sometimes these rehabilitation counselors had been successful where their predecessors had not. So we had much more movement from the unemployed and unsuccessful group to the successful than the reverse. However, there were some moves in reverse, often because of emotional instability or health problems.

Training and placment had had a great effect on the group who were not employed at the time of the original study and give ample reason to keep on trying. If there is any message in the adjustment study follow-up, I think it is "keep on trying." If one counselor cannot succeed, try another counselor because the interpersonal relationship between a counselor and his client can at times get pretty strained. They are both human beings and even though the counselor is taught to keep his feelings out of it, it is a little difficult when he has tried so many things and the person will not move. The counselor gets to feeling that it has to be his fault. Yet, it is not anybody's fault except that maybe a new view, a new personality, can have success. One must beware of saying, "That fellow will never be successful," because it is much more likely to be untrue than if one says, "That one is a good worker and will continue to be employed."

There was also a great deal of evidence that blindness, as such, is a stress situation. If we think of the behavior that blind people produce as a general stress reaction, we can understand it and them a lot better, instead of just thinking of them as being difficult clients. Indeed, as a teacher or counselor, we may be one of their pressures; we may be pushing them toward doing things they fear, toward doing things which are sources of anxiety to them. Maybe somebody else just has to come in and push them in a little different way.

There are other studies of what blind men are made of. I should like to mention a couple that relate to war-blinded persons because excellent financial support has produced detailed descriptions of these people. Gowman's study of the war-blind chiefly emphasized questions of social adjustment, and described blind men who are pretty similar. It is a very homogeneous group because they could all see previously and they were all adventitiously blinded under service-connected circumstances at a fairly narrow age span. The study shows how they related to the culture to which they returned and gives a great deal of detailed information. He found that employment and, therefore, rehabilitation success related very much to the support of the family, the family's attitude toward this war-blinded person as he came back, and to the amount of education he had which inevitably related to the amount of education he could profit by. It is not a clear one-to-one relationship because a lot of people who could profit by education do not choose to get it or do not have the opportunity to get it, but there is a strong relationship to IQ there. Emotional stability has also had a tremendous effect on whether the individual was rehabilitated or not.

More recently, Graham has gone back and studied 851 men who had service-connected visual loss of 70 percent or more, including some of the same people that Gowman studied. He found that although 93 percent of them had worked at some time, by the time he studied them, only 41 percent of them were employed. Therefore, by rehabilitation standards of employment, less than half of them were successfully rehabilitated. He did find that a big cause of not working was general poor health. A person who has suffered blindness from any accidental cause, whether related to a war or not, has usually been subjected to a circumstance which could have caused other kinds of damage, e.g. brain damage, neurological damage, etc. So poor health had a lot to do with it. A lot of these people chose to retire early, apparently in part because they sensed an inability to compete. Blindness and health problems offered an escape which was made even easier by the fact that a person who is blinded in service receives a rather good disability payment and it is possible to manage on this.

All of these are factors and it is important to know about them because they are factors in any of the clients the counselor works with. The counselor needs to recognize that the extent to which our culture provides for, and subsidizes, a blind person does have something to do with his motivation to work. It need not be a work-connected subsidy. Suppose one is working with a person who is very limited in ability, perhaps mentally retarded, has little education, and has been struggling along in a marginal job when he loses his vision. It may be that the subsidy for blind people in his state is more secure and better (because he can be sure of it) than what he makes as an unskilled worker. A good many clients fear rehabilitation and fear the counselor because they are more sure of what they have on blind pension than in the job he can reasonably hope to get them.

There is one more study that I feel I should mention. This is the follow-up of teenagers by the author, Geraldine Scholl, and Marie Chrissy. The states involved are Pennsylvania, Maryland, New Jersey, Virginia, and Michigan. We followed teenagers whom we had seen roughly between 1947 and 1960. These dates allowed enough time to pass so we could see what had happened to the teenagers. Much of our reason for doing this was that most of our teenagers were blinded early (many of them were congenitally blind), which differentiated what we were doing from what Gowman and Graham did and, to some extent, from the adjustment study where some but not most were congenitally blind. We found that 84 percent of the boys, who now are men, are employed as are 36 percent of the women. We did not call the housewife employed; if we had, the percentage for women would be higher. We decided upon three criterion variables: The percentage of time worked, the income made, and the socioeconomic index of the occupations. By this last criterion we mean the status of the occupation. For example, a physician is usually regarded as on a higher socioeconomic level than the salesman, the salesman on a higher level than the telephone operator and so on.

The predictors for percentage of time worked were, in order of strength of prediction, IQ, travel ability, sex (the men worked more than the women), amount of education, and not having other disabilities. All the other items were so low that they were not really predictors at all. Travel ability is a very important factor in how much of the time a person is employed. Of course, one would expect IQ to have something to do with it, and I think we can understand that the men in general are going to work more of the time than the women. Women take themselves out of the work force to get married.

For income, the predictors were: (1) IQ, (2) sex—men make more than women do, and (3) amount of vision. If a person has helpful vision, he can make a little bit more in essentially the same job than if he does not. A fourth predictor was being married, and here I am not sure whether being married motivates one to make more, or when one does make more, he can afford to get married! A fifth predictor was freedom from other disabilities; one makes more if he does not have a secondary disability. Education proved to have an important relationship to how much of the time the individual was employed, but a rather weak relationship to income.

Finally, the predictors for socioeconomic index. Again, the highest predictor is IQ; a professional job relates to the IQ necessary to get through professional education. Other predictors of the socioeconomic index are amount of education, absence of other disabilities, and the amount of money spent on the individual by the agency. The cost factor probably relates to sending the client through college and graduate school so naturally he is going to be able to go into the higher level of socioeconomic occupations. A very weak predictor of socioeconomic index is sex; women are almost as likely to get into a profession as men are if they are appropriately educated for it. Finally, travel ability shows a mild relationship. Professional workers could get away with being poor travelers when salesmen could not.

What is the environment of the blind man made of? Real study of the environment requires a tremendous amount of time and consideration of a great number of factors; until we had computers into which to feed enormous numbers of variables, study of the environment was an almost impossible task. Now, with the use of computers, several people have been studying the effect of the social environment upon blind people. Siller at New York University has been concerned with the relationship between the personality of a nonblind person and his acceptance of, and attitudes toward, a blind person. His findings show that the people who are least likely to accept blind people, the people who are prejudiced against them, the people who do not want to be around them, are the people who have personality problems themselves. The more secure a sighted individual is, the more ready he is to accept the blind person as a fellow worker, to accept the blind person as an employee, or to accept the blind person in the student-teacher relationship. Where prejudice appears, the trouble may be very deep within the personality.

Lukoff and Whiteman (1970), also working in the New York area, attempted to determine why some blind people reacted dependently while others reacted independently. The special emphasis in this research was upon how aspects of the environment affected dependence and independence. Interviews with about 500 blind persons were examined in detail with independence particularly evaluated through employment, travel competence, and skill in eating and shopping.

It was found that environmental expectations do have a great effect upon the dependence or independence of the blind person, but that the standards encountered by any one blind person vary greatly and elements within his own makeup cause him to react more strongly to some stimulae than to others. The dependently oriented blind person is very much affected by his environment, and when that environment expects independent behavior of him, he will try to produce it, contrary to his own inner wishes.

On the other hand, the independently oriented blind person is likely to defy the expectations found in his environment, no matter what those expectations are. Perhaps most interesting of all is the finding that "the blind who do not accept friends and organizational activity within the blind community, despite personal and normative pressures for independence, are less often in the most independent social-role categories. While blind persons who avoid sustained contacts with other blind are often aggressively independent in interpersonal relations with sighted persons, they have low rates of employment and consequently fewer appear in the more independent social-role categories. Those who make their peace with the blind community—through friendships and organizational activity or through the latter alone—are more likely to be employed and to be independent in social-role performance. Without some accommodation to the organized blind community, the likelihood that the blind person will achieve maximum independence is seriously diminished."

REFERENCES

Bauman, Mary K.: *Adjustment to Blindness: A Study as Reported by the Committee to Study Adjustment to Blindness.* Harrisburg, Pennsylvania, Office for the Blind, 1963.

Bauman, Mary K. and Yoder, N. M.: *Adjustment to Blindness—Reviewed.* Springfield, Thomas, 1966.

Cutsforth, T. D.: *The Blind in School and Society.* New York, American Foundation for the Blind, 1951.

Gowman, A. G.: *The War Blind in the American Social Structure.* New York, American Foundation for the Blind, 1957.

Graham, M. D., Robinson, R. L., Lowrey, A., Sarchin, M. M., and Tims, F.: *851 Blind Veterans: A Success Story.* New York, American Foundation for the Blind, 1968.

Lukoff, I. F. and Whiteman, M.: *The Social Source of Adjustment to Blindness.* New York, American Foundation for the Blind, Research Series No. 21, 1970.

Mac Farland, D.: *A Study of Work Efficiency of Blind and Sighted Workers in Industry.* New York, American Foundation for the Blind, 1956.

Nolan, C. Y. and Morris, June E:; Development and validation of the roughness discrimination test. *Int. J. Educ. Blind, 15*:1-6, 1965.

Scholl, Geraldine T., Bauman, Mary K., and Crissey, Marie S.: *A Study of the Vocational Success of Groups of the Visually Handicapped.*

Ann Arbor, Michigan, The University of Michigan, School of Education, 1969.

Siller, J., Chipman, A., Ferguson, Linda T., and Vann, D. H.: *Attitudes of the Nondisabled toward the Physically Disabled.* New York, New York University School of Education, 1967.

Worchel, P.: Space perception and orientation in the blind. *Psychol. Monogr., 65*:15, 1951.

Worchel, P. and Dallenbach, K.: Facial vision: Perception of obstacles by the deaf-blind. *Am. J. Psychol., 60*:4:502-553, 1947.

9

Psychological Adjustment to Blindness

John G. Cull, Jr.

It is true that our clients are much more like us than unlike us, but they differ in one major respect. They have suffered the psychological impact of disability and have adjusted or are in the process of adjusting to this impact. In this chapter we shall discuss the factors which affect the psychological adjustment to blindness and the mechanism by which an individual adjusts to his blindness.

During the first and second world wars, behavioral scientists noticed an increased incidence in conversion reactions. Conversion reactions are (APA, 1965) a type of psychoneurotic disorder in which the impulse causing anxiety is "converted" into functional symptoms in parts of the body rather than the anxiety being experienced consciously. Examples of conversion reactions include such functional disabilities as anesthesias (blindness, deafness), paralyses (aphonia, monoplegia, or hemiplegia), dyskineses (tic, tremor, catalepsy).

The study of these conditions along with other studies led to the development of a discipline known as psychosomatic medicine. Psychosomatic medicine is concerned with the study of the effects of the personality and emotional stresses upon the body and its function. This psychological interaction with physiology can be observed in any of the body systems.

After the establishment of psychosomatic medicine, behavioral scientists (psychiatrists, psychologists, social workers, etc.) began observing the converse of this new field. Instead of studying the effects of emotional stress on bodily functioning, they studied the effects of physical stress on emotional functioning. Their concern was directed toward answering the question, "What are the emotional and personality changes which result from physical stress or a change in body function or physical configuration?"

ROLE OF BODY-IMAGE IN ADJUSTMENT TO BLINDNESS

This new area of study became known as somatopsychology. The basis for this study is the body-image concept. The body-image is a complex conceptualization which we use to describe ourselves. It is one of the basic parts of the total personality and as such determines our reaction to our environment. According to English and English (1966) the body-image is the mental representation one has of his own body.

There are two aspects of the body-image concept—the ideal body-image (the desired body-image) and the actual body-image. The greater the congruity between these two images the better the psychological adjustment of the individual, and conversely, the greater the discrepancy between these two parts of the self-concept, the poorer an individual's psychological adjustment. This is very understandable. If an individual is quite short and views himself as such but has a strong ideal body-image of a tall person, he is less well adjusted than he would be if his desired image were that of a short person. This is a simplistic example, but it portrays the crux of the psychological adjustment to blindness.

In order to adjust to the psychological impact of blindness, the body-image has to change from the image of a sighted person to the body-image of a blind person. Early in the adjustment process the actual body-image will change from that of a sighted person to the actual body-image of a blind person; however, for adequate psychological adjustment to the blindness the ideal body-image must make the corresponding adaptation. Therefore, in essence, psychological adjustment to a disability is the acceptance of an altered body-image which is more in harmony with reality.

FACTORS ASSOCIATED WITH ADJUSTMENT

There are three groups of factors which determine the speed or facility with which an individual will adjust to his disability. They help an individual understand the degree of psychological impact a particular disability is having on a client and the significance of his adjustment.

The first of these three groups of factors are those directly associated with the disability. Psychological effects of disabilities may arise from direct insult or damage to the central nervous system. These psychological effects are called brain syndromes and may be either acute or chronic. In this instance there are a variety of behavioral patterns which may result directly from the disability. In disabilities involving no damage to brain tissue the physical limitations imposed by the disability may cause excessive frustration and in turn result in behavioral disorders. For example an active outdoorsman and nature lover may experience a greater psychological impact upon becoming blind than an individual who leads a more restricted and physically limited life since the restrictions imposed by the disability demand a greater change in the basic life style of the first person. Therefore, factors directly associated with the disability have an important bearing upon an individual's reaction to disability.

The second group consists of those factors arising from the individual's attitude toward his disability. An individual's adjustment to his disability is dependent upon the attitudes he had prior to his disability. If his attitdues toward the blind were quite negative and strong he will naturally have a greater adjustment problem than an individual with a neutral or positive attitude toward disability and the disabled, or specifically the blind and blindness. A part of this attitude formation prior to blindness is dependent upon the experiences the client had with other blind individuals and the stereotypes he developed.

The amount of fear a client experiences or the emotion he expends during the onset and duration of the illness or accident leading up to the disability will determine the psychological impact of the disability. Generally, the greater the amount of emotion expended during onset the better the psychological adjustment to the disability. If an individual goes to sleep a sighted person and awakens a blinded person, his psychological reaction to the disability is much greater than if a great deal of emotion is expended during a process of becoming blinded.

The more information an individual has relating to his disability the less impact the disability will have. If the newly blinded individual is told about his blindness in a simple, straightforward, mechanistic manner, it is much easier to accept and adjust to the disability than if it remains shrouded in a cloak of ignorance and mystery. Any strangeness or unpredictable aspect of our body associated with its function immediately creates anxiety and if not clarified rapidly can result in totally debilitating anxiety. Therefore, it is important for psychological adjustment to a disability that the individual have communicated to him, in terms he can understand, the medical aspects of his disability as soon after onset of disability as possible.

When we are in strange or uncomfortable surroundings, our social perceptiveness becomes keener. Social cues which are below threshold or are not noticed in comfortable surroundings becomes highly significant to us in new, strange or uncomfortable surroundings. Upon the onset of blindness, the client will develop a heightened perceptiveness relative to how he is being treated by family, friends, and professionals. If others start treating him in a condescending fashion and relegate him to a position of less importance, his reaction to the psychological impact of the blindness will be poor. Professionals can react to the client from an anatomical orientation (what is missing) or a functional orientation (what is left). The anatomical orientation is efficient for classification purposes but is completely dehumanizing. The functional orientation is completely individualistic and as such enhances a client's adjustment to his disability.

Perhaps a key concept in the adjustment to blindness is the evaluation of the future and the individual's role in the future. In many physical medicine rehabilitation centers, a rehabilitation counselor is one of the first professionals to see the patient after the medical crisis has passed. The purpose of this approach is to facilitate the patient's psychological adjustment. If he feels there is a potential for his regaining his independence and security the psychological impact of the blindness will be lessened. While the counselor cannot engage in specific vocational counseling with the patient, he can discuss the depth of the vocational rehabilitation program and through these preliminary counseling sessions the counselor can help the newly blinded person evaluate the roles he might play in the future.

The last factor which determines the adjustment process is based upon the individual's view of the purpose of his body and the relationship this view has with the type and extent of disability. The views individuals have of their body may be characterized as falling somewhere on a continuum. At one end of the continuum is the view that the body is a tool to accomplish work; it is a productive machine. At the other end is the view that the body is an esthetic stimulus to be enjoyed and provide pleasure for others. This latter concept is much the same as we have for sculpture and harks back to the philosophy of the ancient Greeks. Everyone falls somewhere on this continuum. To adequately predict the impact of a disability upon an individual, one has to locate the placement of the individual upon this continuum and then evaluate the disability in light of the individual's view of the function of this body.

As an example of the above principle, consider the case in which a day laborer and film actress sustain the same disabling injury—a deep gash across the face. Obviously, when considering the disability in conjunction with the assumed placements of these two upon the functional continuum, the psychological impact will be greater for the actress; since we have assumed the day laborer views his body almost completely as a tool to accomplish work and the disability has not impaired that function, the psychological impact of the disability upon him will be minimal. However, if the disability were changed (they both sustained severe injury to the abdomen resulting in the destruction of the musculature of the abdominal wall) the psychological impact would be reversed. In this case the actress would view her disability as minimal since it did not interfere with the esthetic value of her body, while the day laborer's disability would be overpowering since it had substantial effects upon the productive capacity of his body.

The most obvious conclusion to be drawn from the above three factors is that the degree of psychological impact is not correlated with the degree of disability. This statement is contrary to popular opinion; however, disability and its psychological impact constitute a highly personalized event. Many counselors fall into the trap of equating degree of disability with degree of psychological impact. If the psychological impact suffered by a client is much greater than that considered "normal," the counselor will often times become impatient with the client. It should be remembered that relatively superficial disabilities may have devastating psychological effects. The psychological impact of total blindness is not necessarily greater than partial blindness or, for that matter, more anatomically superficial physical disabilities.

ROLE OF DEFENSE MECHANISMS IN ADJUSTMENT

While the three groups of factors discussed above determine the length of time required for adjustment to blindness, the path to adjustment is best described by defense mechanisms. Defense mechanisms are psychological devices used by all to distort reality. Often reality is so harsh it is unacceptable to us. Therefore, we distort the situation to make it more acceptable. Defense mechanisms are used to satisfy motives which cannot be met in reality; they reduce tensions in personal interactions; and they are used to resolve conflicts. To be effective they must be unconscious. They are not acquired consciously or deliberately. If they become conscious they become ineffective as defenses and others must replace them. For the major part of the remainder of this chapter we will look at the defenses most often employed by the disabled in the general order of their use.

Denial

Denial is an unconscious rejection of an obvious fact which is too disruptive of the personality or too emotionally painful to accept. Therefore, in order to soften reality the obvious fact is denied. Immediately upon onset of disability the individual denies it happened. Then, as the fact of the disability becomes so overwhelming its existance can no longer be denied, there is a denial of the permanency of the disability. The newly blinded individual, while utilizing the defense of denial, will adamantly maintain that he shall see again. There will be a miraculous cure or a new surgical technique will be discovered.

While there are few steadfast rules in human behavior, one

is that rehabilitation at best can be only marginally successful at this point. Rehabilitation cannot procede adequately until the client accepts the permanency of the disability and is ready to cope with the condition. This is what is meant by many professionals when they say a client must accept his blindness. Most clients will never accept their blindness, but they should and will accept the permanence of the blindness. Denial is the front line of psychological defense but it may outlast all other defenses.

Withdrawal

Withdrawal is a mechanism which is used to reduce tension by reducing the requirements for interaction with others within the individual's environment. There are two dynamics which result from withdrawal. In order to keep from being forced to face the acceptance of the newly acquired blindness, the individual withdraws. As a result of the client's changed physical condition—blindness—his social interaction is quite naturally reduced. His circle of interest as determined by friends, business, social responsibilities, church, civic responsibilities and family is drastically reduced. Thus, the client becomes egocentrically oriented until finally his entire world revolves around himself.

Rather than functioning interdependently with his environment to mutually fulfill needs as our culture demands, he is concerned exclusively with his environment fulfilling his needs. As his world becomes more narrowed, his thoughts and preoccupations become more somatic. Physiological processes heretofore unconscious now become conscious. At this point he begins using another defense mechanism—regression.

Regression

Regression is the defense mechanism which reduces stress by avoiding it. The individual psychologically returns to an earlier age that was more satisfying. He adopts the type of behavior that was effective at that age but now has been outgrown and substituted by more mature behavior—behavior which is more effective in coping with stressful situations.

As the newly blinded individual withdraws, becomes egocentric, and hypochrondriacal, he will regress to an earlier age which was more satisfactory. This regression may be manifested in two manners. First he may, in his regression, adopt the dress, mannerisms, speech, etc. of contemporaries at the age level to which he is regressing. Secondly, he may adopt the outmoded dress, mannerisms, speech, etc. of the age to which he regressed. This second manifestation of regression is considerably more maladaptive since it holds the individual out to more ridicule which, at this point in his adjustment to his blindness, quite possibly will result in more emphasis on the defense mechanism of withdrawal.

While utilizing the first three defense mechanisms, if reality is being harshly pushed on him and his defenses are not working, he may as a last resort become highly negative of those around him and negative in general. This negativism is demonstrated as an active refusal, stubbornness, contradictory attitudes and rebellion against external demands. He may become abusive of those around and may become destructive in an effort to act out the thwarting he is experiencing. This negativistic behavior is an indication that the defense mechanisms he is employing are not distorting reality enough to allow him to adjust to his newly acquired disabled status. If, however, he is able to adjust and the defense mechanisms are effective to this point, he will employ the next defense.

Repression

Repression is selective forgetting. It is contrasted with suppression which is a conscious, voluntary forgetting. Repression is unconscious. Events are repressed because they are psychologically traumatic. As mentioned above the attitudes the client had relative to blindness and the blinded has a major bearing upon his adjustment. If these attitudes are highly negative the client will have to repress them at this point if his adjustment is to progress. Until he represses them he will be unable to accept the required new body-image.

Reaction Formation

When an individual has an attitude which creates a great deal of guilt, tension, or anxiety and he unconsciously adopts the opposite of this attitude, he has developed a reaction formation. In order to inhibit a tendency to flee in terror a boy will express his nonchalance by whistling in the dark. Some timid persons, who feel anxious in relating with others, hide behind a facade of gruffness and assume an attitude of hostility to protect themselves from fear. A third and last example is that of a mother who, feeling guilty about her rejection of a newborn child, may adopt an attitude of extreme overprotectiveness to reduce the anxiety produced by this guilt of rejection. This example is seen more often in cases of parents with handicapped children.

In this new, dependent role the blinded individual will feel a varying degree of hostility and resentment toward those upon whom he is so dependent—wife, relatives, etc. Since these feelings are unacceptable he will develop a reaction formation. The manifest behavior will be marked by concern, love, affection, closeness—all to an excessive degree.

Fantasy

Fantasy is daydreaming. It is the imaginary representative of satisfactions that are not attained in real experience. This defense mechanism quite often accompanies withdrawal. As the client starts to adjust to a new body-image and a new role in life, he will develop a rich, overactive fantasy life. In this dreamworld he will place himself into many different situations to see how well he fits.

Rationalization

Rationalization is giving socially acceptable reasons for behavior and decisions. There are four generally accepted types of rationalization. The first is called blaming an incidental cause: the child who stumbles blames the stool by kicking it; the poor or sloppy workman blames his tools. Sour grapes rationalization is called into play when an individual is thwarted. A goal to which the individual aspires is blocked to him; therefore, he devalues the goal by saying he did not really want it so much. The opposite type of rationalization is called sweet lemons. When something the individual does not want is forced upon him, he will modify his attitude by saying it was really a very desirable goal and he feels quite positive about the new condition. The fourth and last type of rationalization is called the doctrine of balances. In this type of rationalization we balance positive attributes in others with perceived negative qualities. And conversely, we balance negative attributes with positive qualities. For example, beautiful women are assumed to be dumb, bright young boys are assumed to be weak and asthenic and the poor are happier than the rich.

The blinded individual will have to rationalize his disability in order to assist himself in accepting the permanence of the blindness. One rationalization may be that he had nothing to do with his current condition, but that something over which he had no control caused the blindness. Another dynamic which might be observed is the adherence to the belief on the part of the client that as a result of the blindness there will be compensating factors. He will develop in other areas such as additional senses or aptitudes and talents he previously did not possess, e.g. an aptitude for music.

I once had a client whose rationalization of his disability ran something like this: All of the men in his family had been highly active outdoors types. They all had died prematurely with coronaries. He, the client, was a highly active outdoors type; however, now that he was severely disabled he would be considerably restricted in his activities. Therefore, he would not die prematurely. This logic resulted in the conclusion that the disability was positive and he was pleased he had become disabled. Granted, rationalization is seldom carried to this extreme in the adjustment to blindness, but this case is illustrative of a type of thinking which must occur for good adjustment.

Projection

A person who perceives traits or qualities in himself which are unacceptable may deny these traits and project them to others. In doing so he is using the defense mechanism of projection. A person who is quite stingy sees others as being essentially more stingy. A person who is basically dishonest sees others as trying to steal from him. A person who feels inferior rejects this idea and instead projects it to others; i.e. he is capable but others will not give him a chance because they doubt his ability. These are examples of projection. With the blinded person many of the feelings he has of himself are unacceptable. Therefore, in order to adjust adequately, he projects these feelings to society in general. "They" feel he is inadequate. "They" feel he is not capable. "They" feel he is inferior and is to be devalued. This type of thinking, normally, leads directly into identification and compensation which are in reality the natural exits to this maze in which he has been wandering around.

Identification

The defense mechanism of identification is used to reduce an individual's conflicts through the achievement of another person or a group of people. Identification can be with material possessions as well as people. A person may derive his social adequacy and psychological adequacy through his clothes ("The clothes make the man"), his sports car, his hi-fi stereo paraphernalia, etc. People identify with larger groups in order to take on the power, prestige, and respect attributed to that organization ("our team won"). This larger group may be a club, lodge, garden club, college, professional group, etc.

In adjustment to his blindness, the client will identify with a larger group. It may be a group of other blind persons, an occupational group, a men's lodge, a veterans' group, etc. But at this point in the adjustment process, he will identify with some group in order to offset some of the feelings he has as a result of the projection he is engaging in. If successful, the identification obviates the need to employ the mechanisms of denial, withdrawal, and regression.

Compensation

If an individual's path to a set of goals is blocked and he finds other routes to achieve that set of goals, he is using the defense mechanism of compensation. A teen-ager is seeking recognition and acceptance from his peers. He decides to gain this recognition through sports. However, when he fails to make the team he decides to become a scholar. This is an example of compensation.

Compensation brings success; therefore, it diverts attention from shortcomings and defects, thereby eliminating expressed or implied criticism. This defense mechanism is most often used to reduce self-criticism rather than external criticism. As the individual experiences successes he will become less preoccupied with anxieties relating to his disability and his lack of productivity.

Identification and compensation usually go together in the adjustment process. When the client starts using these two defenses he is at a point at which he may adequately adjust to the new body-image and his new role in life.

IMPLICATIONS FOR PROFESSIONALS WORKING WITH THE BLIND

Almost everyone in our society views handicapping and disabling conditions from an anatomical point of view rather than functionally. It is imperative that the newly blinded be helped to view their disability functionally rather than anatomically. The client should gain an appreciation for the abilities he has left rather than classifying himself with a group based solely upon an anatomical loss.

The worker with the blind should make sure the information which the client has is factual, concise, and clear. He should be sure the client's perception of his disability is correct and the cause is completely understood. This understanding greatly enhances the adjustment of the client to his blindness.

The client should be helped in exploring his feelings regarding the manner in which he is currently being treated by family and friends. Help him to understand the natural emotional reactions he will have resulting from his newly acquired blindness; and help him to understand that the feelings of family and friends are going to be different for a period of time while they adjust to his disability.

Do not fall into the trap of thinking that the degree of blindness is correlated with the degree of psychological impact. Realize that each individual's disability is unique unto that individual and his reaction to his disability will be unique.

Lastly, in summary, the most important role anyone can play

in assisting a client in the adjustment to blindness is to be a warm, emphatic, accepting individual who is positive in his regard toward the client and who is pragmatic in counseling and planning efforts with the client.

REFERENCES

American Psychiatric Association: *Diagnostic and Statistical Manual of Mental Disorders.* Washington, D. C., American Psychiatric Association, 1965.

English, H. B. and English, A. C.: *A Comprehensive Dictionary of Psychological and Psychoanalytical Terms.* New York, McKay, 1966.

10

Eye Health and Prevention of Blindness Services

Margaret Bowers Gill

It is important for those working with blind persons to know something about the causes of blindness and how they can be attacked. Certainly those of you who are counseling the blind are among the first to recognize the economic and human gain which could be ours if we could prevent the one half of all blindness which is unnecessary.

NATIONAL SOCIETY FOR THE PREVENTION OF BLINDNESS, INC.

The sole purpose of the National Society for the Prevention of Blindness, Inc., and its affiliates is prevention. The society is a volunteer organization started by volunteers, governed by volunteers, and supported by voluntary contributions.

Established in 1908 to Eradicate Ophthalmia Neonatorum

Miss Louisa Lee Schuyler had read a report of a committee investigating blindness in New York State and was irresistibly drawn by a picture of blind children captioned, "Needlessly Blind." In 1908, with the help of the chairman of that commission, Dr. F. Park Lewis, a prominent New York physician and chairman of the American Medical Association's Committee on Prevention of Blindness, Miss Schuyler formed the New York State Committee for the Prevention of Blindness, the forerunner of the National Society for the Prevention of Blindness. It is the second oldest of the national volunteer health agencies, being preceded only by the Tuberculosis Association.

The New York State Committee for the Prevention of Blindness proceeded immediately toward eradicating ophthalmia neonatorum, known as "babies' sore eyes," the cause of blindness in the children of that unforgettable picture. As is often the case even now with other causes of blindness, a method of prevention was known, but was not being widely applied. The prophylactic measure of applying a dilute solution of silver nitrate to the eyes at birth could kill the bacteria which had been transferred from a mother with gonorrhea to the baby's eyes.

Through the efforts of these dedicated volunteers, New York State passed legislation making the application of such drops mandatory. Other states followed, so that in all but three of the states a prophylactic for this purpose is required by law or regulation. A cause of 10 percent of blindness among children in schools for the blind in 1908 has been reduced to less than one tenth of one percent.

Comprehensive Program of Community Services, Public and Professional Education, and Research

The concerns of the Society now span all causes of blindness in all circumstances and all age groups. Because one half of all blindness can be prevented, the society concentrates on early detection and public and professional education.

Research is not neglected by the Society, however, for its operational and statistical research program still produces the best source of reference on the incidence and causes of blindness and vision problems. Other forms of this type of research establish reporting methods, study special population groups, determine the status of eye health and safety regulations and set up conferences for study of special vision problems. Grants for basic and clinical research are made to promising young investigators who are pursuing studies pertinent to the interests of the Society. Other organizations, including agencies of the United States Government, specialize in support of research.

Early Detection Program

Prominent among the Society's early detection programs are preschool vision screening and glaucoma screening. The voluntary nature of the organization is evident in these programs which are sponsored locally by civic groups. The public health aspects of the work are recognized through the approval and cooperation given by state and local health departments. Medical authority and guidance are obtained through national and state medical advisory committees, approval of local medical societies, and active and advisory participation of medical practitioners of appropriate specialties, such as ophthalmology, pediatrics, and family practice.

Follow-up of cases referred for examination is essential and is built into the plan of each of these programs. Reports from these services serve as a basis for information and statistics on etiology and incidence.

The civic group sponsors of these two early detection services provide local organization, volunteers, outlets for public education and public information and some of the materials used. The Society offers its experience, authority, training, supervision or direction, literature, forms, and vision screening charts.

Preschool Vision Screening

Eight hours of training are required of the volunteers who screen the vision of preschool children. The volunteers are given a background of information to give more meaning to their service of vision screening and to enable them to answer many of the questions which may come to them in their work. They must be aware of proper physical surroundings, including such conditions as proper lighting and an uncluttered wall for the eye chart. The volunteers are taught to communicate with the children, and often are more successful than professionals in getting the small child to cooperate.

To the child, the screening is a game. The Snellen illiterate E chart is employed. The tester pretends with the child that the E is a three-legged table, asking him to show with his arms in which direction the legs point away from the table. A young or immature child may need to hold a large E and match it to the one he is shown. Adding to the game aspect is an outline of a pair of feet drawn on a tile which is placed 20 feet away from the chart. When the child stands on these "magic feet" the volunteer can be assured that he is the proper distance from the chart. The occluder used by the tester to block the vision of one eye while testing the visual ability of the other is often in the form of a smooth-nosed "fish" cut from colored construction paper. The "tail" gives a convenient handle which is curved over the finger in such a manner as to keep the "fish" from touching the open eye. The fish and a coloring chart are given as prizes for playing the game.

Since it is a game, there is no "passing" or "failing" so far as the child is concerned, but he is asked to "play the game" on another day if his vision does not meet the passing criteria. These are established by the local project advisory committee, chaired by an ophthalmologist, and are based on criteria set by the National Society's Committee on Eye Health of Children and the State Society's Medical Advisory Committee. Included in the criteria for passing are the critical line on the Snellen chart for each age, as well as a difference in readings between the two eyes.

Observation of the child's behavior, appearance, and complaints during the screening, and a knowledge of such observation by parents and teachers are extremely important. Signs of eye trouble or the fact that one eye sees better than the other can overshadow "passing" the line. A child will not use both eyes if each receives a different image, which is the case with a cross-eyed or walleyed child, or if there is a line difference between the two eyes.

Crossed eyes are not outgrown, as was often believed in the past. On the contrary, possibilities for correction grow dimmer as time passes. The brain shuts out the vision from one eye which has not learned to see as well as the other or the child may use the eyes alternately, but not together. In time there may be no useful vision in the poorer eye. Furthermore, if the good eye becomes blinded through accident or disease, the person is blind for most intents and purposes.

The National Society for the Prevention of Blindness states that amblyopia ex anopsia (dimness of vision from disuse), commonly called "lazy eye," can rarely be corrected after age six. In some instances, orthoptists are able to produce improved vision after this age. Best correction is directly related to the youth of the child. A child with an obvious deviation by the age of six months should be seen immediately by an ophthalmologist. Treatment consists of patching the better eye to force use and development of the poorer one. Surgical correction is used when necessary.

A supervisor of plant safety for the Celanese Fibers Company has a wife and two children with amblyopic vision. His two grandchildren were found as toddlers to need treatment. The two-year-old, after the good eye had been patched for six months, was wearing glasses at 18 months of age. She now has 20/40 vision in the poorer eye without correction. The four-year-old has been treated for two years. The formerly weaker eye is now seeing better than the "good" eye. Her ophthalmologist says that a balance can be expected after treatment of the former "better" eye.

One in 20 children between the ages of three and six has a vision problem. Parents, family, physicians, pediatricians, and others responsible for children of this age should be aware of the signs of eye trouble in children. Personnel in physicians' offices, teachers, and school nurses need training in vision screening and good eye health and safety practices. Some signs of eye trouble are as follows: rubs eyes excessively, shuts or covers one eye, tilts head or thrusts head forward; has difficulty in reading or in other work requiring close use of the eyes; blinks more than usual or is irritable when doing close work; stumbles over small objects; holds books close to eyes; is unable to see distant things clearly; squints eyelids together or frowns; crossed eyes; red-rimmed, encrusted, or swollen eyelids; inflamed or watery eyes; recurring styes; eyes itch, burn, or feel scratchy; cannot see well; dizziness, headaches, or nausea following close eye work; blurred or double vision.

Glaucoma

Glaucoma screening programs under the auspices of the society are designed to find those persons over 35 years of age whose intraocular pressure is suspiciously high and direct them to an ophthalmologist for a thorough examination. The screening test, called tonometry, is performed by ophthalmologist and eye service residents with local family practice physicians experienced in the use of the Schitz tonometer sometimes participating.

Volunteers, given a one-session training by the society, greet, register, and guide applicants through the screening. When visual acuity tests precede the tonometry test, trained volunteers are used. The use of this test is left to the medical members of the local advisory group. It does not help in finding glaucoma patients, but does find persons who need correction or treatment who might not know it. Volunteers, including registered nurses, assist the ophthalmologists and interpret normal pressure findings.

It is important that the person who has been tested knows that this single test cannot rule out glaucoma and that periodic tests are advisable. A medical professional (physician or nurse) is best suited to advising the referred person that glaucoma has not been found but that the high tension found at this time warrants a thorough examination for glaucoma by an ophthalmologist.

Overall direction of the actual screening is given by the society, which is also responsible for follow-up on referred persons. The local health department is helpful in the follow-up of the most difficult cases to reach.

Two of every 100 persons over age 35 have glaucoma, which ranks second among all causes of blindness. Half of the 1,718,500 Americans afflicted with glaucoma do not know it. Chronic glaucoma can be robbing sight without pain or obvious loss of vision to its victim. Acute glaucoma, on the other hand, is characterized by intense pain and immediate loss of vision so that professional help is and should be sought immediately.

While much is yet to be learned about the cause of the increased pressure, glaucoma is characterized by elevated intraocular tension. The inflow and outflow of the aqueous humor (the fluid giving shape to the front of the eye) are out of balance. Either the secretion of fluid is increased or the absorption is blocked, with the result that more fluid is flowing in than is flowing out, rendering the surface less flexible, as in a tire with too much air.

The fluid in the rear of the eyeball, under increased pressure from the front, pushes against the retina. The nerve cells and fibers of the retina constitute a major link with the brain in the process of seeing. It is this link which glaucoma attacks by reducing the blood supply which nourishes the cells and fibers.

The small capillaries which feed the nerve cells and fibers affecting peripheral vision are the first to be destroyed. The field of vision is gradually restricted, resulting in tunnel vision and finally blindness, unless the glaucoma is treated.

Stumbling over low-placed obstacles or stepping out into the path of a moving vehicle without prior realization of its presence can result from the loss of peripheral vision. Other symptoms of glaucoma include seeing rainbow colored rings around lights; blurred or foggy vision; difficulty in focusing on closework; frequent changes of glasses, none of which is satisfactory; and inability to adjust the eyes to darkened rooms, such as theaters.

Sight lost to glaucoma cannot be regained, but its progress can be slowed and blindness averted if it is found in time and kept under constant treatment and observation. Treatment usually consists of self-administered drops and routine visits to the ophthalmologist. Surgery is sometimes indicated.

The best defense against blindness from glaucoma is a regular visit to the eye physician at least every other year, yearly if blood relatives have glaucoma. Studies indicate that 10 of every 100 persons with known cases of glaucoma in the family also have the disease.

Many corporations are now including a test for glaucoma in routine examinations of their employees over 35 years of age. Some family physicians are including it in annual physical examinations of their patients. The Society continues to encourage these and other sources of help in finding the glaucoma victim early enough to prevent further loss of sight. Hospitals, nursing homes, and homes for the aged could all be helpful in ferreting out glaucoma before blindness occurs.

Public and Professional Education through Early Detection Programs

These two early detection services of the society not only find potentially blinding disorders in time to save vision and find those whose vision can be corrected, but are vital means of both public and professional education. The publicity essential to glaucoma screenings and "open" preschool vision screenings warn of the need for these tests and regular eye examinations. Often, following a community glaucoma screening, local ophthalmologists will see patients who did not attend the public screening but were reminded by the notices of it to visit their own ophthalmologists. Many patients are now requesting regularly that their eye physicians check for glaucoma by tonometry.

Student nurses working with registered nurses at glaucoma screening programs are learning "on the job" about glaucoma. Public health nurses exposed to this experience are becoming more aware of the disease, as are family practice physicians serving on steering committees or in the screenings.

Physicians and nurse members of preschool vision screening project advisory committees not only increase their knowledge but carry information to their colleagues informally and through professional meetings. Local public health nurses are invited to training sessions.

Parents and teachers of preschool children become aware of the need for early detection for early correction and apply their new knowledge to other children for whom they are responsible. Even in screening projects serving only in nursery schools, kindergartens, day care centers, and clinics, where there is no need for publicity to bring in the children for screening, the volunteer sponsoring group is eager to have the story told publicly. Thus, even those not reached directly benefit from the information.

School Eye Health

A complete, competent, professional eye examination is the ideal goal for every child before entering school and at stated strategic intervals during school life. Until this goal is attained, vision screening programs during the preschool and school years are necessary to locate children who may be in need of eye care, so they can be directed toward adequate professional attention.

One of every four children of school age has an eye problem. If not found as early as possible and corrected, the problem can produce emotional and social, as well as educational handicaps. Furthermore, good vision is a prime factor in physical safety. Yet a young child does not know that he is not seeing as well as another child because he has no means of comparison. Furthermore, since seeing is a developmental process, a child whose vision is adequate when he enters school may have an eye problem at a later date.

Vision screening should be utilized in classroom activities for teaching eye health. Proper follow-up procedures, essential to detection of vision problems, constitute one means of parent education. Both parents and children can be educated through dramatic skits with the children as actors, assembly and PTA programs with lay or professional speakers and/or films, as well as distribution and discussion of pamphlets and literature. Poster contests can involve art classes. English, social studies, and typing classes may include assignments for study and writing on eyes and vision.

A comfortable and healthful environment should include lighting which is adequate in quantity and quality. Carefully planned policies should be set to prevent eye accidents. Medically approved first aid procedures must be instituted with proper facilities immediately available. Special educational and teaching services must be provided for children whose vision is limited.

Helping the partially seeing child—a responsibility long assumed by the National Society for the Prevention of Blindness—is now one of the programs of the American Foundation for the Blind. Literature and counseling services are available. In Virginia, teachers and local school systems look to the Virginia Commission for the Visually Handicapped for guidance in educating this child. The National Society for the Prevention of Blindness, with its affiliates such as the Virginia Society, continues to be interested in finding this child as well as the chld whose vision can be corrected to a more nearly normal degree.

Responsibility for eye health and safety of school children may rest with the superintendent, the principal, or the school physician. Usually, the teacher, with the help of the school or public health nurse, must screen the vision of the children. With many demands on the teacher's time and thought as well as lack of training in this area, often only a perfunctory screening is done. It is recommended that an eye health committee be extablished to plan all phases of the school's eye health program, give guidance in methods of screening and follow-up, and evaluate the program. The committee should consist of eye specialists, school health personnel, and school administrators.

Those persons screening the vision of the children should be carefully prepared. Teachers, nurses, technicians, or volunteers can be given adequate preparation and a thorough understanding of the tests used. A minimum of six hours of instruction is recommended in addition to supervised screening of children.

Educational materials available from the society include general recommendations, literature on various vision problems and safety measures, guides for vision testing, a vocabulary of terms relating to the eye, vision testing charts, other aids, and films. The society also offers counseling service.

Vision screening is an essential part of a well-rounded school eye health program which should be a part of the total school health program. It can be useful in teaching about eye care and should be followed up to insure that those referred actually receive competent eye examinations. This is the ultimate goal of screening.

Eye Safety

Among persons under 65 years of age, injury is the major cause of visual impairments. United States industry reports an average of 1,000 eye injuries per working day. During 1969, an estimated 169,400 American school children suffered eye injuries.

School Eye Safety

School eye safety laws, promoted and encouraged by the National Society for the Prevention of Blindness, have been passed in 30 states. These laws, which make eye protection mandatory for students, teachers, and visitors in chemistry laboratories and industrial arts classes, are not only protecting eyes exposed to hazards in schools but are developing safety habits in future industrial workers.

The Wise Owl Club—Industrial and School Eye Safety Incentive Plan

One of the ways in which the society has encouraged implementation of these laws is to extend to schools the industrial eye safety incentive plan, "The Wise Owl Club of America." Schools and industries which become chapters of the Wise Owl Club receive publications and information to encourage eye safety. When a student or worker in a Wise Owl Club chapter is saved from a potentially blinding accident by the use of proper eye protection, he is publicly awarded a Wise Owl Club membership. His certificate, pin, and badge serve as reminders to himself and his fellow workers to protect the gift of sight at all times.

Honorary Wise Owl Membership. It is hoped that the same eye safety consciousness being developed in schools and industrial work will carry over into the home and community.

A one-eyed man in Radford, Virginia, was working in his home workshop without eye protection when a friend happened by. The friend noticed that the man was preparing to punch holes in a hacksaw blade. Having his safety glasses in his pocket, the friend offered to perform this work. The hacksaw blade broke in the hands of the friend and one piece struck his safety lens. Neither man suffered injury. It is sobering to think what would have happened if the one-eyed man had proceeded without eye protection. His friend received an honorary Wise Owl Club award given for avoiding blindness by the use of proper eye protection in an off-the-job accident.

Safety Glasses for General Wear

Following intensive education by the National Society and its affiliates on the necessity for safety eyewear for all persons wearing glasses at any time, the Federal Food and Drug Administration has proposed a regulation which would require all lenses, except contact lenses, to be impact-resistant—that is, heat-treated, tempered, plastic or laminated, unless otherwise prescribed by the examiner. Sunglasses are included. This regulation will be a major step in prevention of blindness.

A Massachusetts housewife was blinded from her own glasses in an automobile accident from which she suffered no other physical injury. This is but one of many documented cases of eye injury caused by ordinary glasses. An informal survey of ophthalmologists in 1969 to determine the extent of this problem in Virginia produced reports of 76 eye injuries, five persons with visual loss, and one enucleated eye—all because of broken eyeglasses.

This campaign of the Society will not be complete without a similar regulation governing safety, nonflammable frames, and a requirement that the Department of Defense issue impact-resistant glasses to military personnel wearing corrective lenses.

Eye Safety at Home and at Play

Hazards to eyes of children and adults at home and at play are innumerable—hazards from which there are protective measures. Home chemicals such as aerosol sprays and cleansing agents should be stored out of the reach of children. Safety glasses can protect one not only from hazards posed by power equipment in home workshops, as shown by the honorary Wise Owl award cited, but from stones tossed up by a power lawn mower or even branches displaced or unnoticed in the process of pruning shrubs and bushes.

B.B. GUNS. B.B. guns are weapons, not toys, and should be used only by those trained to use them safely. In investigating Christmas eye accidents, the Virginia Society for the Prevention of Blindness was told by one ophthalmologist that he had spent five of the seven days between Christmas and New Year's Day in the operating room removing eyes because of injury from B.B. shots.

TOYS. Prominent among the hazards cited by ophthalmologists at that time were chemistry sets. Missile-type toys, easily breakable plastic toys, and those with removable parts which expose sharp-pointed areas, should be avoided. The society's safe toy campaign has influenced legislators to ban toys which pose a thermal, electrical or mechanical threat to children, extending the categories (pressurized and flammable) banned by the Child Protection Act of 1966. All toys should be appropriate to the age and maturity of the child. Scissors, pencils, and sticks can be dangerous weapons in the hands of a small child. An older child should be taught to avoid danger to others, especially smaller children, in the vicinity of his activity.

FIREWORKS. A continuing concern of the society is the sale and use of fireworks. Its 1969 survey in cooperation with the Fire

Protection Association and the Fire Marshals' Association revealed 1,330 injuries, including over 200 eye injuries. Class C category of fireworks (i.e. small firecrackers, sparklers) which are still permitted in interstate commerce and within some states, caused 46 percent of these injuries. States which permit class C fireworks are running the risk of eye injury caused not only by these "harmless" fireworks but also by "Roman candles," "cherry bombs," and more dangerous explosives which are being sold illegally at the stands handling the legal issue.

Industry

Industrial Eye Safety

Eye safety in industry does not mean donning a pair of safety glasses when a worker thinks his vision may be in danger. It means full-time door-to-door protection for everyone entering a hazardous arca, and it mcans thc proper protection for the job being performed. Often it is the fellow worker or passerby who is hit; furthermore, safety goggles do not protect from all industrial hazards. Face shields and other equipment may be needed.

The society's industrial eye safety program dates back to 1917 when the first report on industrial eye hazards with recommendations for safety practices was published. Many large industries owe their established eye safety practices to the intensive educational program which has been a major emphasis of the society for over half a century. Yet many still need to be persuaded. When every person entering a hazardous area puts on eye protection to protect his own vision and not just to show the supervisor he is following regulations, the educational job will have been accomplished.

Vision Needed for the Job

Besides safety, employers should be concerned about proper vision needed for the job. Color-blind persons have difficulty sorting color film or working with telephone cables of multiple hues among other problems. One-eyed persons have difficulty in adjusting to jobs requiring depth perception. Clear vision is needed to distinguish one numeral from another. There are jobs which require close vision in a limited field and others in which the breadth of field is more important. Periodic in-plant vision testing, followed by proper correction, if needed, and by proper placement, will improve efficiency, effectiveness, and job satisfaction.

Eye Health in Industry

Business and industry could provide, or at least encourage, periodic tests for glaucoma for all employees over age 35. Some do. Concern for total eye health and safety of his workers would move an employer to be interested in providing good visual environment, including cleanliness and proper lighting.

Aging

As a person ages, a normal change takes place in power of accommodation, starting at age 15 and becoming noticeable around the age of forty when corrective lenses may be necessary for sharp vision at near distance.

Regular medical eye examinations become more important as one grows older.

The Elderly Glaucoma Patient

Glaucoma, the second leading cause of blindness in the United States, has been treated extensively earlier. Because it may not affect visual acuity in its early stages, and because the drops used are for prevention of further loss of sight and do not improve vision lost, an elderly person may discontinue using them, especially if he is dependent upon someone else to apply them. Interpretation of the essential nature of this treatment is necessary to the person who does not like to feel dependent and does not understand the nature of this "sneak thief of sight." When the home situation of an older person with glaucoma is changed by "visiting" with several different relatives, each of those with whom he lives or who are responsible for him should be thoroughly acquainted with the ophthalmologist's instructions and see that they are carried out.

Cataract

The leading cause of blindness among adults in the United States today is cataract. Forty percent of the vision problems among people over 65 are caused by cataract. So-called "senile" cataract may occur at a much earlier age.

Cataract is a clouding of the lens of the eye. The clouded lens can be removed surgically, the only cure. A cataract lens in spectacles or a contact lens is prescribed to replace its focusing ability.

The prevention of blindness challenge here is an educational one. In more than 95 percent of the cases this treatment is successful, yet many older people still hesitate to follow medical advice for cataract surgery.

The Elderly and Safety

Safety takes on a new dimension in dealing with the aged. Their eyes do not adjust to changes of light as quickly as they did at a younger age. More light is required for a given task. Passageways and steps should be well lighted and free of objects over which a person might stumble. Because of a stronger possibility of falls at this age, safety lenses in sturdy frames assume an even greater importance.

Blindness as a Result of Disease

Blindness has many causes. Preventing it leads to concern for many factors including systemic diseases such as rubella, diabetes, and vascular disorders.

Rubella

Rubella (German measles) during pregnancy can cause a variety of abnormalities in the infant. Among them are congenital cataracts and other eye defects. All children in the highly susceptible age groups should be given the vaccine for rubella which was recently made available, so that women in the child-bearing age will have less exposure to this disease.

Diabetes

Diabetes is the third leading cause of blindness. All who are interested in preventing blindness must have concern for the control of this disease in those who suffer from it, and must stress the importance of good eye care for diabetics.

Vascular Disorders

Vascular problems lead to vision problems unless kept under good control. Again, the best defense is strict adherence to medical advice in the control of the disease.

Professional Education

There are many areas of professional concern in preventing serious eye problems and in improved treatment methods for serious eye disorders.

Retrolental fibroplasia (RLF), a leading cause of blindness in children in the 1940's and early 1950's, was found by various researchers, including those working under the auspices of the National Society of the Prevention of Blindness, to be related to the high level of oxygen administered to premature infants. Though greatly reduced, this problem is still not conquered. Continued study, interpretation and application of knowledge in this area is essential.

Detached retina strikes 20,000 persons a year but now can be controlled in approximately 85 percent of the cases.

Congenital and hereditary conditions account for 17 percent of all blindness. A professional working with the blind may be questioned concerning the possibility of blindness in the client's or patient's children. A helpful reference will be found in *Advising Patients about Hereditary Eye Diseases,* publication P-3 of the National Society for the Prevention of Blindness.

The society also encourages eye examinations at birth before the baby leaves the hospital. Such a routine procedure could be responsible for the saving of vision in many children.

Physicians, nurses, schoolteachers, and counselors can do much to help those for whose well-being they carry some responsibility by being aware of causes of blindness, signs of eye problems, and hazards to vision, along with measures for preventing blindness and loss of vision. Teachers, school nurses, and pediatricians and their assistants should be thoroughly trained in vision screening. It is to be hoped that glaucoma screening in the offices of family practice physicians will become routine for patients 35 years of age or over. Professional workers have a responsibility for the overall well-being of those with whom they work. The importance of good vision to the total person cannot be overemphasized.

The National Society for the Prevention of Blindness and its affiliates stand ready to help through publications, films, and consultation.

REFERENCES

Pamphlets

Advising Patients About Hereditary Eye Diseases. New York, The National Society for the Prevention of Blindness.

Another Eye Saved—The Wise Owl Story. New York, The National Society for the Prevention of Blindness.

Cataract—Fact and Fancy. New York, The National Society for the Prevention of Blindness.

Causes of Blindness in School Children. New York, The National Society for the Prevention of Blindness.

Estimated Statistics on Blindness and Vision Problems. New York, The National Society for the Prevention of Blindness.

Eyes in Industry. New York, The National Society for the Prevention of Blindness.

Glaucoma—Sneak Thief of Sight. New York, The National Society for the Prevention of Blindness.

Organization of Glaucoma Screening Programs. New York, The National Society for the Prevention of Blindness.

Pre-School Vision Screening. New York, The National Society for the Prevention of Blindness.

Progress in the Management of Detached Retina. New York, The National Society for the Prevention of Blindness.

Signs of Eye Trouble in Children. New York, The National Society for the Prevention of Blindness.

Standards of Low Vision Aids Facilities. New York, The National Society for the Prevention of Blindness.

Vision Screening of Children. New York, The National Society for the Prevention of Blindness.

Vocabulary of Terms Relating to the Eye. New York, The National Society for the Prevention of Blindness.

Article

Hevey, Lena A.: Vision and aging. *Nurs. Outlook, 12*:6, 1964.

Part Three

Rehabilitation Services For The Blind

11

The Rehabilitation Process

Keith C. Wright

Rehabilitation means many things to many people. It has been referred to in some circles as the third phase of medicine—a concept, as most of us realize, that is quite limited. We have heard rehabilitation alluded to as being basically a philosophy, a belief in people. In this context we recognize such concepts as the dignity and worth of the individual and the importance of attaining personal happiness through acceptance, healthy independence and usefulness.

Rehabilitation has also been defined as an investment. From this viewpoint we view rehabilitation basically on economic factors. In this context we are concerned about the conservation of human resources—our country's most valuable resources. We are concerned with efficient manpower utilization, earning power, tax savings, and reduction of disability costs.

Rehabilitation often is seen merely as a series of services by some people, while others view rehabilitation primarily as a restorative or corrective process. To some persons it is looked upon as a privilege for a select few, while others view it as the right of all citizens. Yet, to others, rehabilitation is equated to the creation of equal opportunity.

Rehabilitation has also been discussed in relationship to the ecological movement—the relationship between disabled handicapped man and his environment. This would include the concept of recycling: the recycling of an unproductive person to one of productivity, the recycling of a person from a state of dependence to one of healthy independence, the recycling of a person from a status of disfunction to a functional status.

All of these concepts are valid. The purpose of this chapter is to discuss rehabilitation as a *process*. Perhaps in this way we can give meaning to all the above-mentioned concepts of rehabilitation.

In discussing the rehabilitation process, perhaps the most effective method would be, first, to identify typical steps in the process. These steps would necessarily include those activities which are usually entered into with every rehabilitation client. Such steps in the rehabilitation process would be as follows:

1. Case-finding (including application and/or referral).
2. Diagnostic and case study procedures.
3. Planning (with client).
4. Provision and/or arranging of necessary services.
5. Placement and follow-up.

At this point it might be well to point out that such a process has some unique characteristics, characteristics which distinguish the rehabilitation counseling profession from most others. First, there is the *continuity of client-counselor relationship* which permeates or pervades the entire rehabilitation process. In many professions, the professional worker is primarily concerned with his client at a particular point in time. For instance, the psychologist is often involved only during step two (the diagnostic and case study procedures). The physician is often involved in only steps one and two (referral and/or diagnostic and case study procedures). The occupational therapist or physical therapist and other members of a rehabilitation team often find their involvement with a client at a specific point in step four (provision of services). Rehabilitation team concepts and team practices have essentially modified the role of the rehabilitation counselor. Perhaps one of his most important professional concerns in present day practice is to give meaning to the disabled client in all steps in the rehabilitation process and to give meaning and interpretation to the client as to the purposes and concerns for all other members of the team who will be actively involved in the client's rehabilitation program. It is the rehabilitation counselor, most often, who has the global picture of the client and his problems, and the plan for solving problems and achieving goals. It is to the counselor, therefore, that the client must turn for interpretation of relationships in services. Therefore, this characteristic concerning continuity of client-counselor relationship is perhaps one of the most unique and important aspects of the counselor's role in the process.

The second unique characteristic of rehabilitation would be that of *discriminatory selection and use of services.* This is not to say that other professions do not discriminate in their selection of services. Perhaps the unique aspect insofar as rehabilitation counseling is concerned is the wide variety of services that the rehabilitation counselor has available.

The third unique characteristic of the rehabilitation process is the *comprehensiveness of the diagnostic and case study procedures.* The rehabilitation client is evaluated from several vantage points, and these will be discussed later in this chapter.

Finally, a fourth unique characteristic would be the *goal orientation* in the rehabilitation process—the goal of work. This orientation, therefore, is definitely concerned with function. It is a positive orientation. It means that the diagnostic and case study procedures must become much more involved with assets, rather than with mere certification of disability and handicaps. It means that every aspect of the case study must not only identify problems and obstacles, but each must also identify assets, strengths, and resources.

CASE-FINDING

Case-finding is a necessary and logical step with which to begin the rehabilitation process. It might be defined as "the activity of locating persons who may be in need of and eligible for vocational rehabilitation services." It includes interpretation of objectives and services of the agency to the disabled, to interested agencies, and to the public—through personal contact and through public information media. It also includes the development and maintenance of regular channels of referral and early agency attention to those referred.

Case-finding as an initial step in the rehabilitation process is very important because there are several factors which indicate a real need for case-finding activities. We know, for instance, that the present rehabilitation program reaches only a small fraction of the total number of prospects in need of rehabilitation services. Secondly, statistics confirm the fact that many persons apply for or are referred to rehabilitation agencies many years after the onset of their disability. Thirdly, many persons do not know about rehabilitation services. Since an application is necessary for almost all of the governmental helping services it becomes very important that the helping agencies and the professionals serving them conduct an ongoing case-finding program.

There are several characteristics of an adequate case-finding program. Some of these are as follows:

1. Referrals should occur early in the period of disablement.
2. Referrals should be representative of the disabled population (in blindness, referrals should be representative of the many types of eye problems).
3. Referrals should come from all potential sources.
4. There should be a close coordination and exchange of services by all agencies serving the handicapped.
5. There must be a mutual respect, courtesy, and reporting back to referral sources.
6. Good casework.

Some counselors have a tendency to work in those locations and with those types of problems in which they have experienced the most success. This situation usually results because of insufficient manpower to serve the needs of all persons in need of assistance; this shortage of trained professional persons forces adoption of a priority or selection system. A shortage of good cases in an area can usually be attributed to lack of an effective case-finding program rather than to a scarcity of eligible applicants.

DIAGNOSTIC AND CASE STUDY PROCEDURES

As mentioned earlier in this chapter, one of the unique characteristics of the rehabilitation process is the comprehensiveness of the diagnostic and case study procedures. The rehabilitation counselor, in his efforts to be comprehensive, evaluates his clients from six major vantage points, as follows:

medical
psychological
social
educational
economic
vocational

A medical evaluation is required of all applicants to rehabilitation for several reasons. The counselor wants to establish the nature and extent of the disability, as well as to appraise the total health of his client in order to determine capacities and limitations. He also wants to ascertain if physical restoration services could remove, correct, or minimize the disabling condition(s). The medical evaluation is also utilized to contribute a sound medical basis for a selection of a vocational rehabilitation objective. In blindness and visual handicaps, of course, additional special examinations are given—ophthalmological and often audiological.

A rehabilitation counselor utilizes a psychological evaluation of his client for a variety of reasons. It is used as an aid for counseling to help the client better understand himself and for making reasonable plans and decisions. Psychological evaluation will also aid the client in identifying problems and understanding his relative strengths and weaknesses. This evaluation is often necessary to provide information or confirmation of a client's abilities, aptitudes, achievements, interests, and personality patterns. It is important when data on the client's capacities and abilities are lacking, or are ambiguous or contradictory.

Social evaluation is another major area of concern in which more counselor expertise is needed. This fact has been reinforced in our attempts to work with the socially and culturally deprived. We have failed many times to understand the social values and the value systems often imposed on our clients because of disability, environment, or family influence. We must recognize the fact that as rehabilitation counselors, we do not necessarily have the most influence on the client. Family relationships are most important. Actually, rehabilitation is essentially a family concern, and many rehabilitation plans fail because we have not evaluated and utilized properly the attitudes and support of family members. The attitudes of family and friends have often conditioned the behavior of the disabled and therefore must be considered when developing a rehabilitation plan. Home visits can be very important, as well as counseling sessions with other persons directly involved with the client.

Educational evaluation provides the counselor with important information for rehabilitation planning. It is important to know how the client functioned in the educational setting, i.e. in what subjects did he do best and in what subjects did he perform poorly. Here we can get an idea as to learning ability, ability to accept instruction, and some social data such as ability to get along with others. Perhaps the counselor can build on these educational experiences and attainments. Contact with the teachers, the principal, guidance counselor, or school nurse can often result in information that could be helpful to the counselor and client. An educational evaluation becomes even more important when development of a training plan is being considered.

Economic evaluation is for the purpose of determining what investment the client can make toward his own rehabilitation. This evaluation is directly related to a long-standing rehabilitation concept that we as rehabilitation counselors should not do for a disabled client those things that he can do for himself. This concept also recognizes the fact that most clients do better when they have an investment in their own program. Generally speaking, insofar as economic need is concerned, rehabilitation services are basically intended to supplement and compliment the existing resources of the client.

Vocational evaluation can be defined as the activity of gathering, analyzing, interpreting, and then synthesizing all of the vocationally significant data regarding the client, and relating this information to occupational requirements and opportunities. The concept of vocational evaluation is much more than mere collection of a work history on an individual. In essence, the vocational evaluation is a process in itself, whereby all of the above-mentioned evaluations are synthesized toward a meaningful vocational choice for the client.

An additional aspect of vocational evaluation is "work evaluation." For years, the rehabilitation counselor has been collecting data on his clients—and has been, in many instances, building impressive case folders. Yet, when he has arrived at the point of vocational evaluation, he finds that he does not know the client as a person. He is unable to answer such questions as are often put to him by an employer, such questions as "How does the client get along with his fellow co-workers?" "How does the client accept and profit from supervision?" "What are the client's work habits?" and many more. A well-organized and developed work evaluation, often secured at a sheltered workshop or other rehabilitation facility, can provide the counselor with answers to these kinds of questions. This will then permit him to represent the client more adequately to an employer, and also will provide the opportunity to counsel more appropriately with the client concerning some of the problems which might be identified in the work evaluation.

Following evaluations in the six above-mentioned categories, the rehabilitation counselor and his client can then proceed to step three in the rehabilitation process—the rehabilitation plan.

THE REHABILITATION PLAN

The rehabilitation plan is a statement of the ways and means by which the client is to overcome his handicap and regain his competitive capacity to work. It is a comprehensive, businesslike, organized statement of the problem(s) and the resources and methods for solving them. The plan contains a statement of the goals sought in each of the major components of the client's handicap. It identifies the services needed and indicates by whom they will be rendered and in what sequence. The plan provides a valid estimate of the length of time needed as well as an indication of anticipated costs. In addition, the rehabilitation plan indicates a vocational objective.

It is important that the rehabilitation plan be jointly formulated by both client and counselor. This is necessary for client acceptance. As rehabilitation counselors, we must keep in mind that we do not really rehabilitate anyone; instead, we help them to rehabilitate themselves.

It is also important that the rehabilitation plan be based on a sound rehabilitation diagnosis, and that it state how and to what extent the handicap can be lessened or removed. It should involve individualized, coordinated, and discriminating use of a variety of resources when necessary.

Counseling pervades the entire rehabilitation process. It should be pointed out, however, that when the rehabilitation plan is being developed—by the client and the counselor—the counseling relationship is of prime importance. It is at this point that the several evaluative areas are synthesized in a meaningful manner. It is at this point that interpretation of the evaluations in order to effect planning becomes essential. It is at this point in the rehabilitation process that the counselor and the client reason together in a problem-solving situation in an effort to determine the ways and means by which the client will overcome his handicap. It is at this point in the rehabilitation process that the client will be counseled as to the services he will be receiving, by whom, and in what order. It is at this stage in the rehabilitation process that the responsibilities of both client and counselor are determined.

PROVISION AND/OR ARRANGING OF NECESSARY SERVICES

The rehabilitation counselor may provide any goods and/or services necessary to render an eligible individual fit to engage in a gainful occupation. In addition to evaluation, counseling and guidance, and placement services, the counselor can, when indicated, arrange and provide for physical restoration services, training (including prevocational and personal adjustment), books and training materials (including tools), maintenance during provision of other services, equipment, initial stocks and supplies, transportation, business and occupational licenses, services to family members, and other goods and services. This wide array of possibilities gives the rehabilitation counselor and the client the opportunity to effectively develop an individual rehabilitation plan specifically suited to the client. It also requires that the rehabilitation counselor be community-oriented as well as client-oriented.

Physical restoration services can be defined as medical or medically related services necessary to correct or substantially modify, within a reasonable period of time, a physical or mental condition which is stable (static) or slowly progressive. In this instance we would include psychiatric treatment and psychotherapy under this category. Physical restoration services would include medical or surgical treatment, dentistry, nursing, hospitalization, convalescent care, drugs and supplies, prosthetic devices, physical therapy, occupational therapy, and other medically related rehabilitation services such as speech and hearing therapy.

Rehabilitation training services can be defined as any type of training that may be necessary in order to rehabilitate a disabled individual. This would include vocational, prevocational, personal adjustment, and other training which contributes to the individual's vocational adjustment.

The general rehabilitation counselor or counselors serving the blind can provide or arrange for several types of vocational training; for instance, institutional training such as at a college or university, business school, or rehabilitation center. He could arrange for employment or on-the-job training, as well as correspondence training and tutorial training.

Prevocational training would include any form of academic or basic training given for the acquisition of background knowledge or skills which are prerequisite or preparatory to vocational training or to employment where the primary occupational knowledge and skills are learned on the job. Personal adjustment training could be provided for a variety of reasons—to assist the individual to function more effectively, to assist him in developing an increase in work tolerance, to assist him in the development of good work habits, and to assist him in the provision of compensatory skills or techniques.

The rehabilitation counselor must advise each trainee at the beginning of a training program, what is expected of him, and inform him that the service will continue only if progress, attitude, and conduct are satisfactory. The counselor must require periodic progress reports and promptly call the trainee's attention to evidence of unsatisfactory progress or attendance before such conditions become serious. The counselor should provide encouragement to the trainee with due commendation for effective efforts. He should also make certain that the trainee enrolls in the courses necessary to qualify for the job objective. During the training program the counselor must continue a close counseling relationship with close supervision.

PLACEMENT AND FOLLOW-UP

The final stage in the rehabilitation process is placement and follow-up. This involves assisting a person to find suitable work and a remunerative occupation and following up entrance into employment so as to assure that vocational rehabilitation has been achieved. This activity depends on much more than referral to employers. It is at this stage in the process that the counselor reevaluates the client in relation to the vocational objective. The counselor must determine whether or not the client is ready for work. He has to assure himself that all necessary services under the rehabilitation plan have been provided, and that the client has sufficient work tolerance. He must also be assured that the client understands his performance abilities and limitations in terms of his disability, and that the client knows his job objective in terms of performance standards, usual wages and benefits, working conditions, and opportunities for advancement. The counselor must also be assured that the client has the skills and knowledge required for the vocational objective and the attitude of a desirable employee.

In arriving at an evaluation of job readiness, the counselor must consider such factors as physical readiness, psychological readiness, occupational readiness, and placement readiness. The counselor might prepare the client for employment interviews and refer him; he might refer the client at an appropriate time to the state employment service, or he might accompany the client to the employer for direct placement.

Several purposes for follow-up become evident. For instance, follow-up can provide the occasion for the giving of emotional support to the client when needed. It also provides the opportunity to effect needed adjustments, and often forestalls the client's quitting without attempts at such adjustment. It indicates the counselor's continuing interest in his client and affords the counselor the opportunity to determine whether further counseling or training is necessary or desirable. Follow-up is necessary to determine if a revised plan is needed. It allows for ventilation of client feelings.

Not only is follow-up concerned with the client, but it also provides evidence of interest in the employer's welfare. It provides the counselor an opportunity to determine the employer's satisfaction with the client and with information concerning the possibility of future placements. It will also help to determine the employer's satisfaction with rehabilitation services. It is at this point that the counselor determines if employment is suitable, whether or not the work might aggravate the client's disability, and if additional training or other rehabilitation services are needed.

Prior to closing the case record, the counselor must consider at least three basic criteria. If these are determined as satisfactory, he can then complete the rehabilitation process with his client. These criteria are as follows: (1) the program of rehabilitation services has been completed insofar as possible, (2) substantial rehabilitation services have been rendered the client by the counselor, and (3) the client is suitably employed.

12

Special Problems in the Psychological Evaluation of Blind Persons

Mary K. Bauman

What is a test? Many people who know little about psychology seem to feel that tests have some magic about them. Many clients come into the testing situation with anxiety about how they are going to manage with this mysterious standard that is called a test. A test is merely a standard piece of material, used in a standard way, resulting in some behavior which can be measured. This measure, a set of numbers in most cases, is compared with the results of a standard group which has also been subjected to this same test administered in this same way. Projective techniques may be a major exception to this description, but even in these tests counting of responses often plays a part.

How does this relate to blind people? Little material is devised specifically for blind people at this point. Usually, the same material as is used with sighted people becomes the test of the blind person with minor adjustments in how it is administered. With the Turning test of the Minnesota Rate of Manipulation Test (Betts and Ziegler, 1946) and the Pennsylvania Bi-Manual Work Sample (Roberts, 1945), an assembly and disassembly of nuts and bolts, the adjustment made is giving blind people more chance to practice. In the end the test is done exactly as by sighted persons. Most employers will accept the idea that it might take a little longer for a blind worker to learn his job; the important question is whether he can do the job as well as the sighted worker beside him. The above procedure of testing with the same material as was used with sighted workers not only represented an acceptable way to measure the blind person's abilities but also could be a selling point with employers, showing that the same job can be done with a little extra time in which to learn it.

In measurement of dexterity, we made early strides that were quite significant during World War II but which have come to be less and less important with the passage of time, largely because there are fewer assembly lines. Machines tend to do the work of people on assembly lines. Also, our view of the appropriate job for a blind person has greatly changed in the last 25 years. When I first came into this field, we were pretty glad to get any job for a blind person. We now are by no means glad to get a job that is not appropriate to the interests and abilities of the blind person.

INTELLIGENCE TESTING

At any rate, it is possible to use some test materials without change. "One of the best illustrations of the test we can use without change, is the verbal scale of the Wechsler Adult Intelligence Scale (Wechsler, 1955) and in part for this reason is the most used of all the mental measures with blind clients." There are two sections to the Wechsler: a Verbal Scale and Performance Scale. The Verbal Scale consists of six kinds of subtests and is easily used with a blind person because it is done in a face-to-face, one person-to-one person context, and the client need not read or actually perform any task. The six subtests are (1) information, or facts about the world around us, (2) comprehension, which is a kind of common sense reasoning, (3) arithmetic, which consists of quite simple arithmetic problems, (4) similarities, which represents a somewhat more abstract perception of relationships, (5) digit span, and (6) vocabulary. Going back to our definition of a test, these materials can be used in exactly the way they would be with sighted persons, the responses are given in the same way, and the results are counted in the same way. Finally, to fit the definition of a test, it is necessary to compare the resulting number with a standard group. Here we may run into difficulty in our application to blind clients. The implication of a standard group for the Wechsler is that the individual has had normal opportunity to learn and has been through what in this country is called a normal educational process. Not all blind people have had normal opportunity to learn or have been through a standard educational process. Consequently, when we interpret the IQ's of blind clients we have sometimes to make adjustments. For example, we may have a child who has grown up in very protected environment and who has not experienced what most children of his age would have experienced. We must find out what the opportunities in this child's environment have been by getting an excellent history in order to determine whether his family setting offered normal background for learning. Even as the child grows older, there are some possibilities that his educational opportunities are not "normal." For example, the partially sighted child may sit in a public school classroom with little extra attention, consequently learning little. Unfortunately, it is quite possible to be passed from grade to grade without having learned a great deal and it is even possible to graduate nominally from high school and to hold a diploma that is almost meaningless. This is not normal educational opportunity. If as counselors or as psychologists we are convinced that the individual before us did not have normal educational opportunity, we must make some allowance with regard to interpreting his IQ.

To some extent, the Wechsler Verbal Scale helps us to do this because from the list of the six subtests one can see that three of them are closely related to schooling: information, arithmetic and vocabulary. These can scarcely help being affected by the individual's schooling, so if a child has gone through 12 years of school with books he could not read and if he has not been able to see the arithmetic problems that were put on the board, these subtests will be lower than the others. The pattern of the Wechsler Verbal Scale results can point to problems in the individual's background, but one must substantiate the presence of these problems through an excellent history.

The Performance Scale of the Wechsler requires doing things with materials, and is much affected by vision. For a great many years, those of us who were doing psychological work with blind persons complained bitterly about the lack of performance material appropriate to them. A few of us tried to invent ways in which we could get around this problem, and I very early adapted a test usually used with sighted children which I called the Non-

Language Learning Test. It is a board containing four kinds of holes into which a varying number of blocks can be fitted. The administration of the test is such that learning can be measured by repeated trials. However, because the test is much affected by variations in vision, I have been reluctant to set up firm standards and have been inclined to call it a clinical instrument rather than, strictly speaking, a test. Yet, it does tell us a great deal about how people learn when words are not involved in the learning.

The Federal Government has also subsidized several efforts to develop performance test materials for blind clients. One of these is the Haptic Intelligence Scale for the Adult Blind (Shurrager and Shurrager, 1964). Its content largely duplicates the concepts, and in part the materials, of the WAIS Performance Scale. An effort was made in developing norms for the Haptic Intelligence Scale to duplicate the normative group patterns of the WAIS, and a generally excellent job was done. However, there are several disadvantages to this test, the chief of which may be that, at this time, norms are available only for totally blind persons. Also, norms go down only to age 16, and one section of the test, the abacus, is invalidated if the client is familiar with the abacus as an arithmetic tool.

In another project supported by the Federal Government, Suinn and Dauterman (1966) borrowed from a group of Japanese (Ohwaki, Tanno, Ohwaki, Hariu, Hayasaka, and Miyake, 1960) an adaptation of the Kohs Block Design Test (Kohs, 1919). The client is asked to copy patterns of increasing complexity by appropriate arrangements of blocks. These can prove quite difficult and a considerable spread of ability can be measured by this test. My own feeling is that it has been extremely valuable to me, although the higher and lower norms may need some improvement.

TESTS OF SOCIAL ABILITY

Another approach to nonacademic evaluation is through measurement of social competency. This is a measure of what people do day by day, not in a test situation but in an actual life situation. For young children we have used the Maxfield-Bucholz Scale of

Social Maturity for use with preschool blind children (Maxfield and Bucholz, 1958) for a number of years. It has its foundation in the Vineland Social Maturity Scale (Doll, 1953) and is used in the same way which means that the test is not given to the child but results from conversation with an adult who knows the child well. This procedure overcomes many of the difficulties involved in testing young children where the fatigue of a trip, fright at meeting a stranger in a strange place, and sheer immaturity can block effective testing. In the past several years, I have developed the Overbrook Social Competency Scale which starts at the age of six, where the Maxfield-Bucholz stops, and goes through the high school level. Eventually, it is planned that this will go to a superior adult level. A measure in this area is important because the social competency of a client does greatly affect his acceptability to employers and fellow workers and of course to the public. The results of the scale may also be useful in counseling the individual or the family, particularly when they have been overprotecting the blind person or limiting his opportunities for social development.

OTHER TESTS OF VERBAL SKILLS

Some other verbal tests are used. Psychologists who are comfortable with the Stanford-Binet Intelligence Scale (Terman and Merrill, 1960) have for many years used the Hayes adaptation of the Binet and will probably be very interested in the Perkins-Binet, a much newer version which will soon be available. My own opinion is that psychologists should use tests which are familiar to them and with which they are therefore comfortable. Also, the less the psychologist knows about blind people the more it is important for him to have the security of a familiar test instrument when he is asked to evaluate a blind person.

MEASURES OF VOCATIONAL INTERESTS

All of the preceding measures relate chiefly to general learning ability in either a verbal or a performance setting. We have also mentioned to a slight degree the dexterity tests through which the speed and smoothness of hand movement are evaluated and the results of which of course relate very much to the performance of manual tasks where speed is the important measure. However, from the point of view of the happiness of the client himself, one of the most important things for us to evaluate is his interest. All of us want to do the things we like best. We are motivated by the opportunity to do such things. The various interest inventories give at least a broad guideline to the direction which will most interest the given client. The most used inventories in this field are the Kuder Preference Record-Vocational (Kuder, 1956) and the Strong Vocational Interest Blank (Strong, 1959). The latter has two forms, one for men and one for women, and in my experience is most useful for individuals who are at least high school graduates and are considering professional or semiprofessional goals. However, it does include some scales below that level. The Kuder presents activities in groups of three and the individual is asked to say which in each group he likes best and which he likes least. It has the value of forcing a choice; as life itself forces choices for most of us, it is relatively realistic. However, the client's own choice may not be very realistic by comparison with his abilities and opportunities. Also, both the Kuder and the Strong interest inventories contain some items which are not readily imagined as jobs for blind people, and both present some difficulties in administration. Consequently, in the last several years I have developed an interest inventory, the items of which come from the professional and clerical, industrial and service studies and therefore represent work content of legally blind persons. This has been designed for easy administration with a visually handicapped person and also has the advantage of evaluating generally negative or generally positive feelings. The general negative yields too low scores while the generally positive reaction yields too high scores. This can be measured and adjusted in this particular test. It also has the very great value that one can tell the client that all of these items represent things blind people really can do.

MEASURES OF ADJUSTMENT

The final major area of measurement is adjustment or personality. Here the whole concept of adjustment to blindness itself plays an important part, for no personality evaluation of a visually handicapped person can be regarded as complete without considering this particular facet. At the adult level and also at the adolescent level, I have developed adjustment inventories largely on the basis of recorded discussions of blind people in which they listed problems they saw themselves and their friends as having. Thus, the content of the scale is relevant to blind persons and the norms are also based on blind persons. Long years of use of these two scales has disclosed certain patterns as characteristic of certain problems, such as the problem of recent visual loss. A validation score helps us to determine with what frankness the client has responded and how dependable the results therefore are.

Th above listed tests are the heart of our battery as used with visually handicapped clients. However, special tests such as measures of sales apititude, supervisory insight, etc. can be administered by reading to the client and recording his response for him. If such tests are used, the test administrator should be extremely careful to be sure the reading is both clear and impersonal in nature, and should be especially sure that where multiple choice items are involved, the choices are read slowly, carefully and with as much repetition as the client may need in order to keep them clearly in mind. It is our experience that multiple choice tests administered by reading to the client can place the blind client at considerable disadvantage and every effort must be made to overcome this either by repeated readings of the choices or by putting those choices into braille form so that the client can refer to them as he makes his decisions.

REFERENCES

Bauman, Mary K.: *The Non-language Learning Test.* Philadelphia, Personnel Research Center.

Betts, G. L. and Ziegler, W. A.: *Manual for the Minnesota Rate of Manipulation Test.* Chicago, Educational Test Bureau, 1946.

Doll, E. A.: *The Vineland Social Maturity Scale.* Chicago, Educational Test Bureau, 1953.

Kuder, G. F.: *Kuder Preference Record-Vocational.* Chicago, Sci. Res. Assoc., 1956.

Maxfield, K. E. and Bucholz, S.: *The Maxfield Scale of Social Maturity for Use with Preschool Blind Children.* New York, American Foundation for the Blind, 1958.

Ohwaki, Y.: *Manual of the Ohwaki-Kohs Tactile Block Design Intelligence Test for the Blind.* Japan, Ohwaki Institute of Child Psychology. U. S. Distributor: Los Angeles, Western Psychological Service.

Roberts, J. R.: *Manual for the Pennsylvania Bi-Manual Work Sample.* Minneapolis, Education Test Bureau, 1945.

Shurrager, H. C. and Shurrager, P. S.: *Manual for the Haptic Intelligence Scale for the Blind.* Chicago, Psychology Research Technology Center, Illinois Institute of Technology, 1964.

Strong, E. K.: *Strong Vocational Interest Blank, revised.* Palo Alto, Consulting Psychologist Press, 1959.

Suinn, R. M. and Dauterman, W. L.: *A Manual for the Stanford-Kohs Block Design Test for the Blind.* VRA Grant RD 1625-S-65, Vocational Rehabilitation Adminstration, U. S. Dept. HEW, 1966.

Terman, L. M. and Merrill, M. A.: *The Revised Stanford-Binet Intelligence Scale, 3rd revision.* Boston, Houghton, 1960.

Wechsler, D.: *Manual for the Wechsler Adult Intelligence Scale.* New York, Psychological Cooperation, 1955.

13

Orientation and Mobility: A Symposium

BACKGROUND DISCOURSE

Russell C. Williams

Father Thomas Carroll's book, *Blindness: What It is, What It Does and How to Live with It,* classified among the losses in blindness the loss of mobility. And he categorized it as a reality loss along with loss of written communication, loss of techniques of daily living and the like. His exact words were that the loss of mobility was on a "reality level—without inclusion of the neurotic whatsoever." This is one point of view.

Here is another. Dr. Leslie Kay of New Zealand, who has brought his electronic device for detecting obstacles to the United States for testing, was speaking at Airlie House before the newly established National Academy of Engineering. He said that problems in mobility can be boiled down to difficulties in environmental sensing and that if blind people were able to sense the environment there would be no trouble insofar as mobility is concerned. I think I know what his point was. He is suggesting what every teacher of the blind knows: blind people without additional handicaps have the muscular wherewithal to be mobile. I shall return to this later. But meanwhile I would like to take another approach, suggested in part by thinking of how ophthalmology is related to blindness.

BLINDNESS AND MOBILITY

In talking to people about the problems of mobility, I think the point to tackle first is the question of what the eye does for people who *see,* so that we can more clearly understand what kind of information and assistance they are getting through eyesight. I cannot begin to name all the things eyesight does. But it does provide us with distance and direction from one thing to another, from me to things. It gives motion, color, contrast, parallel, perspective, and depth—all used ordinarily by people involved in mobility, in movement from one place to another.

I was a seeing person for 26½ years of my life—a normal seeing person who drove automobiles, ran through the woods, waded across "cricks," fired guns (not much of that, but some), ran, played in athletics (basketball, football), all things where the eye is an extremely important part of the activity. I played football, and forward passing was a part of my responsibility. If there is any place where the use of the eye, especially its peripheral vision, is important, it is there. If you throw that ball where you have been looking, somebody else has got you spotted and (if he can) is going to get it before your receiver does. Basketball is the same way. There is not much point in looking at a player and then passing directly to him. You had better be passing to the teammate you see in the peripheral field.

Since the eye does so many things in sensing the environment in which we are functioning, a good deal of modification seems to be necessary when sight does not exist. To emphasize this a little further, consider how much the glance gives us in an instant. A slight turn of the head and the glance can satisfy the movement needed to leave a crowded room, go around tables, chairs, cash registers, hatracks, and out. Several glances, coming quickly together, would satisfy much more difficult mobility needs, needs which would be much more complex for me as a person who does not see at all and who must get out of rooms and buildings into public places where determinations as to directions must be made. This is what Dr. Kay means by sensing the environment.

I have often thought about what the eye does in controlling the environment and in acting on the environment. Man evolved using the values of sight. He was able to run and protect himself, go toward things which attracted him. The eye played an even greater part of this than the ear or nose. With the eye, a man could very quickly find a limb when a bear was chasing him. He could see across a stream to see if it was too wide to tackle, could possibly even see if there was a ford across which he could go. He developed into the kind of person who had quite a lot of control over the environment. Then, it seems to me, he began to modify his environment to make looking more efficient. Arrows were developed to reach what the eye could see but the arms and hands could not reach. Guns and their sights were the same sort of extension of power, not only made possible by the eye but suggested by the eye.

Automobiles and the speed at which they go not only requires eyesight for operating, but eyesight to imagine them and the kind of roads on which they run. What I am trying to get at here is that environment becomes more complex because mankind is constantly making changes—suggested by the eye—for maximum use of the eye. This in turn makes sight increasingly important in seeing the environment and controlling it.

With all this in mind, then, let us go to the subject of orientation and mobility without the use of the eye. In the histories I have read on blindness, I have found anecdotes as far back as the story goes showing that blind people were mobile; that is, *some* blind people were. I have read of blind people who traveled extensively over Europe and so on. Even half of what we read of the exploits of "Blind Jack" Metcalf of Knaresborough, England's pioneer road builder, would lead us to conclude that he had his environmental sensors or he could not have accomplished what he did. In his case, we think we know what one of these was. An old portrait of him shows him holding in his hand a cane which seems to be rising even higher than his hat. Whether or not it was actually that long we do not know. It is a three-quarter picture which does not show how far the cane went to the ground. But it is told of him that he had an extra long cane, and he is holding it with obvious pride. The thing that sticks in my mind is that there were not very many Metcalfs, that he was a legend in his own time because he differed so markedly from what the world expected of blind people.

The first truly organized program to teach orientation and mobility to blind people in this country was guide-dog training at Seeing Eye, founded by Mrs. Dorothy Harrison Eustis. Following on the heels of this development was the landmark program which gave me much useful experience. This was the Army program of training in orientation and mobility during World War II. In this I participated first as a trainee and later as a staff person.

MOBILITY TRAINING

My observation was that the people who tackled the question of how to deliver orientation and mobility at Valley Forge General Hospital, Dibble Army General Hospital and Avon Old Farm had some very real problems, but they also had some very well put together circumstances with which to work.

The basic, very real problem was that blind people began to flow out from a source which made them a national responsibility; moreover, it was the kind of responsibility on which it was possible to focus the attention of the power complex concentrating on the war. Back from the conflict for all kinds of reasons (injuries from training, from fighting against the enemy, and diseases of all kinds) came a problem for the Army Medical Corps, to deal with: this was blindness. So the Army, having set up its centers to deal with ophthalmology, established its new rehabilitation programs.

The Army program with which I was most familiar was that at Valley Forge. This hospital had 100, then 150 blinded soldiers, collected together, many of whose blindness was permanent and who knew it. There were some morale factors that could have gotten out of hand. Amputations were not unusual. Brain damage was something seen quite often. Hearing losses were almost the rule rather than the exception. This caused feelings about themselves which were very strong. They had in the past been doing things that were extremely masculine, and then blindness intruded itself so that strong, well-conditioned arms and legs, did not work. Many of them were confronted by the fact that they might have been able to run a hundred yard dash just about as fast as they ever had only if they had some idea of where to go once they started. I was in that position. I had an Army injury, but was not injured badly enough to have any residual disability. My legs were all right. I never could run very fast by track standards. But I could have run just as fast at this time after injury as I could before *had I just been able to see.*

One of the harrowing experiences of early blindness came to me not long after I realized it was true that I was blind and, as far as medical science knows, blind forever. I was wrestling around with the tremendous feelings that accompanied this realization, and I was on a bed in England under which there were some flimsy slippers. I knew they were down there somewhere, so I slid down after them. I fished around for quite a while, and finally came up with one or both of them and the bed was gone! It was *gone.* It had just slipped out of existence. This made such a distinct impression on me that I remember it to this day very clearly. Of course, somehow the bed was recovered, with whose assistance I do not remember; but before that I was sure that the bed was not where I thought it ought to be. In my mind then, this world had undergone a change all of a sudden, and I had not. I had gotten out of orientation with the world. And I had begun to appreciate some of the problems I would run into because I could not see.

As I have said, confronted with problems like this the men had begun to show some real morale problems while the completion of their medical treatment was taking place at Valley Forge Hospital (e.g. ophthalmic and plastic surgery, treatment for burns). Treatment had to be completed, as well as all the administrative procedures attendant on getting out of the service and away from the medical corps. This was why, after the encouragement of a directive from President Roosevelt, who understood these things, the Army was obliged to provide rehabilitation of a kind which would make possible transition from blindness into readiness to undertake community life.

Right away some imaginative people got into the act. I have often struggled for words to describe them. They did not seem to worry too much about tradition, though some of them were familiar with it. And one tradition they ignored entirely—the tradition that blind people learn the common skills of blindness "naturally," and that it is only special vocational skills which require much formal training. Along with this went the notion that if there are tricks and lore of daily living for a blind person, these are best learned from an old hand who is blind himself.

The Valley Forge group was in a position to ignore this because they were in an Army situation, and the Army is basically rather arbitrary and thick-skinned toward outside interference. If a person can get permission on the inside to innovate, he does not have to worry so much about civilian interference for quite a time, as one would in a country school system for instance. The War Blind Service from the start had its critics, but it was not so easy for them to get control of the facts. The result was an entirely new approach to patient care of blind people in hospitals with a regime that had no counterpart which even faintly resembled it, except the pioneering of Seeing Eye with guide-dogs.

The approach included strong attention to physical activity in every conceivable way, but particularly to mobility. And this physical activity and mobility were perhaps in the one of the best traditions of teaching blind people, inasmuch as they concentrated on the use of the remaining senses even though this required a method which made the individual look blind; he was nevertheless in charge of his situation and his life. Against tradition, a formalized training program and regime of teaching common skills was set up. The firm foundation of this was mobility, called at Valley Forge, *foot travel*—a rather good old-fashioned term. Ways to get us mobile within the hospital and within the hospital environment were gotten under way rather rapidly, at first on a somewhat experimental basis. The experiment shaped up fast into an active program which when formalized involved a staff of 50 persons. Later, when I was a staff member myself, I counted the patients on the eye service who were to some extent in the blindness services and there were 360. It was the job of the 50 to get the 360 in motion without too much discouragement. Very soon they were doing it with definite techniques, and an instrument—the cane. That cane, the way that it was used and the canes that came after it were to cause no small stir. It represented a break with tradition, but a conscious break by people who knew what tradition was.

Some of the people who formed the Valley Forge program had worked in schools and agencies for the blind for a long time. Paul Conlan had been in charge of the Michigan School Program for the Blind. Richard Hoover and Warren Bledsoe had both been at the Maryland School for the Blind; Martha Miller with the state program in Ohio, Rosalie Cohen with the New York State program; Louisa Walker Kirby with the South Carolina School for the Blind; Ilah Ojah with the New York Institute; L. P. Howser with the Kentucky School for the Blind. Whatever their various initial reactions were to the new training and the cane involved in it, this group developed a remarkable concensus which supported the innovation. The innovation itself was certainly out of the brain of Richard Hoover, but had the very strong support of these other people and the staff of 50 GI instructors they helped to influence and train. Since the cane which had formerly been used was not long enough to do what the Valley Forge people wanted done, they made it longer. As making it longer made it heavy, they sought some material to make it lighter. This resulted in the manufacture of 300 light steel canes, weighing only six ounces, but which were very strong with a handle like a shepherd's crook. The whole business was dubbed "bo-peep" by its godparent, Hoover. And it served. It served to sense the environment with something which was much closer to being an antennae than a club, showing with a good deal of subtlety what to back off from politely and what to take hold of with the hand. Also, as it was wielded it told with great accuracy that a man was on the edge of a staircase or a bottomless pit, told him in time for him to take stock of his situation and decide what to do next, provided he was willing to let bystanders see him use the cane in a way which only a blind person would use it.

The environment of Valley Forge was conditioned to favor all this. For example, if I had an appointment at the eye clinic, which was six or seven hundred yards down the corridor, I was expected to go there. When I got to that clinic and was finished with what I was doing, the clinic people were pretty much aware that I could go back. If I seemed to demonstrate a disposition to go back on my own resources, they let me do it. More than that, they expected me to do it. This was not only in the eye department. It was all over the hospital—a big one of two or three thousand beds with all kinds of services: plastic surgery, psychiatry, medical. I can remember distinctly having an appointment in the medical service. When I was finished, the doctor said, "Are you all set to go back?"

There was an expectancy operating here that people would do things, and the hospital did not intrude on the efforts of blind men to go places to go all over town in fact.

There was an environmental imperative which said to the administration, "If this man is in a position to walk up here and get eye drops or something, do not load all the medicine and stuff in a cart and take it around, requiring him and his like to sit on the edge of the bed. That is the pursuit of efficiency, and might enhance the nursing efficiency. But it does not respect the efforts that are being made by blind people and the staff people working with them. While a patient may walk up here and flounder around and cause some commotion as he gets ready to receive medicines, in the long run this is the most efficient way in which to get this responsibility discharged, a way of paving a sort of transition from new blindness and all that that means, into readiness for community life.

THE AVON PROGRAM

There was a special hospital at Avon, Connecticut, whose responsibility was primarily, not secondarily, to provide the rehabilitation program for the man to go home. At Valley Forge, rehabilitation was secondary. If a man had an eye ready for surgery just as the right time came for some rehabilitation step, the surgery came first. At Avon the situation was reversed. Rehabilitation was primary, and if a man had a medical condition he was transferred to a neighboring hospital. This was understood when he went to Avon. Between the two places there were some differences in philosophies, mainly where the cane was concerned.

At Avon there were areas staked off for the purpose of training blind people. These training areas lessened the need for external aids. In my terminology, I classify external aids as such things as canes, dogs, other people, electronic machinery—anything outside my own mental and physical resources. Avon, at the outset of its establishment, held that a cane was not necessary, modifying this doctrine to some extent as time went on with regard to downtown travel, but always appearing to ascribe some particular virtue to avoidance of its use whenever possible.

Now the environment of Avon was five or six hundred yards

in one dimension, four or five hundred in the other three. The building was of four floors and made in the strangest way. It had been modeled after an English school built hundreds of years ago, and there were some real dandies in the way of architectural barriers to get acquainted with—spiral staircases with steps shaped like pieces of pie, designed mainly to give the invader fighting his way up as much trouble as possible. At least one could always be sure the wide side was on the right when coming down. This was to give maximum cutting swathe to the swordsmen defending the castle. The principle was literally medieval and not even especially good Army booby trap training.

No canes were employed, and my own feeling at this stage of the game was that while the idea could be sound around a person's office, home, or yard where perhaps no external aid is needed, this environment can get too large. The requirements, the problems, the lack of security in movement were too great to expect that people would have a positive learning situation. I think that perhaps this tended to kill a lot of interest in movement and in traveling by one's self. This point is important as I take up the next great development in rehabilitation programs for the war-blinded.

THE HINES CENTER

In 1947, the Veterans Administration was assigned by Presidential directive to pick up blind center services which the Army and the Navy were allowed to drop. This was a legitimate shift of responsibility to the Veterans Administration because most of the people blinded during wartime were out of the service; however, the government's consultants on blindness were pointing out that not all of the blindness coming from wartime had occurred yet. So we were allowed to set up a very small blind rehabilitation center. This was the Hines Center in the suburbs of Chicago. It fell upon me to be the chief.

In getting the program under way, the thing that I was especially interested in advancing was mobility. Long before Father Carroll wrote his book, mobility was in my judgment one of the primary loss areas in blindness. But it was loss which could be used during the therapeutic segment of the program in order to get men thinking in the ways they have to think and perform, ways which are different now that they cannot see. These constitute reorganization to blindness; personal adjustment, some of us say. Mobility is crucial in a readiness program, readiness to return to community life and do a creditable job with regard to performance, responsibility, emotional control and all the other things that make a person's life; in short, to enable him to play his role through the next 30, 40 or 50 years of life remaining. We wanted the blind person to realize that the extent to which he managed his problems was the extent to which other people around him would not have to. If he simply ignored them, most of them would not go away. Someone would have to deal with them.

We also wanted the blinded veteran to think reasonably about performance on his part. If he decided to be one of those people who just picked himself up and ran across streets on sheer nerve, that would not be the answer, because the whole town would have to devote itself to keeping him from getting killed. We decided to put emphasis on the cane. This was different from the policy at Avon and more like that of Valley Forge where a respect was created for the external aids, regarding them not as crutches but as instruments and as therapeutic devices. So we used canes in the Hines program from the beginning.

We had a program that started under the simplest of circumstances, giving some early work to the blind person without any use of an external aid; this was done under extremely secure circumstances. One of the things we wanted to build into the mobility program was an awareness that if a certain amount of security can be provided, the remaining senses begin to operate more efficiently; the hearing antennae are out further because one is freed from insecurity and worry about what may be underfoot. So we employed this external aid—the cane of unusual length—and we employed it a lot, hour upon hour. I think if we averaged it out, it would probably be about 150 hours of time devoted to this with lots of repetition.

What we were mostly interested in was evidence that the man felt secure, that this instrument, if manipulated and held in the right way, could offer a great deal of security, thus allowing his hearing to be used in seeking any sort of information in the environment which would guide him to where he wanted to go.

In addition, the cane does a great deal of environmental sensing itself. If a cane is held right and if it is light and wieldy, one learns that if it touches nothing but solid ground, it is a *go* sound. If it touches a fire plug or a sappling, it is a signal to pause and *go around.* If it touches something that growls, that is another matter. But it can do much more subtle sensing than that, e.g. sensing of mud, grass, or asphalt. The same manipulation that provides for security, allowing other senses to rise up like antennae and range about, also gives the tangible sense of drops, shorelines, curbs. All these are things that guide us.

Mobility, I should add, was only part of a larger process going on. Our complete program involved communication skills, manual skills, and counseling, which was a kind of readying program for the vocational counseling, which came after the men left the hospital. The relationships with the staff and other blind people were important, very important. But what started the whole process off and bound it together was the mobility program.

Neither the simplicity, nor the complexity, nor the subtlety of this program are easy to put into words. We find this out again every time we have to attempt it with a new high-level public official up the line who finds he is responsible down the line for one of our programs. This came up again with the recently developed architectural barriers program sponsored by the Federal Government. We had to explain that we had never thought it wise to count on the world changing its ways too much for blind people, that we wanted blind people to learn to take things as they were, that for this reason we had not thought too much about how to modify buildings to make it easier for those of us who could not see. We also, when pressed further, had to point out that truly effective modification would include such things as building square pillars in front of buildings so one could take a direction from them (everything that is round offers a special problem in orientation and this is true also for curbs at corners). Of these there would be quite a number to modify.

The psychological subtleties are difficult to describe plainly. For example, it may seem rather unbelievable that at least one of our trainees had to be very carefully watched because we were quite certain he suddenly crossed a busy street on an angle, on purpose. He was an embittered soul with a double handicap, having both hands amputated, and we could hardly blame him for the self-destructive feelings he had. But it was the business of our mobility instructor to be enough of a psychologist to stay on top of this, to do a great deal of careful observation and diagnosis to know what might happen before it ever did happen, and to stay with the situation whatever occurred. Stanley Suterko was the instructor in this case, a past master at the art: right behind the trainee, protecting life, but letting the man work through the difficulty he had made for himself.

Suterko has been called the "St. Peter" of the mobility development, and certainly his rocklike stability combined with great sensitivity commands widespread respect. I saw him demonstrate perfectly the subtlety and simplicity of a good mobility program when he was asked to demonstrate a diagnostic procedure. This was with a youngster—a girl who was very much shut in on herself. Suterko took her into a wide open area (a gymnasium), and walked ahead of her talking with her about things only he and she heard. As he made a path, all of a sudden she began to babble and chatter as no one had heard her do before. This opening up was enough of itself to convince those who had been working with her that the mobility instructor knew what he was about, but more than that it told the mobility instructor that she had potential which had not been uncovered by anyone previously. This was an especially valuable demonstration—an occasion on which we were lucky with regard to our larger diplomatic mission. Almost at the start, a small group of people had come into the room. Suterko looked for signs of nervousness in the trainee when this occurred. Such signs did not appear, and he did not ask the intruders to leave although he might well have if they had appeared to be affecting the situation adversely. Later, he discovered one of the visitors was the superintendent of schools in the area.

We have already mentioned the increased effectiveness of the senses when mobility techniques produce relaxation of tension. I would like to cite a further example of this which I myself helped to observe. This was with a boy of about 10 or 11, whom I saw before mobility training, picking his way, watching every step in a kind of duckwalk, but finally getting to school. After the boy's lessons, the mobility instructor reported that he came bouncing into the house, dropped his books and violin case and set off in search of a friend named Pete. On the way, what we call obstacle perception asserted itself when off to his side he noticed something unusual, a large crate. Far from being upset, he stopped to explore it, his only comment being, "It wasn't too smart to leave that there." What this meant to the instructor was that a great deal of security was operating now out in front underfoot, freeing his attention and allowing it to range out further and enable him to detect change.

We were not set up as a training establishment at Hines Hospital. We did do in-service training with our own people, but there was no provision in our law for training people from outside. We did have the responsibility of government, under the right conditions, to let people observe and audit our programs. Not too long after we began operating smoothly, we did begin to let outsiders observe. Our method was to put them through some pretty tough paces, but we could not tell them what to do when they went back home because we did not know their situation. We were not familiar with the circumstances under which they were operating. We explained what ours were, the part in the therapeutic programs played by mobility, the solution of problems of mobility and the realistic appraisal of how a person is going to manage mobility problems under blindness. This is much easier to demonstrate than it is to put into words.

Anecdotes help to illustrate. For example, we had a very intelligent and articulate Wall Street lawyer who worked for the Securities Exchange Commission and who came to us at the age of 50 after becoming discouraged by failure to secure paid guides despite all kinds of advertising. He lived in New Jersey and had to commute, crossing on the ferry. A year after he had left Hines he got on the tape recorder and talked to me.

He said, "Think about this. When I advertised for guides, as I told you, I got no takers. Now I start out each morning, and it isn't long until I run into somebody, and I go with people most of the way, and the same is true at night. I'm getting assistance from other people for free. And I couldn't even pay for it before." He also said, "What's the difference? What happened? I have boiled it down to 'a changed point of view'." That point of view came from the knowledge that he could start out with some efficiency and security if nobody came along. He had the knowledge that enabled him to get into the swim of things, where he could come across the kind of assistance that would help. He had the knowledge that if he encountered someone he would not take them out of their way in order to satisfy his needs. But he went each morning and each evening. He started out. That is the big thing. He had what it took to start out, and he carried with him the security that whenever the other person had to go *that* way, he had what it takes to go *this* way. He worked for 18 years on Wall Street, and he told me when he retired at 68 that though he had learned all kinds of techniques—the use of recorders, phoning, shaking hands and parting his hair if he had any—it was the management of mobility problems on a realistic basis that was, in his particular case, the keystone of the program we gave him at Hines.

Having cited a very able and active citizen, something should be said about those of lesser abilities. In this connection, mention should be made of our program in the Veterans Administration for psychiatric patients who are blind. There are 35 psychiatric hospitals in the Veterans Administration system. It is estimated that 25 out of every 1,000 such patients are blind. We now have some on-going programs for these people who have been hospitalized as much as 15 or 20 years. These are the kind who will be seen in utterly inactive fetal positions, or who upon being led to a chair will stay there for the rest of the day. I have been advised by at least one chief of psychiatry that as we get to them, and as they get some control of their physical circumstances, they have less need for their psychiatric illnesses. In this case the work is extremely hard, and far from requiring something less in the way of mobility teaching skill actually requires more.

One nurse said to me, "Appreciate this! It is mightly helpful when the nursing staff no longer thinks about going down and getting a fellow out half a dozen times a day and taking him to the bathroom. Bladder and bowel control are dramatically improved, as well as dressing and things like that. They are eating better, sleeping better. The response to people is improved." At our Northhampton psychiatric hospital, the men started to go home on weekends for the first time in years.

Mention has been made of our visitor observers at Hines. They came from everywhere: Korea, Japan, Finland, South Africa and many states. Certainly this contributed to the application of mobility methods as we saw them, and news of our doings infiltrated into larger programs of reorganization to blindness. But we saw over those years that we were not doing as well as we wanted to. We had no formal way to do it. We thought that in many ways this was a disservice to the country. We wanted to share what we did. People were welcome, but we also thought that we were misleading some of them. We saw that ever so many of the people who visited us went back to their home programs and did not last long. We checked into this, and had feedback from enough of them to believe that they had not really had the opportunity to explore the validity of the methods.

In 1959 we got together with the Rehabilitation Services Administration of HEW, the American Foundation for the Blind, and other interested people to decide how to put the method on a more formal basis. Out of this grew very generous support financially from RSA for the splendid graduate training programs established at Boston College, Western Michigan and Los Angeles State. I am proud to say that many of the personnel resources came from the Veterans Administration, and we have been paid back in return because a great part of our blind rehabilitation staffs are now composed of university-trained people, many of them trained under Stanley Suterko who went from our program to Western Michigan.

A few more words are in order about how the usefulness of these graduates of universities can be extended by subprofessionals. It seems to me that there are a great many needs of blind people which require the mobility instructor or peripathologist to function only in a supervisory capacity, for instance, people who require a driver, someone to go into the voting booth, or a shopping guide. This is in the form of assistance for the individual who must go somewhere either before he has had mobility training or because he is not a candidate for it due to age and infirmity. There are a great many mobility needs of this kind which agencies should try to meet. And this type of program would function best under the "eye" of the graduate mobility instructor. There is no preparation for orientation and mobility training which excels the experience of being expertly guided.

Many things have been left unsaid here because this paper is a companion piece to those of Stanley Suterko and Donald Blasch. Nevertherless, something more must be added to sum up what I have to offer in the way of experience.

When I became blind in 1944, there were just a few newly organized (and by our standards crude) mobility programs operating, other than the guide-dog training schools. Now there are a great many operating in a great many places. And the skill has moved to other countries. It has come to the attention of the National Academy of Sciences, and more recently to the new Academy of Engineering. They are thinking about it as part of their responsibility. But as they get into it we find—by the questions they ask and by the rather extensive answers our instructors are able to give—that science, in order to help us, must first absorb what is already a rather sophisticated body of knowledge. This is one indication of how far we have come in 26 years.

PRACTICAL PROBLEMS OF ORIENTATION AND MOBILITY

Stanley Suterko

The greatest practical problem confronting practitioners is how to provide good quality mobility services. By good quality mobility services I mean the kind in which the blind individual will elicit the unsolicited comment of "How much can he see?" When this degree of sophisticated movement by the blind individuals is achieved with regularity, the practitioners can then assume that they are providing the best service that is attainable. Some may question this goal as being an unrealistic one; however, I feel this is a realistic goal to strive for.

At the other end of the continuum is the kind of mobility instruction given to a Commander Buckley when he lost his vision. He said that they gave him a cane and led him out the front door to the porch, and with a hearty slap on the back told him to "go to it old chap." What irritated him most was the fact that they went back into the house and shut the door. He further stated, "They didn't even have the guts to stay around and see if I would fall down the stairs situated at the end of the porch."

This latter approach to mobility instruction has no real problems, for it tends to be self-liquidating in the very early stages; however, the former approach has many practical problems and I shall try to present a few of these.

Administration Problems

For this paper I have categorized the practical problems in two groups. They are first, the problems inherent in planning and administering a mobility program, and second, the problems emanating as a result of direct client service. Some of the most obvious practical problems in the administration of mobility programs are as follows:

1. The mobility instructor should receive the approval and support of the agency administrator to institute an orientation and mobility in-service training program for all staff members. This in-service training program should include all of the basic mobility skills. This will not only ensure a uniformity of approach to the client, but also will begin to acquaint him with a philosophy which indicates that the agency is practicing what it preaches—independence of the blind individual. How many times have you witnessed a new blind client enter an agency's door and be guided by the elbow by the first staff member to meet him; the next staff member pulls him by the hand, and a third staff member or perhaps the office help places a hand in the middle of his back and propels him to another destination. Can you imagine what attitudes are being formulated in the mind of this new client concerning his personal independence and the unique independent approach each staff member has toward this goal?

2. The mobility instructor needs to solicit the cooperation and support of all staff members to ensure that all blind clients move about their respective classrooms with efficiency and grace through the employment of the basic orientation and mobility

skills. The staff should also be made aware of the need to make realistic demands of clients that are consistent with their mobility capabilities. By this I mean that when the client is ready and capable, he should be expected to navigate on his own to the next classroom, dormitory, or dining room. To impose this growing responsibility, the staff will naturally have to keep currently informed of the progress the blind person is making with his mobility.

3. The practitioners need time to survey the town or city so that they may select geographical areas which lend themselves to the development of a sequential outline of mobility lessons. In many instances this will mean beginning the outside travel lessons at a farther distance from the rehabilitation center than some of the later lessons.

4. The practitioners will also need time to develop an outline of lesson plans for different categories of blind clients. These are (a) the congenitally blind, (b) the adventitiously blind, (c) the geriatric blind, (d) those with useful residual vision, (e) the blind with additional disabilities.

5. The mobility instructor should be given time to study and revise the mobility lesson plans at least yearly so that he may incorporate changes which will ensure a consistent success pattern on the part of his clients. These revisions may also be dictated by changes in routes resulting from construction, altered traffic patterns, and so forth.

6. One very real practical problem the instructor has to cope with is to have sufficient time to offer a complete mobility program at the client's assimilation rate and not at the administration's predicted rate. This naturally leads to another problem of deciding whether the practitioner should continue moving the client at his assimilation rate and omit giving him mobility experiences in the advanced complex areas, or, accelerate the client beyond his present capacities at the risk of setting him back psychologically.

7. The practitioner should also be able to provide follow-up services to clients. Some clients will not need this service, but there are some who would profit immensely from having the mobility instructor visit them a week or two after they arrive

home. At this time, any unusual mobility problems confronting the client can be worked out, and fears of the family can be eliminated when they understand how the blind person is able to function. Along this same vein, I always encourage my client to give me a call anytime after he arrives home in the event he experiences any difficulties with mobility in his community.

8. The mobility instructor should also have time in which to counsel or give guidance to parents and family members of the blind individual. The practitioner will need to emphasize to parents the need to permit, if not request, the youngster to go on errands. The child should be encouraged to go to the local stores, mail letters, visit relatives' and friends' houses; in fact, he should be encouraged to travel in any areas that are within his capabilities. If the person is a blind husband, it may prove beneficial to inform the wife of the therapeutic value in permitting her husband to travel alone to the local pub so that he may visit with his old buddies.

9. The practitioner should have time for public education, especially if the mobility program is new to the community. He should be prepared to give demonstrations and talks to church groups, Lions Clubs, and other civic clubs so the community has some understanding of what the agency and he are attempting to accomplish.

10. The mobility instructor also needs time for professional growth in the area of new research and developments as well as mobility devices for the blind. No doubt, as news releases come out regarding the development of visual prostheses or electronic mobility devices, he will be expected to be fully knowledgeable about them. As these devices become available, he should not only get information on their operation but also should have an opportunity to evaluate their effectiveness. This information need was vividly demonstrated when the ultrasonic torch was made available in this country, which according to the newspaper releases "would replace Seeing Eye and the cane." I am certain that all family members of a blind person would become intensely interested in getting further information on a device with these potentialities.

11. The mobility instructor will also need time for the de-

velopment of teaching aids such as tactual maps of communities, aids to develop concepts, and so on.

Client Service Problems

Without a doubt, the most pressing and urgent practical problems that will tax the knowledge and ingenuity of the practitioner are those stemming from direct client service. These problems are as numerous as there are clients to work with, and they become further complicated and multiplied as we begin to serve the geriatric blind, retarded blind, cerebral-palsied blind, and other similar groups.

In teaching orientation and mobility skills to congenitally blind children, practitioners have recognized some common problems. Many of these youngsters lack adequate body-image and, therefore, do not understand how to control their body in space or in relation to objects in space. It is essential that blind children be put on a program of body-image training.

Another problem posed by many of the congenitally blind is a lack of understanding space and geometrical patterns found in the physical environment. Many can verbalize the dictionary definition of a square, rectangle or triangle; but, when getting them to walk around a square block, they are unable to explain how many turns need to be made to complete this circuit. And far too often these youngsters are unable to explain the relationship of the wall or street on their left after they have made a 90 degree right turn. All of this indicates an urgent need for additional training before formalized cane travel is instituted.

Practitioners have also discovered that a number of children do not fully understand many of the common words used to describe relative positions in space. Such words as "above," "below," "ahead," "behind," etc. are used by youngsters in daily conversation but are not really understood. Many feel that "above" denotes the space at ceiling height and do not know that above could also refer to space below their waist level as in the case of a footstool. Thus, practitioners need to test the child's understanding of spatial terms and institute training if it is needed.

A very common problem that has been with us for some time is poor or abnormal posture and gait. However, it has been only relatively recently that professionals in other disciplines have become interested in studying these problems and in sharing their expertise in ameliorating these difficulties. We have been fortunate to have such individuals as Dr. Siegel, an orthopedist, and Josephine Miller, a physiotherapist, carry on an extensive study in this area. These studies have borne some fruit as they have both postulated treatment methods designed to minimize postural and gait deficiencies. Dr. Siegel advocates resistive exercises, reflex splinting, and the use of weights on extremities as treatment methods to be instituted in a training program. Josephine Miller feels these treatment methods are not sufficient in themselves as they tend to treat the symptoms and not the cause. In addition, she believes there is a strong need to provide the blind youngster or adult with effective and adequate mobility methods as this will eliminate the fear aspect which is probably the primary cause of postural and gait abnormalities.

Then there are the subskills of nonvisual locomotion that present problems to the practitioner when the client is not functioning effectively. And it may well be that the client is having difficulties with only one or a combination of subskills. One of the most common of the subskills is linear movement versus rotary movement. This is especially crucial when street-crossing, or in negotiating large paved areas such as gasoline stations, parking lots, etc. In attempting to eliminate rotary movement the practitioner needs to become a diagnostician to determine which of the influential variables are the causes in this specific individual's case. Is it the type of imagery this person is employing, is it due to an excessive lateral shift of the center of gravity as he commences his street-crossing, or is it a conscious or unconscious overcompensation due to a fear of the parallel traffic? Hopefully, the practitioner will identify the causative factors and institute remedial activities which will eliminate the problem. Progression of the individual into more threatening and complex areas without eliminating these problems will tend to ensure that he give up independent mobility because it is too difficult and ineffective.

Some other subskills of nonvisual locomotion are perception of gradients, perception of lateral tilts, perception of lateral curvature in pathways, and the aftereffects of just-prior movements.

I list these subskills to acquaint the reader with the fact that we must be cognizant of the factors that are influential and need our attention if many more blind individuals are to achieve effective, safe, and graceful mobility.

Another area of mobility training that presents practical problems to the practitioner is the training of the remaining senses. We recognize the importance of maximum use of the remaining senses. My feeling is that inherent in every mobility experience should be a maximum utilization of all of the senses. Rather than go down the list enumerating all of the senses, I have selected one sense to illustrate some of the problems identified with it.

I selected the sense of hearing since it is generally recognized as one of the most important senses. The practitioner is confronted with the problem of fully understanding where and when are the optimum conditions for teaching the following aspects of audition: sound localization, sound shadows, echolocation (or, echodetection), masking sounds, and selective listening. In order to teach these aspects of hearing properly, he needs to understand some of the physics of sounds. He will need to know about sound frequencies, wavelengths, intensities, pitch, and the reflective characteristics of low frequency waves versus high frequency waves. He should also have access to, and be able to interpret, the client's audiogram so that he will establish realistic expectations concerning his clients' auditory abilities.

Here again the practitioner is not the only one who has been concerned with the hearing ability of blind persons. Some very notable experts in the field of audition and psychology have turned their attention to some of these same problems. Dr. Worchell and Dr. Dallenbach have studied and attempted to identify the most important frequencies needed to identify objects in one's path or to one side. Doctors Rice and Finestein from Stanford University have done considerable work in identifying the most common human sounds used in detecting various-sized targets. They have also given us knowledge on the influence of target parameters on echodetection.

Another significant contribution to the area of audition is that of Dr. Kohler of Austria. He has provided much information concerning the use of hearing by the blind through his experiments and studies with the pseudophone and subcutaneous Novocain® injections.

Dr. Kellogg from Florida has also enhanced our knowledge through his studies of the blind person's ability to determine the effectiveness of human echolocation on tasks such as size discrimination, density discrimination, and determination of relative distance to objects.

There have also been numerous others who have contributed knowledge to this area and who are worthy of mention. These are Dr. Harris from Schilling Laboratories and Dr. Griffin from Harvard. It is good to know that experts from other disciplines are helping us with some of the problems confronting the practitioner.

We have also looked to other disciplines and experts in the areas of tactual sense, the kinesthetic sense, the sense of smell and the sense of vision. This last area, the sense of vision, has not been delved into as much as I think it should. I do not mean to imply that nothing has been done in this area; however, we have not fully focused on it. What we need to do is bring together the expertise of those concerned with low vision and the mobility practitioner and have them engage in a brainstorming session.

The last area I would like to discuss is that of electronic mobility and sensing devices. I know of a number of practitioners who have been repeatedly confronted by friends or family members of a blind person with the question, "I read in the paper about a new device that enables a blind person to go all over with no difficulty." As the family or the blind person anticipates, the practitioner needs to be knowledgeable in this area so he may explain the device to their satisfaction. To do this he will need to know about passive environments, sensors, sensory enhancement devices, active energy radiating systems, electronic linear walking aids, and the electronic sound beacons. Of these general categories of aids, he should be well acquainted, if not experienced, with the ultrasonic torch, the Russell travel path sounder, and the Laser cane.

In summary, then, I would like to reemphasize that the real problems confronting the practitioner are not his alone; they have also come to the attention and interest of some very knowledgeable people in other disciplines. We have had the benefit of studies by an orthopedic doctor, physiotherapists, and persons in the areas of psychology, audition, the human senses, electrical engineering, mechanical engineering, biophysics, psychomotor skills, and even one who has designed the satellite tracking system for the space program. Some of these individuals are members of the rather elite group of persons who constitute the National Academy of Sciences. Before closing, I would quote one of the recommendations made by the National Academy of Sciences in their most recent publication, entitled *Sensory Aids for the Blind*:

> A concerted attack on the mobility problem should proceed concurrently with that on the reading problem, but owing to our ignorance of human mobility (compared to reading) and the need for experience with man-device interaction, research and small scale evaluation should be emphasized.

ORIENTATION AND MOBILITY FANS OUT*

Donald Blasch†

Previous issues of the A.A.W.B. *Blindness Annual* have treated the beginnings of orientation and mobility training at Valley Forge Army General Hospital, in "The Valley Forge Story" by R. E. Hoover, M.D., 1968; the transfer to the Veterans Administration Hospital, Hines, Illinois in "From Valley Forge to Hines" by Warren Bledsoe, 1969; and the development of the Hines program in "The First 15 Years at Hines" by John Malamazian, 1970. A general view of the subject by Martha J. Ball Rosemeyer appeared in *Blindness 1964*. Full documentation of the teaching system begun by Hoover requires a description of action and events by which it fanned out to agencies beyond the Veterans Administration system.

Enough has been written, perhaps, concerning Hines as a culture for orientation and mobility. However, the degree to which it accumulated respect during the 1950's may be further illustrated by the stream of visitors—observers from work for the

---

*This article appeared in *Blindness 1971* (A.A.W.B. Annual).

†Mr. Blasch was assisted in the research for this paper by Ruth Kaarlela.

blind—who made arrangements to view the program at first hand for several days or weeks. Significant among these were Mr. William Champion (1950) and Mr. Frederick Silver (1952) from the Catholic Guild for All the Blind, then in Boston, Massachusetts; Miss Anta Ryman from the School for the Blind in Stockholm; Mr. Albert Asenjo from the American Foundation for the Blind (1953); Dr. William Thompson from the Blinded Veterans Association (1954); and Mr. Carl McCoy from the Kansas Rehabilitation Center (1956). There were many more. These visits served chiefly to whet the appetites for a much more thorough indoctrination and training. Often, the agency heads who had arranged for their staff to go to Hines had hoped they would return, having mastered whatever techniques were in use and able to mold them into the agency program. Almost invariably these hopes were doomed to disappointment. A healthy unrest about the exacting nature of the necessary background and skills for teaching orientation and mobility thereby was generated and slowly spread in work for the blind.

This unrest culminated in a conference held at the American Foundation for the Blind in June 1959. The catalyst for the conference was Father Thomas J. Carroll, supported by Mr. Louis Rives, Chief of the Division of Services for the Blind, Office of Vocational Rehabilitation, Washington, D. C. The purpose of the conference related to the prospect of professional preparation of orientation and mobility personnel: to establish criteria for the basic selection of orientation and mobility personnel; to develop a well-balanced curriculum, and to recommend length of training and appropriate sponsorship.

The conference coordinator was Arthur Voorhees, American Foundation for the Blind; conference recorder was C. Warren Bledsoe, Assistant Chief, Division of Services for the Blind, OVR; the conference secretary was Helen Isaac. Conference participants included educators of the blind, directors of rehabilitation services, practitioners in orientation and mobility, and Mr. William Debetaz, Vice-President of The Seeing Eye, Inc. The following speakers addressed the conference; Mr. Robert Barnett, Executive Director, American Foundation for the Blind; Kathern F. Gruber, Director, Division of Research and Specialist Services, A.F.B.; Dr.

Richard Hoover, Ophthalmologist, Baltimore, Maryland; and Dr. Frederick M. Jervis, Director of Counseling, University of New Hampshire.

It was the consensus of the conference that it would be very necessary for mobility instructors to have a graduate training period of at least one year in an established and recognized setting. Practitioners at the conference, without animus, declared they could not support the training of mobility instructors on a short-term basis, however concentrated. Necessary emotional conditioning was so intricate a process, the ingraining of principles through time-consuming laboratory experience so necessary, that the needs of the situation could not be met in a compressed teaching program of two weeks, two months, or even four months.

This stand gained something from its relation to a second point which was firmly made by the majority of the group. This was that the teaching of mobility was a task of a sighted, rather than a blind individual. Aware of the fact that this was opposed to classic theory of pioneers in the field, the great majority of the conference maintained that all experience indicated a revision of the theory. When discussion had established this principle, the need for a year's training gained substance, as the necessity for practical laboratory experience was taken into account. Obviously, the demands of the situation would be a deep identification with blindness and something of what it entailed on a basis so intimate and particular that the instructor would gain the habit of thinking all the time about how to manage problems of living without sight. This would entail living through a number of stages of identification while acquiring techniques.

It was concluded that the following standards should govern the selection of personnel: (1) Academic—Bachelor's degree, majors preferably in education, biological sciences, psychology or sociology, (2) Physical; (a) vision—no visual impairment not correctible to 20/20, no errors in the vision under all common circumstances, and no evidence of pathology contributing to progressive deterioration; (b) hearing—normal; (c) physical condition—good; (3) Personal characteristics—a character capable of meeting the demands of emotional stresses in a creative, realistic and optimistic way appeared to be the consensus.

It was recommended that five broad areas of study be included in the curriculum. This included (1) physical orientation and mobility; (2) dynamics of human behavior related to blindness; (3) function of human body in relation to blindness; (4) the sensorium and its relation to blindness; and (5) cultural and psychological implications of blindness. The entire learning process should be geared to real life situations through concurrent laboratory experiences and clinical practice. Physical orientation and mobility were to be conducted on a one-to-one basis with a master orientor.

Later that year, at a meeting of the National Council of State Agencies for the Blind, a report of the Orientation and Mobility Conference was given. It was positively received. Subsequently, Mr. Rives announced that OVR would support the establishment of such a program.

John Malamazian, in the article mentioned above, referred to the establishment of graduate training for orientation and mobility instructors as the "landmark event in the story of Hines." This was indeed a landmark event in all work for the blind. It brought to the field a degree of professionalism that was unique and certainly long overdue.

The peripatology program at Boston College was inaugurated in June, 1960. Much of the credit for the establishment of this program belongs to Father Thomas Carroll. Hines personnel were not available at that time, and Father Carroll generously allowed members of his own staff to serve on the faculty. The program coordinator was Joseph M. Runci. In charge of the orientation and mobility aspects of the curriculum was Frederick A. Silver, on leave from St. Paul's Rehabilitation Center. He was assisted by Bernard E. Hickey. Dr. John Eichorn was appointed coordinator in 1962. The program began with eight students.

This was followed by the establishment of an orientation and mobility specialists program at Western Michigan University in June, 1961. Dr. George G. Mallinson, Dean of the College of Graduate Studies, who had long been interested in the establishment of this type of program, had been working closely with the Division of Services to the Blind, OVR, and the Veterans Administration. Securing qualified personnel had been the major obstacle. He finally secured Donald Blasch, operational assistant of the Central Blind Rehabilitation Center at Hines, as director, and Stanley Suterko, supervisor of orientation and mobility, as chief of orientation and mobility. Mr. Lawrence Blaha, assistant supervisor at Hines, was also part of the staff. The program began with twelve students.

Throughout the process of establishing the program there was excellent cooperation between the officials of the schools involved and the personnel from the division of Services to the Blind of OVR. They in turn received a great deal of support and encouragement from Mr. Russell C. Williams, chief of the Blind Section, Physical Medicine and Rehabilitation Division, and other personnel from the Veterans Administration. Without all of their enthusiastic and dedicated support this venture may have been delayed for many more years.

Coincident with the evolution of the educational programs, an integrated cluster of RSA projects supporting orientation and mobility training for blind clients of rehabilitation services enhanced the breakthrough in three ways: (1) by demonstration of the clear-cut value of the methods which were carried to the grass root programs; (2) by the development of an equally clear-cut relationship between the research and demonstration programs and the personnel training programs of RSA; and (3) by the high level of cooperation with other government agencies and voluntary organizations for the blind.

One of the pilot demonstrations was carried out by the Society of St. Vincent dePaul of St. Louis, in 1962. Guidelines were issued in 1963 by RSA,* stating the objectives of the projects as follows:

General

1. To reemphasize the basic mission of work for the blind; namely, to discover how things are done without sight and make these methods available to blind people who need them.

2. To establish a means of demonstrating to the field validated skills in mobility which have lately been organized.

---

*Formerly OVR.

Specific

1. Through systematic teaching by a competent, trained instructor, to show blind people themselves the possibilities of cultivating maximum capability in getting about without sight, thus helping them to discover and capitalize on latent aptitudes in mobility skill and become as free as possible to come and go.

2. To give key officials who make decisions with respect to programs for blind people, as well as working practitioners functioning in direct personal contact with blind people, a realization of the increased capability which can be achieved through the above-mentioned type of instruction.

3. To implement the demonstration project by the employment of a fully qualified instructor, either from one of the two university training courses in mobility, or an instructor with five or more years of experience at a recognized training center working full-time as a mobility instructor.

Since 1963, 30 demonstration projects were carried out, in 22 states and the District of Columbia:

Arkansas–1	Missouri–1
California–3	New Hampshire–1
District of Columbia–1	New Mexico–1
Florida–1	New York–1
Georgia–1	North Carolina–1
Illinois–3	North Dakota–1
Indiana–1	Ohio–2
Maryland–1	Rhode Island–1
Massachusetts–1	South Dakota–1
Michigan–2	Tennessee–1
Minnesota–1	Texas–2

West Virginia–1

The supporting agencies included public and private agencies for the blind, as well as residential schools and public and private day schools.

One of the greatest unsuspected sources of employment was the residential and day school programs for blind children. Initially, the programs were set up to train students primarily to work with the productive blind adult population. At workshops, conducted by Hines personnel, it was discovered that many of the techniques employed were equally applicable to blind children. Although the skills and techniques were basically the same, the methods of presentation differed and the building of experiences and concepts that correlated with the reality of the environment and, in many cases, corrective exercises to improve gait, posture and body-image were necessary to ensure a meaningful orientation and mobility program for the blind student. Much of this was substantiated by an RSA demonstration grant to Catholic Charities, Archidiocese of Chicago, in 1962. This program was directed by Miss Marian C. Quinn, Director, Department of Vision and Hearing Services; Mr. Robert Gockman was the mobility instructor. Educators of blind children were eager to secure this type of service as it appeared to help fill a large void in the education of the blind student. At the present time almost all colleges and universities training teachers for blind children have a course in orientation and mobility for the classroom teacher. Approximately 45 percent of the graduating orientation and mobility instructors were being hired by residential and day schools.

The interrelated performances of the instructors and the success of the learners in the demonstrations produced a demand for orientation and mobility instructors from rehabilitation centers, private and state agencies for the blind, residential schools, special classes and school systems. The programs of professional preparation were not able to meet the demands.

Consequently, in cooperation with the RSA, the Department of Rehabilitation Counseling, Virginia Commonwealth University, sponsored an "Ad Hoc Committee Concerned with Mobility Instruction for the Blind" meeting in Washington, D. C., April 18-20, 1966. The purposes of the meeting were:

1. To review and evaluate existing training programs for mobility instructors.

2. To explore ways to recruit and train more young people for the field of mobility instruction.

3. To make recommendations for future training programs.

A total of 40 persons, representing RSA, Office of Education, the Veterans Administration, Virginia Commonwealth University, private agency and state agency administrators, residential school personnel and the spectrum of educators, were in attendance.

Miss Mary E. Switzer, then Commissioner of the RSA, identified the major problem as the need to acquire the largest number, the most talented, and the best trained mobility instructors in the shortest period of time. She urged greater use of new resources, scientific research and technology, as well as more effective use of our current knowledge and skills to insure that each blind person in need of mobility instruction could be trained to get about as efficiently and safely as possible.

This conference brought to a head a question which had been festering over a period of time: Should orientation and mobility be offered at the undergraduate level? There was also discussion of short-term and crash programs. The statistics presented by Boston College and Western Michigan University with respect to the summer programs which had been offered by them, showed that out of 50 trainees so prepared, only four were still employed as full-fledged instructors.

With respect to the level of preparation of professional orientation and mobility instructors, the group was not in total agreement that graduate programs were necessary, although they found no short-cut to preparation time—even if programs were offered at the undergraduate level.

It was at this conference that Mr. John Jones, Coordinator, Unit of Education for the Visually Handicapped, Office of Education, expressed the interest of his office in supporting the preparation of orientation and mobility personnel for blind children in residential schools and day schools. A graduate program was to begin, with Office of Education support, in September 1966, at San Francisco State College. Much of the credit belongs to Miss Georgie Lee Abel, who secured the services of Mr. Berdell Wurzburger and later Mr. Richards as mobility instructors. A pilot program was also to be supported at Florida State University, at the undergraduate level. This was established under the guidance of Dr. Gideon Jones; the first mobility instructor was Mr. William Goodman, later replaced by Mr. Purvis Ponder and Mr. Everett Hill.

RSA helped to establish a graduate program at California State College at Los Angeles in the fall of 1966, and the program director was Mr. Lawrence E. Blaha. After his untimely death he was succeeded by Mr. Robert Eisenberg.

In addition to identification of manpower shortage, the problem of level of professional preparation, the announcement of support for orientation and mobility by the Office of Education, and the establishment of a pilot undergraduate program, there was acknowledgement of the need for interest in mobility assistance for the person with useful sight.

The year 1966, in addition to the assessment of the "state of orientation and mobility," was a landmark year with the publication of the report of the Commission on Standards and Accreditation of Services for the Blind. One of 12 technical committees had been appointed to establish standards of practice in the area of orientation and mobility. The committee included the following:

Chairman

George Werntz, Jr., Morristown, N. J., Executive Vice-President, The Seeing Eye, Inc.

Members

Donald Blasch, Kalamazoo, Mich., Director, Blind Rehabilitation Programs, Training Center for Orientation and Mobility, Western Michigan University.

John R. Eichorn, Ed.D., Chestnut Hill, Mass., Department of Education, Boston College.

Richard E. Hoover, M.D., Baltimore, Md.

William F. Johns, San Rafael, Calif., Executive Director, Guide Dogs for the Blind.

A. Ryrie Koch, Boston, Mass., Regional Representative, Vocational Rehabilitation Administration, U. S. Department of Health, Education, and Welfare.

Russell C. Williams, HH.D., Washington, D. C., Chief, Blind Rehabilitation, Department of Medicine and Surgery, U. S. Veterans Administration.

Commission Representatives

Louis H. Rives, Jr., Washington, D. C., Special Assistant

to the Commissioner, Vocational Rehabilitation Administration, U. S. Department of Health, Education and Welfare.

McAllister Upshaw, Detroit, Mich., Executive Director, Metropolitan Society for the Blind.

Staff Associate

Arthur M. Dye, Jr., Moylan, Pa.

In addition to describing the orientation and mobility instructor's place within the agency structure, the standards listed those skills to be taught and the general information which was to be imparted. It was stated that active travel training requires one instructor to one trainee. Physical and personal qualifications include the following:

1. Vision: no impairment not correctible in each eye to 20/20, no restriction in the visual peripheral field under all common circumstances, no evidence of pathology contributing to progressive deterioration.
2. Hearing: normal in both ears.
3. General physical condition: no physical impairments or organic mental deterioration that would limit the instructor's capacity to perform effectively or prevent him from protecting his client from imminent danger.
4. Ophthalmological, otological and general physical examinations are required every two years.
5. Personality makeup capable of meeting the demands and emotional stress of the job in a creative, realistic and optimistic way.
6. Ability to effect relationships of a courteous professional nature.
7. Keen observation and the ability to interpret observations.
8. Ability to organize work.
9. Ability to accept supervision in a constructive manner.
10. Flexibility, patience, unpossessiveness, prudence, tolerance and integrity.

Professional qualifications were listed as follows:

1. Graduation from an accredited graduate level program for training teachers of orientation and mobility.

2. Alternatively, approval by an appropriate body to be established for certification of teachers qualified by experience who meet all but the academic standards.

The accredited gradaute level program, as described, included the following major requirements: the setting should be within an education department, the curriculum should include course work regarding sensory deficiencies, physiological, social and emotional aspects of visual impairment, history of services to the blind, orientation and mobility services to the visually impaired, legislation, low-vision aids and practice.

The Commission on Standards and Accreditation of Services for the Blind (COMSTAC) further recommended the establishment of a certifying body to consider the applications of those instructors in the field who did not meet the standards, but who wished to be accredited.

Subsequently, under the auspices of the American Association of Workers for the Blind, and in cooperation with the Association for Education of the Visually Handicapped, a certification committee was established. Group IX of A.A.W.B. became the orientation and mobility group and has become one of the largest and most active groups within the organization. Since the inception of this committee in 1969, a total of 201 applications have been received.

Since 1966, orientation and mobility programs have been established in the University of Northern Colorado, Greeley, Colorado (1970), where Mr. Robert Crouse was appointed as chief mobility instructor, and at the University of Pittsburgh, Pittsburgh, Pennsylvania (1969), with Mr. Bruce Blasch assuming the responsibility for teaching orientation and mobility.

Prior to this time, the long cane technique had received very little favorable notice in England. In 1964, Dr. Alfred Leonard, a research psychologist on the staff of Nottingham University, was assigned by the Medical Research Council of England to investigate and make recommendations concerning mobility for the blind in the United Kingdom. Dr. Leonard scoured the literature, interviewed leaders and workers in the field, and studied the mobility habits of many blind individuals. Much of his knowledge was acquired from two of Britain's largest organizatons—St.

Dunstan's and the Royal National Institute for the Blind. His attention then focused on the United States and he succeeded in raising funds for the sole purpose of exploring mobility services in the United States. Two of the many places he visited were Central Blind Rehabilitation Section, Veterans Administration Hospital, Hines, Illinois; and the Institute of Blind Rehabilitation, Western Michigan University, Kalamazoo, Michigan. Upon his return to England he reported his findings, stating that he was greatly impressed, and recommended that a blind person be sent over for training in the spring of 1966.

In the meantime, Mr. William Goodman, then with the Metropolitan Society for the Blind, Detroit, Michigan, under the joint auspices of the American Foundation for the Blind, The American Foundation for Overseas Blind, and the Royal National Institute for the Blind, conducted a study of mobility in educational institutions and rehabilitation centers, conferred with teachers, and exposed blind youths to use of the long cane in the United Kingdom. This occurred in the summer of 1965, and in 1966 Mr. Lee Farmer of the Blind Center at Hines spent some time teaching at the Assessment Center at Torquay. The British remained skeptical and apparently wanted further evidence in order to be convinced.

In 1966, St. Dunstan's selected and sponsored Mr. Walter Thornton, a totally blind World War II veteran, with the expressed purpose of subjecting him to the "American traning methods" for evaluative purposes. Mr. Thornton, a senior executive with Cadbury Chocolates, Bournville, England, was personally very interested in mobility for blind persons and was a capable and willing student. He received one week of intensive experience at Hines and three weeks of intensive work at Western Michigan University. His progress was excellent and he apparently recognized the value of systematic training methodology and the merits of the long cane. He submitted a favorable report upon his return to England, and in collaboration with Dr. Leonard, was able to secure a one year's grant from the Viscount Nuffield Foundation to establish a nonresidential mobility training center. Nottingham University was to be the fiscal administrator of the project. Mr. Stanley Suterko, Western Michigan University, was requested to develop the program and was granted one year's leave of absence from the university—August 1966 to August 1967.

Mr. Suterko listed his accomplishments as follows: (1) The blind individuals who were trained demonstrated the effectiveness of the long cane and its associated training methodology in England; (2) mobility instructors who were trained initiated mobility programs in residential schools (England and Scotland), in agencies, and community mobility programs; (3) establishment of the training of teachers of the blind in the United Kingdom was accomplished so that they could all receive at least the basic skills in orientation and mobility; (4) creation of a demand for mobility instructors as evidenced by the requests from agencies and residential schools; (5) creation of a desire on the part of another local authority in England to develop a similar mobility center in their area.

The commitment of England to orientation and mobility methods was underscored by the continuation of the Viscount Nuffield Foundation grant for two more years. Mr. Robert Crouse, an American instructor and a graduate of Western Michigan University, replaced Mr. Suterko for the next two years. Upon the completion of his tour, Mr. Crouse noted, "The most intriguing facet of the progress of the Midlands Mobility Centre has been its fantastic growth. In a little over two years it has grown from inception to a fully functioning Centre with a professional staff of four." The Midlands Mobility Centre has become a permanent service in England.

Additional fan-out to England was provided by Robert LaDuke, then an instructor at Western Michigan University, who spent six months establishing orientation and mobility courses at the Royal School for the Blind and the Saint Vincent's School for the Blind in 1968-69.

Under the auspices of the American Foundation for Overseas Blind, Mr. Suterko conducted two workshops in Paris, France, in 1968 and 1969. Representatives of 14 nations from four different continents participated in the workshops. He was replaced in 1970 by Mr. William Walkowiak of Boston College. Concurrent with the workshops in Paris, similar workshops were conducted in the Far East by the American Foundation for Overseas

Blind, under the direction of Mr. Jeakle, a graduate of Boston College.

Rodney J. Kossick has provided a detailed description of his contribution in Vietnam, 1966-1968, in his paper, "Activating A Program for the Blind in South Vietnam," *Blindness 1970.*

The most recent developments are now taking place in Australia. Mr. Holdsworth, Executive Director of the Royal Guide Dogs for the Blind Associations of Austrialia, has long been interested in improving mobility services to the blind of Australia. Mr. Holdsworth has made several trips to the United States to evaluate our mobility training programs. He has requested and received the services of Mr. Suterko to evaluate the services in Australia and New Zealand and to discuss our methods of training. These visits were conducted in August and September of 1970. As a result of these contacts the Institute of Blind Rehabilitation, Western Michigan University, has been requested to help them initiate a program similar to the one established in England. The program is scheduled to start in July of 1971.

Mention should be made of students from foreign lands who have come for professional preparation. Unfortunately, it has not been possible to accept all who requested admission because of various regulations. However, students from Norway, South Africa and Canada have been admitted to our professional sequence and undoubtedly will make an impact on services to the blind in their respective countries. In retrospect, it is truly phenomenal how the discipline of orientation and mobility has spread throughout the world in such a relatively short time. We are sure that it has exceeded by far the fondest hopes of its originators.

The fan-out of orientation and mobility services throughout the world has been gratifying. It lends some credence to an old adage, "Develop a superior product and the world will beat a pathway to your door." It has had an enormous impact in the rehabilitation process of blind individuals; it has brought about changes in the educational process of blind children; it has helped raise work with the blind to a professional status; but it has also fanned out in adjacent areas.

More and more orientation and mobility instructors are being consulted by developers of aids for the blind; some have developed aids on their own initiative. This is particularly true in the development of collapsible canes. Within the past five years more functional collapsible canes have appeared than were available in the past three decades and all of the new ones are far superior from a functional standpoint.

More and more orientation and mobility instructors are being asked to supervise and carry out the field testing of new aids. In addition to various types of canes, tips, grips, etc., they have been field testing the Laser Beam Cane that was developed and produced by the Bionic Instruments, Inc., Bala Cynwyd, Pennsylvania. At the present time they are in the process of field testing the Binaural Ultrasonic Sensor, developed by Dr. Leslie Kay of New Zealand. The blind have long been subjected to exaggerated claims for many aids, and, hopefully, this type of field testing will eliminate or validate these claims for the benefit of the blind consumer.

Another barometer of fan-out is literature. *The Long Cane News,* a joint publication of Boston College and Western Michigan University, is becoming more sophisticated. Initially, it was intended only as a newsletter for the graduates of the two schools. Later it was extended to the graduates of all seven colleges and universities with orientation and mobility programs. The content now includes meaningful professional articles. Requests for the publication come from all parts of the country and some foreign countries so that at the present time there is a mailing list of approximately 1200. Concurrently, articles about orientation and mobility have appeared in professional journals and publications in ever-increasing numbers. For example, three articles on this subject appeared in *The New Outlook for the Blind* in 1960. In 1970, 16 articles appeared in this publication.

No discipline fans out at this exceptional rate without evoking some criticism, and the discipline of orientation and mobility is no exception. Some of the criticisms are as follows: (1) Highly trained mobility specialists did not remain in the field; (2) they would not be content just teaching mobility. In 1970, Mr. Bruce Blasch, University of Pittsburgh, and Mr. Berdell Wurzburger, San Francisco State College, made a survey of all graduates of orientation and mobility programs, inclusive of April 1970. Their findings were published in the *Long Cane News,* Vol. IV, No. 3, January, 1971. They found that there were 332 graduates. Of this total number, 87 percent, or 289, are still working with the visually handicapped. Of this number (289) 95 percent are directly involved with orientation and mobility. Of the 13 percent that are not working with the visually handicapped, 3.3 percent are females who, due to family responsibilities, are unable to work at this time. This does not mean that they will not return to teach at a later date—some have already gone through this cycle. Another 3.3 percent are working in an area other than the visually handicapped. Approximately 2.5 percent have returned to universities for advanced degrees. Two percent are unaccounted for due to lack of communication and may be working in this area. Another two percent have either retired or are in the military services. If we were to include all of the 2 percent unaccounted for and the 3.3 percent not working in this area, this would make 5.3 percent who did not find themselves suited to teach orientation and mobility. Other professional training areas would envy this record as it is far superior to most other professional programs. Compared to other nonprofessional methods of training orientation and mobility instructors, it has proven itself the most economical and efficient; but most important, it assures the blind client he is receiving the best service available.

If this has instilled any complacency in the graduate orientation and mobility instructor, let us get rid of it now. We have barely scratched the surface of what needs to be done. We have fanned out into the area of training residual vision but we have not, as yet, come up with good programs in that area. We have fanned out into working with the multihandicapped blind person but we have not consolidated our efforts in that area. We have fanned out into the area of the geriatric blind but this has been only a token gesture and we have not really attacked the many problems existing in that area. We have fanned out to working with additional mobility aids, but we have not incorporated them into a total program. We have done very little with the preschool blind child and much less with the parents. All in all, it has been great, but it can, and should, be better.

14

Providing Counseling Services to the Blind and Severely Visually Impaired

Richard E. Hardy

WHAT IS COUNSELING?

Counseling has been defined in various terms and by many experts. Gustad (1953) has written that "counseling is a learning oriented process, carried on in a simple, one-to-one social environment in which a counselor, professionally competent in relative psychological skills and knowledge, seeks to assist the client to learn more about himself, to know how to put understanding into effect in relation to clearly perceived, realistically defined goals to the end that the client may become a happier and more productive member of his society."

While definitions vary according to the orientation of the counselor, certain truisms have resulted from the enormous amount of research concerning the effectiveness of counseling. These will be explained in the following paragraphs.

No matter what particular school or theory of counseling is accepted by the practitioner, the most important factor determining the outcome of counseling effectiveness is the "personality" of the counselor himself. In other words, whether he counts himself as Rogerian, Ellisonian, or eclectic, the personality of the counselor will come through in counseling sessions and affect the outcome to a degree which will determine whether or not the counseling session is effective. Just as teachers can bring about enormous growth and changes in students by modifying their attitudes toward various subject matter, the counselor can bring about substantial changes in his client for better or worse.

Effective counseling requires certain basic ingredients. As the strength or weakness of these ingredients vary so does the ability of the counselor to help the client. There are three basic prerequisites to effective counseling. First, the counselor must accept the client without imposing conditions for this acceptance. He must be willing to work with the client and become actively involved with him as an individual no matter what the counselee's race, attitudes, or mode of life may be. This is necessary in order for the counselee to gain the knowledge that the counselor as a person wishes to help him with his problems and is not prejudging.

The counselor must be "genuine" in that he must function in a way which indicates to the client that he is being true to his own feelings and to himself. To be otherwise is to present a facade to the client—a false image which will act as a deterrant to a successful relationship. Counselors must avoid artificiality in their relationships. If the counselor hides behind a professional mystique, he may find that the counselee is better at "fooling" him than he is at deceiving the client. The professional worker cannot expect his client to be open, sincere, and genuine if he himself does not represent these characteristics well.

In addition, the counselor must have an empathetic understanding and feeling vis-à-vis the client. He must make a sincere effort to see the client's problem through the "client's eyes" and he must be able to communicate the depth of his understanding.

Counseling can be considered a relationship between two persons which is conducive to good mental health. Inherent in an effective counseling relationship is the absence of threat. The counselor must remove threat if the client is to grow and be able to solve his problems in an uninhibited manner. Counseling as a relationship is also typified by the types of feelings that many of us have for our closest friends. True close friendships are characterized by honest caring, genuine interest, and a high level of concern about helping in a time of need. Real friendships often require one person to put aside his own selfish needs in order to listen long enough and with enough empathy so that a friend's problem may begin to work itself out in a natural and constructive manner.

There are a number of adjectives which apply to various types of counseling (religious, marital, rehabilitation, educational, personal, vocational, and others). Counseling services vary according to the needs of the client, not the counselor. A counselee who comes to the counselor for help will often at first outline a concern which is not the real problem. The counselor must have considerable flexibility and insight to know what is required in each individual situation.

REHABILITATION COUNSELING

Rehabilitation counselors are concerned mainly with individuals who have vocational handicaps. These handicaps may result from physical disability, emotional or mental illness, social or cultural deprivation. In each individual case, the counselor must be able to decide what remedy is required in order to move the counselee toward successful personal adjustment in his family, community, and on the job.

Rehabilitation counseling requires the ingredients mentioned earlier for effective counselor-client relationships; however, much of rehabilitation counseling consists of advice-giving and coordination of services to the client. In a sense, "rehabilitation counseling" can be considered a misnomer when the term is applied across the board. A substantial number of clients need considerable advice and information which the counselor has to offer concerning social and rehabilitation services from which they can profit. When the counselee needs advice and information, the rehabilitation counselor must be able to recognize this need and provide what is required. There also will be many instances in which the client and counselor must enter into a number of counseling sessions in depth. The counselor must make the judgment concerning what type of help is needed for the client to solve his particular problems. Rehabilitation counselors need appropriate training that will enable them to decide whether or not they are qualified to do the kind of counseling which is necessary.

Many counselors fall into the trap of wanting to play the role of "junior therapist" and involve high percentages of their clients in in-depth counseling sessions. This is particularly true of the graduates of many rehabilitation counselor training programs. Some workers hide behind "counseling" (as synonomous with quality) in terms of their justifying low numbers of rehabilitated clients. There is much talk of quality services and in-depth counseling which require considerable time. The rehabilitation counselor who is an effective manager of his caseload can "rehabilitate" the number of persons required by his agency administrator and while doing so can provide counseling services as needed to his clients.

Rehabilitation work requires a broad definition of counseling which includes the offering of some, and coordination of other professional services to clients. Generally, agency administrators —especially those trained in counseling—do not accept the explanation of "the time required and quality services" for a low client rehabilitation rate. Any agency administrator or supervisor knows that some cases require much involved counseling, and that these cases in many instances are the most difficult ones. They are time-consuming, and they can test the fiber of the rehabilitation counselor. Untrained counselors generally cannot handle such cases without help from someone who has had some advanced orientation in counseling. However, counselors who play the role of "junior therapist" in trying to become deeply involved with all of their clients—whether or not this type of service is called for—will be ineffective and probably will not remain long in rehabilitation work.

The rehabilitation counselor will find his coordinating and facilitating role highly rewarding when it is done well and gets needed services. One of the greatest satisfactions that the counselor can have is the assurance that he knows when certain types of services are required and whether these should be more therapeutically oriented or more oriented toward advice, information, and coordination of community resources and professional services.

Rehabilitation counselors should not rank-order their clients in a psychological need hierarchy which places the individual with severe psychological problems at the top of the counselor's list for services. Certainly, these persons should be served immediately upon the counselor's realization that severe psychological problems exist. They should be referred to the appropriate psychologist or psychiatrist if problems are so severe that the counselor cannot handle them alone, or they should be served by rehabilitation counselors who are competent in the type of service required. The point to be made here is that the rehabilitation process is a complicated procedure; the client who may be adjusting normally to a loss and who does not need substantial in-depth therapeutic involvement is as good a case for services as one requiring more therapeutic work. Coordination of services of supportive personnel and professional personnel is a substantial part of the work of the rehabilitation counselor. In many cases, he will have to bring this team together in order that the client can continue to receive effective and necessary rehabilitation services.

The rehabilitation counselor must actively involve himself within the community in order to be fully aware of the many resources which exist that can be of substantial benefit to his clients. Generally, counselors have indicated that so much of their time is taken with counseling and coordination of services that they are unable to put forward enough effort to learn all that the community has to offer. Counselors who utilize community resources effectively are very familiar with the offerings of various agencies and through coordination and cooperation find that their work load is lessened by the support of other social service programs.

The counselor will wish to offer his services to various types of community agencies. For instance, most counselors can give a great deal of useful advice to such programs as the community action and model cities efforts sponsored by the Federal Government. Agencies and organizations such as family service programs and welfare agencies can be of considerable help in getting needed services for the rehabilitation client. The counselor should take a major responsibility in coordinating efforts of agencies and programs that can help in the rehabilitation of clients, and he should volunteer his time and energies to help strengthen other social service programs.

The rehabilitation counselor must keep in mind that he should be moving the client toward end objectives of independence and successful adjustment on the job. Rehabilitation differs from some other social service professions in the regard that a substantial test of the counselor's work is made at the end of the rehabilitation process. That test consists of the appropriateness of the client's behavior in work situation (Hardy, 1972).

REHABILITATION COUNSELING WITH THE BLIND AND SEVERELY VISUALLY IMPARED

No special counseling theory need be constructed in order for the rehabilitation counselor to serve blind persons. There is, however, a substantial body of knowledge with which the counselor should be thoroughly familiar. Topics include the etiology of diseases related to blindness, problems in adjustment to visual loss including mobility, social adjustment, occupational advice and job placement. The counselor serving blind persons has a real responsibility to undertake considerable study in order to acquaint himself with what Father Carroll (1961) has called in the title of his book, *Blindness: What It Is, What It Does, and How to Live with It.*

The rehabilitation counselor serving blind persons has as much or more of a coordinating function as does the counselor in a general agency setting. A counselor concerned with the blind will work closely with the educational services specialist, the social worker, the ophthalmologist, the placement specialist, the rehabilitation teacher, and the mobility instructor who help in the team effort of moving the blind individual toward adjustment to his visual problem and later to adjustment on the job.

Rehabilitation counselors serving the blind, just as counselors working with any other rehabilitation clients, must be certain that their clients are without need of further medical or psychological treatment. In this regard, the counselor helping the partially sighted should make certain that no visual aid or professional service can offer additional help to the client. He should be fully aware of the various problems which go hand in hand with a loss of sight. Persons who are experiencing a severe physical inadequacy lose some ability to be independent. They feel socially inadequate and in some cases may have additional problems which at first might not be apparent to the counselor. Advanced age or other physical incapabilities may add to the blind person's adjustment problems.

The client will be very much interested in the prognosis for his future, and the rehabilitation counselor should make sure that valid information is provided. An effective counselor must be ready to help the blind person understand what his opportunities are for education, employment, social activities. He should also talk with those persons who give information to the blind client, especially professional individuals such as ophthalmologists, to make certain that they have useful information concerning blindness and the services of the state rehabilitation agency.

Bauman and Yoder (1966) have suggested that the rehabilitation counselor must offer

> a combination of several qualities: (1) his own emotional acceptance of blindness (he must be the first person to whom the client has spoken who did not immediately show great pity and anxiety—a helping new experience for the client); (2) formal or informal instruction in procedures which make it easier to live as a blind person (the home teacher and also some adjustment on pre-vocational training can help here); (3) realistic planning for the future, including vocational planning if the age and general health of the client make this appropriate. It is true that all of these may be rejected for a time, in which case the counselor must offer (4) understanding, patience, and a gentle persistence which keeps him available until the client and his family are able to reorient themselves to the future instead of clinging to the past.

In counseling with blind persons, the rehabilitation counselor must remember that he is working with individuals who cannot see or whose sight is impaired. The client will differ from fellow blind persons as much as he will differ from sighted persons. Some blind persons are very healthy; others are sickly. Some are well adjusted psychologically; others are poorly adjusted. In many cases, blindness will have caused severe psychological stress which has not been overcome, just as an accident or some other type of traumatic experience may have caused either a sighted or a blind person severe psychological difficulty.

Often, reaction to partial vision causes as much or more frustration and anxiety than reaction to total blindness. One reason for this seems to be that partially sighted persons are unable to function normally and do not want to accept their loss of sight as a reality. They live in a no-man's-world between blindness and sight.

The rehabilitation counselor serving blind and severely visually impaired persons must be even more planful and thoughtful than the counselor who is concerned with individuals who are sighted. Often it will be necessary to anticipate problems which may arise for the blind client. For instance, simply getting to and from the counselor's office may become a very troublesome and embarrassing task. The blind client may be traveling over unfamiliar terrain with or without the help of relatives or friends. The counselor, in many cases, may want to visit initially in the home and later during the relationship invite the client to the rehabilitation agency.

The counselor must be very much aware that this blind client is "tuned in" to auditory clues (yes's and unhum's may be helpful), since the usual eye contact and other nonverbal communications are not effective with blind persons. For instances, silence over a considerable period of time often takes place in counseling sessions, but when the counselor is working with a blind client, silence may be interpreted at times as disinterest or rejection.

It is respectful and appropriate for the counselor to look directly into the face and eyes of the client just as if the counselee were fully sighted. Blind persons are often aware that sighted persons are not looking at them and they get the impression, which may be true, that the counselor is not listening.

Counselors should be particularly careful about shuffling papers, tapping a pencil on the desk, or making other sounds that are distracting. They should also be aware that many blind persons, especially the congenitally blind, give the counselor little to go by in terms of facial expression. The counselor who is used to reading emotionality in various facial responses may be at a considerable loss with some persons who have been blind for a number of years and who are not nearly as responsive in this respect as sighted people (Jordan, 1962).

A rehabilitation counselor providing professional services to blind persons must avoid fostering unnecessary dependence. Often counselors, unknowingly as well as knowingly, build their own self-esteem by continually allowing clients to rely on them for personal advice and other services. On the other hand, many rehabilitation counselors are afraid to show sufficient interest in the problems of the client because they are concerned about being forced to give a great deal of time and attention to the client. Neither of these extremes will allow the counselor to be effective.

SUMMARY

It has been said that the most important variable for helping people which the counselor brings to the counseling relationship is "himself." The rehabilitation counselor, whether he is working with blind or sighted clients, must make a substantial effort to maintain genuiness, openness, sincerity, honesty, and respect for the client. While techniques and procedures are important in accomplishing goals in counseling sessions, the real key to successful counseling is whether the counselor genuinely cares for the individual. A rehabilitation counselor provides substantial professional and coordinated services from which the client benefits enormously. Most rehabilitation counselors will have certain quotas to meet and the effective counselor, through proper caseload management, will be able to provide quality and quantity services. He will also realize that his coordinative and facilitative function is as important as his counseling function. He must serve clients according to *their needs* and not his own; when this is done, counselees will not claim that his work lacks quality because he will have been much more concerned with them as individuals than with whether or not his services were "professional" in nature.

REFERENCES

Bauman, Mary K. and Yoder, Norman M.: *Adjustment to Blindness—Re-Viewed.* Springfield, Thomas, 1966.

Carroll, Thomas J.: *Blindness: What It Is, What It Does, and How to Live with It.* Boston, Little, 1961.

Gustad, J. W.: The definition of counseling. In Berdie, R. F.: *Roles and Relationship in Counseling.* Minneapolis, U. of Minn., 1953.

Hardy, Richard E.: Vocational placement. In Cull, John G. and Hardy, Richard E.: *Vocational Rehabilitation: Profession and Process.* Springfield, Thomas, 1972.

Jordan, John E.: Counseling the blind. *Personnel and Guidance Journal, 39*:3:10-214, 1962.

Morgan, Clayton A.: Personality of counseling. *Blindness,* AAWB Annual, American Association of Workers for the Blind, Inc., Washington, D. C., 1969.

Truax, Charles B. and Cartkuff, Robert R.: *Toward Effective Counseling and Psychotherapy: Training and Practice.* Chicago, Aldine, 1967.

15

Occupational Information and Career Planning for Blind Persons

George A. Magers

Vocational rehabilitation has been with us 50 years. However, as far as the blind are concerned, vocational rehabilitation has been meaningful only since 1943. If we had to pick a landmark in this period of work for the blind, it would be the Barden-Lafollette Act of 1943. It was one of the real landmarks in the whole aspect of work for the blind, especially in the United States. It was at that moment in time that the blind actually became an accepted part of the state-federal vocational rehabilitation program. Prior to 1943, blind persons had either vocationally rehabilitated themselves or, in rare instances, received vocational rehabilitation services through the formal state-federal program. However, our programs, as we know them today, had their beginning with the expansion of the Vocational Rehabilitation Act in 1943.

Five years before that, in initiating the vending stand program in this country, the Randolph-Sheppard Act set forth some provisions for the development of employment programs. This suggested the carrying out of studies to ascertain what types of jobs and new careers could be developed for blind persons as the primary emphasis of that piece of legislation in 1938. Both the Barden-LaFollette Act and the Randolph-Sheppard Act served to back up acceptance of the idea that blind persons were able not only to be educated but could be vocationally prepared to take their place in competitive employment. Prior to 1943, less than 1,000 blind persons in the United States moved into the competitive labor market each year through the state-federal vocational rehabilitation program. In 1969, the state-federal vocational rehabilitation program for the blind assisted 7,105 blind persons and 13,411 severely visually handicapped individuals (above the legal definition of blindness) to move into gainful employment.

With that introduction, I will base the remainder of this chapter on the state-federal vocational rehabilitation program for the blind as it relates to occupational information.

PROFESSIONAL FIELDS OF WORK

If we used projected estimates for occupational categories from previous years, the breakdown of 7,105 blind rehabilitants in 1969 would show that approximately 900 found jobs in the professions or in managerial pursuits. The range of professional occupations can be seen in careers of teaching, psychology, social work, law, writing, chemistry, physics, math, etc. Although the increase in the number of rehabilitants over the last quarter of the century is certainly important, of much greater significance is the kind of opportunities that are now opening up to blind people; that is, the widening range of job situations in which blind persons are being trained and in which they are finding opportunities to work. More than 2,500 blind people will be in college this September in over 450 colleges and universities throughout this country, and they will be studying in almost every field imaginable. Not long ago I had an occasion to work with an individual who had majored as an actuary. This is a type of profession that one would normally think could not be performed competently without sight. Actuarial work is based almost entirely on the examination of statistics and figures about people. Nevertheless, he finished his undergraduate work, got a graduate degree, and now has a rather good position as an actuary working in the social security program. This is just one example of the type of employment that we are gradually moving into as far as blind persons are concerned. Many more examples can be found in the field of computer sciences. In 1963, one could count on his fingers the number of blind persons who were in the computer sciences. Since that time, we have a listing of over 400 blind persons who are employed as computer programmers. Today we have a hundred more who are in training. There are seven recognized training centers throughout the country. So here is another field that is now open to trained and qualified blind persons.

This does not mean that because this field has opened up, we automatically have access to normal training facilities and can go right along and start opening up another field, assuming that occupational opportunity in the computer field is now available. We must continually work at this because a computer is a highly complex piece of machinery and its technology is moving more rapidly than that of any other professional endeavor. So there has to be a constant follow-up, a continuous observation. A seemingly minor change, especially as it affects hardware, might well jeopardize the continued employment of blind persons in this field.

One of the things we are quite concerned about with computer programmers is the type of feedback that we have access to as far as a program has developed. Blind people are now working with program decks that will give them the print-out in braille, using the regular high-speed printer. In the next few years a generation of computers will be developed to the point where electrostatic printing techniques will serve to give programmers feedback on their input. When this happens, we will have problems as far as blind programmers are concerned because of the difference between securing braille print-out from the chain link mechanical printer and the equipment which will be involved in electrostatic printing. We are involved in a rather substantial program of research aimed at developing new methods and techniques and hardware alternatives which will enable both blind persons now employed and those who are or will bc in training to be flexible to the extent that they can keep in pace with forseeable technological advances. Along with this research we are also planning specific steps to widen the horizons for the training and employment of the blind and visually handicapped within the total field of the computer sciences. New highly specialized positions, i.e. "the software specialist," are already developing; and undoubtedly, there will be other kinds of new careers. While we must continually search for new kinds of jobs, it is equally important to extend and expand career opportunities for trained and qualified people already in the field.

Another field which is fascinating to watch is that of teaching, which has shown marked development over the last 10 to 15 years for blind individuals. As part of our overall efforts to move ahead in opening new opportunities for disabled individuals, a grant was made to the New York Association for the Blind for the purpose of bringing together a national planning institute which had as its goal the promulgation of guidelines for the selection, training, and placement of blind persons in elementary and secondary schools teaching sighted children. Seven successfully employed blind grade and high school teachers participated, as did school administrators, officials from teacher-training institutions, college placement specialists, and experts in vocational rehabilitation for the blind. Just a few years ago, a blind person successfully performing in an elementary or secondary classroom situation teaching sighted children was the rare exception. Last year, more than half of the over 100 newly trained blind teachers found positions in our public and private schools. The remainder pursued other careers in the field of education, including college teaching. There are today several hundred successful blind teachers helping to meet the critical manpower needs in our nation's regular school program.

SERVICE FIELDS OF WORK

We are not limiting ourselves to the professions in developing new opportunities for blind and visually handicapped clientele. I should explain that our efforts ordinarily go forward in steps from research efforts to the initiation of a demonstration program. From these demonstrations, or in some instances, national planning seminars, come the informational material in counseling and guidance tools aimed at making the necessary knowledge available to vocational rehabilitation counseling personnel and others working with the blind and visually disabled.

One of the newest careers to open up is the service representative. When I mention service here it is in a different context from that of the employment of blind persons in service occupations. With the society and our economy becoming more and more complex all the time, the actual provision of services requires professional expediting of a particular plan or pattern that an individual needs—joining that pattern or plan and individuals together so that the job gets done. This requires the type of position now being called "service representative." The Office for the Blind and Visually Handicapped became a part of the new career research in this area as a result of our activities in opening up federal job situations for blind people.

More than three years ago, the Social and Rehabilitation Service and the Internal Revenue Service, in conjunction with the Arkansas Enterprises for the Blind in Little Rock, commenced to explore the possibility of training blind persons to provide information to taxpayers. Originally, the training and employment was planned around the taxpayer assister position in the Internal Revenue Service. However, with refinements in both the training and position responsibilities, the total plan was moved upward to include taxpayer service representative jobs. A number of blind persons are finding a successful new career in this capacity with the Internal Revenue Service, and we understand this number is to increase beyond our original expectations over the next two years.

From all indications, a second important result of this research and demonstration project is the emergence of a wide range of other service representative-type positions in federal, state, and local governmental organizations for which blind and visually handicapped individuals can be trained. Industry, too, will offer new careers in positions requiring similar skills and ability. Such organizations as telephone companies, airlines, and hospitals have service representative jobs, many of which may be successfully performed by trained and qualified blind persons.

I have said very little yet on some of the other occupations. In the area of clerical work, here again, we have felt that it is partly the Federal Government's job first to imagine and then engineer the kinds of innovative approaches and research and demonstrative efforts which open up new types of occupations or expanding job areas in which blind people are being trained and placed.

For many years the employment of medical records transcribers has been no new thing. However, it has been necessary to take an intensive look at this employment program to see where it is, what it is, what it needs to keep it moving, and to keep the actual training abreast with the demands of employers.

We brought together a national planning group. In this planning institute we began to think of a series of conferences looking at occupations in depth. These national planning institutes over the years gradually developed guidelines for the selection, training, and placement of blind persons in particular occupations or jobs.

In developing this overall approach, we felt that on the national level we should try to do several things, one of which was to involve recognized professional organizations dealing with a particular occupation. With the medical records transcribers, we worked out a program with Hadley School for the Blind and with the American Association of Medical Records Librarians; most often, the latter group had the power to actually hire. The medical records librarian is usually the individual who has the muscle to say, "This one I'll take, that one I don't want," as far as medical records transcribers in this department are concerned. We involved these people and then, of course, felt it necessary to involve vocational rehabilitation people because they were going to be in the business of counseling and actually working with the client in maping out a vocational plan involving training and placement.

We also realized the importance of involving the trainers (the people doing the actual vocational training), because vocational preparation is truly at the heart of a successful vocational rehabilitation plan. This is probably our weakest link in the vocational rehabilitation process today—the actual vocational preparation. We have a long way to go yet. We are doing a pretty good job in medical and vocational diagnosis. We are doing a reasonably good job in the adjustment area with mobility, communication skills, activities of daily living, and so forth, either through the rehabilitation teacher or through the adjustment and rehabilitation center. After people are really adequately adjusted or vocationally prepared, we are not doing too badly as far as placement is concerned. But one of the great problems we are running into is the actual vocational preparation itself in the rehabilitation process. That is a different topic from occupations and new careers, but it is certainly very closely akin to the development of the one and the actual understanding of what is available in the other.

We brought conferees together in this national planning institute for medical records transcribers and one of the things we found was that while people have been employed as medical records transcribers for a number of years, there was certainly good reason to believe that this occupation was going to expand. In fact, there was good reason to believe that the demand was going to excede the number of people we could find to go into this work at least in the forseeable future. This has proven to be the case, because even today the demand for trained, really qualified medical transcribers is higher than the available supply of blind and visually handicapped candidates. One of the reasons for this has been brought about by technological advances in communication where new modern hospitals are equipped for the almost instantaneous typing of dictation from a particular station in the hospital, and even out of the hospital from the doctor's car, his home or his office, where he merely dials in to the medical records' room or department and dictates medical case information to be transcribed and made a part of a person's medical records.

Part of the increased workload comes from new state laws and new accreditation requirements as far as hospitals are concerned, concerning the kind of medical records that have to be maintained on individuals. This has expanded the whole process of medical records maintenance. It has resulted in the development of recommendations for both training and new tools for equipment. These efforts involve the development of teaching materials, as well as adequate tools to be used at work. For example, the latest edition of *Dorland's Medical Dictionary* has been put into braille, and almost 200 sets are in use. A medical speller and sections of the *Physicians' Desk Reference* are now being put into braille and should be available within the next few months. These tools will be extremely valuable to the medical transcriber on the job.

SPECIALIZED EQUIPMENT

Once the research is done, part of career development is finding a mechanism whereby we can put the tool in the hands of the blind person who needs it for his particular occupation. This is one of the big problems when one starts working with a small group. However, fortunately the number of blind people in this country in a comparative sense is small: some 420,000 or 422,000. A much smaller number is moving into the competitive labor market.

One of the problems we run into is that when we find the tool needed, how do we make it available to the blind person going into a particular job situation? This problem is greater in some of the adjustment areas than it is in the vocational areas.

Over the past eight years, we have held a number of our "occupation in depth" national planning institutes for switchboard operators, medical records transcribers, computer programmers, teachers of sighted children, and for supportive positions in hospitals. These are the jobs not directly involved with services to patients. These are the behind-the-scenes type jobs in hospitals, in the food and lodging industry, in the recreational activities in general. These, for the most part, are the types of things we have been doing in the occupational depth series and out of each one have come guidelines as mentioned earlier. The switchboard operator publication is obsolete and no longer available. It is an occupation in which blind persons have been employed for at least 40 years, and, of course, originally it was a natural for a lot of blind people in this country. Telephone equipment at that time was what they called the drop-trap board. Many small telephone companies throughout America had the switchboard in the operator's own house. Actually, it was ideal equipment as far as a blind person was concerned because when a call would come in, a shutter would drop down extending out from the board. The operator would hear a click and all she had to do was run the back of her hand across the board, touch the shutter that had dropped, and plug in. Of course, with technological change, this equipment gradually moved out and the regular cord-board came into play in the thirties. What is known as touch pilot equipment was developed to enable blind persons to operate cord-board equipment. This signal cabinet or touch pilot is a little board that sits beside the big switchboard. When a call comes in, a peg jumps up by the particular extension number.

With technological changes in the communication industry, other types of special equipment have been developed for switchboard operators who are blind or visually handicapped. The two primary examples are Bell Laboratory's Seeing Aid® and the Telebraille® device built in Oregon and used in the northwestern part of our country. As communications technology advanced and telephone equipment became more sophisticated, the number of employed blind persons in this field diminished. However, today, we note a change in this trend in that automation is changing job requirements in such a manner that persons with little or no vision are able to perform operator duties successfully in a growing number of job situations. We forsee that in the next few years more training programs will need to be developed to prepare blind and visually handicapped individuals for this occupation. It is already evident that we will need to plan for a new institute in this particular occupation before the middle of the decade.

New careers in which blind people may participate are already becoming evident in the clerical field. The development of both dictating equipment and typewriters is opening up additional opportunities. Somewhat like the telephone industry a few years ago, typing pools were disbanded in favor of the individual's personal secretary. However, many government agencies and business enterprises are now planning to reinstate centralized typing units using highly sophisticated equipment. The magnetic tape Selectra® typewriter is playing an important role in this change in office systems. The operation of this equipment, of course, will require specialized training, but a number of the job responsibilities will not require sight and will, undoubtedly, open a much wider latitude of job opportunities for blind persons.

SHIFTS IN VOCATIONS

In the early 1900's employment in the United States was based on a rural economy. With the development of better tools of production, we have seen this shift to an urban way of life with fewer and fewer individuals required to produce the population's food. The perfection of hybrid seeds and the development of equipment for intensive agriculture have played a part in this change along with plans for mass production of consumer items.

Now we are noting a different shift, or change. Forty-five years ago, relatively few Americans had full-time employment in service occupations. However, today, with the advent of automated means of production, with increased leisure time and an easy flow of money, at least one of ten workers in our country has his primary job in providing service.

It is most probable that this change will continue until the year 2000, when one of every five individuals will be engaged in service occupations or in the service industry. We would like to cite a few examples of occupational areas in which we have already commenced planning, but in which we need to continue efforts, especially in regard to the selection and training of blind persons. In 1960, the service industries stood fourth in rank among employers, providing jobs for more than six and one-half million people. These millions were working in such diverse places as auto and other kinds of repair shops, laundries, dry cleaning establishments, hotels, barber shops, theaters, movie production and advertising firms.

The service industry group has been one of the fastest growing and is now well over three times its size in 1919. This reflects a very important fact about our way of life—that as we grow and prosper, higher and higher proportions of people will be engaged, not in making things, but in performing the multitude of services that make life more pleasant and easy for people generally in the next 10 years.

Today, there are nearly forty thousand identifiable occupations in the competitive field of work, and it is gratifying to note how widely blind people have fanned out into this great industrial complex.

The industrial revolution began approximately 200 years ago and it is not yet complete. Three phases have succeeded each other during this time. First, the bringing together of men into factories;

second, making machines to do the work of men; and third, arranging the work so that the men guiding the machines could do so with the least amount of effort. We are now in the midst of the fourth major step in this industrial revolution, that of making machines that run themselves, feed themselves, and turn out the finished product. This phase in our economy is usually referred to as automation. With an ever-growing sophistication in machinery and its arrangement in our manufacturing, we will move deeper into the era of automation. No one can truly predict the length of time or the nature of the next major step in producing the various items needed and wanted by man.

Much has been written about the twenty-first century as the era of cybernetics and perhaps it will be during that century that this phase of our economy will be recorded in history as having begun. Even though our industrial processes are highly mechanized and extremely sophisticated, and even though automated machine tools come into being, we still have a long way to go before we can say we have moved to this next era. During the 1960's, each year noted an increase in the number of people employed in the United States. At the present time, it is estimated that 76,000,000 people are fully employed in the country. By 1980 we will have reached the 90,000,000 mark and by the beginning of the twenty-first century we should have well over 100,000,000 individuals employed in the nation. Even though the rate of the percentage of jobs in manufacturing concerns is decreasing in comparison to the total number of employment opportunities in the country, this phase of our economy continues to offer employment to the majority of workers in America.

Mechanization, it is true, has enabled our manufacturers to produce more goods with fewer man hours; however, our imagination, ingenuity, and competitive system have created many new products and, with the rising standard of living, demand has kept pace. At the outset of every major phase in our industrial development, there has been the real concern (primarily on the part of labor) that jobs would be eliminated and that machines would replace individuals and create great unemployment. As our society has adjusted to automation, the clamor against this development has eased. However, even today, there is much discussion with regard to new production methods and advanced equipment creating a serious unemployment problem. So far, in every instance, the concern has not been valid. Rather than creating a large body of unemployed workers, industrial know-how has actually increased the number of jobs available in the land. In fact, this year there will be more new jobs created than there are individuals newly coming on to the labor market.

Jobs in industry are changing; old ways of producing materials are giving way to new and more effective resources. Training and skill requirements of workers are more demanding. In many instances, this necessitates retraining of workers for new positions. In other instances, it means an actual shift from one industry to another; however, Americans are generally a highly mobile people and adjust to these requirements as they develop.

The history of the employment of blind persons in industry in large numbers is, of course, short in comparison to the overall industrial revolution. Consistent growth in the ranks of these employed people began in the early 1940's, during the Second World War and thereafter. For example, during the 1960's, the number of blind persons entering competitive employment doubled, and the highest category of employment has continued to be in the industrial or manufacturing segment of our economy. The kinds of jobs they are performing are continually changing and the requirements for performance are on the increase. Thus, if we are to maintain our standing in the competitive labor market, we must constantly plan for improved vocational preparation and must better prepare professional personnel performing the selective placement process for the blind. Our nation is now concerned with the development of more effective trade technical training resources, and strengthened manpower programs for workers in general; thus it is even more essential that we gear our program of services to the blind to keep pace. No longer can we prepare our clients for today's jobs only. We must give them the kind of training and develop the skill needed for employment tomorrow and five years hence.

In 1970, 1,200 individuals were placed in industry through the state-federal vocational rehabilitation program. In fiscal year 1971, this number increased to more than 1,500. In planning our selective placement training program of counselors, one of the more significant changes we had noted is the requirement of flexibility in factory workers.

Personnel practices and sound production management have amply demonstrated the value of moving a worker from station to station rather than requiring him to stay at the same job hour after hour, day after day. This movement of personnel within the plant has increased the productivity of the worker, improved his satisfaction with his job, and lengthened his time of employment with an employer. In noting this trend, we have found it necessary to prepare our clientele to perform a number of operations rather than just the single task. In seeking employment opportunities for blind persons, our counselors are forced to make a careful evaluation of many jobs within a company, choosing those that can be done without sight and which will not create a drastic change in the normal shift of employees during the working day. While this requires a more careful selection of both the worker and the job, it is proving not to be as formidable as we feared a few short years ago. Blind persons, properly trained and placed in the right employment setting, are proving to be as flexible as their fellow workers with the one exception that they still must do those jobs where sight is not an essential factor. Fortunately, there are still more of these openings than we have clients prepared to fill them. The basic secret to success continues to be a vigorous, dynamic selective placement program involving professional people with initiative, imagination, and ingenuity, and above all, confidence in the products they are bringing to employers as well as a belief in the fundamental soundness of this program.

A number of blind persons are being trained and are securing employment in the trade technical areas. For example, a few years ago the School of Science at Wahpeton, North Dakota, undertook a research and demonstration project sponsored by the Rehabilitation Services Administration, aimed at demonstrating the effectiveness of providing trade technical training to blind persons in a particular region. Two courses were initiated, each of two-years duration: one in machine-shop work, and the other in small engine repair and maintenance. The machine-shop course was started during the first year and the small engine mechanics course commenced at the beginning of the second year of the project. The first class of machinists graduated in June of 1965. Five of the six graduates are now employed as machinists in such plants as John Deere, Cessna Airplane, General Electric, and in two instances, in small job machine shops. Seven students graduated in 1966, four from the machine shop, and three from the small engine mechanics course. In each instance, these individuals are employed in accordance with their training. In summary, we have no set list of jobs for the blind nor do we want one since we are firmly convinced that such a list would be much more limiting than helpful with regard to the provision of information on occupations or in the development of new careers. The ever-widening range of jobs in which blind persons are proving successful is ample evidence of both their ability and capacity to cope with future employment demands.

Certainly, many jobs of today will disappear, but there will be completely new jobs for which we must be prepared to train our clientele. Blind persons, like our sighted colleagues, must have a basic educational background which will permit their skills to be readily convertible in retraining programs. If it is true that the sighted worker of the future will require retraining at least six times during his work period, it will be even more imperative for the blind person in the competitive labor market.

We have merely scratched the surface and not given a detailed description of how blind persons are now being trained for and placed in many industrial, clerical, service, managerial, and professional occupations. However, we believe the reader can note the significance of the progress made during recent years. Blind persons at work in many communities throughout our land take pride in their chance to perform, for they know this is the avenue to even greater progress for all blind people now and in the future.

16

Placement in Competitive Employment

Louis Vieceli

Placement of the blind and visually handicapped in suitable employment is still one of the most challenging aspects of the rehabilitation process. It is not a separate or distinct service but is involved in the total rehabilitation process and is an on-going part of the process. Placement begins at the time of the initial interview and continues through putting the blind person on the job and following up to assure job success. It becomes the continuous process of assisting the workers to adjust successfully to a job which will allow the fullest use of his skills and at the same time will agree with him physically.

Placement, then, means putting a blind or visually handicapped person in a job that is most suitable in terms of the individual's remaining abilities. Effective placement includes evaluating a person on the basis of his total capacities including experience, training, aptitudes, skills and physical qualification. The requirements of the job are then carefully analyzed so that the blind individual can be fitted into the job with the best use of his work potential. Placement is thc matching of visual, physical and mental requirements of the job with the visual, physical and mental capacities of the worker.

CAREER PLANNING

Career planning or choosing a vocation is one of the most important and most difficult decisions facing any individual in his lifetime and deserves the most careful individual attention. In present-day society, work determines our way of life. Crawford, in his book, *Career Planning for the Blind,* says: "Career planning requires a thorough analysis and understanding of one's self, including strengths, weaknesses, abilities, interests, and aptitudes. Plans must be made in advance, consultation should be had with others, and education and training are of prime importance." Wise choice is important because it may well determine whether the individual will be employed or not and may determine success or failure and influence almost every aspect of his life.

In the past we have been either unwilling or unequipped to examine what jobs demands there will be one, three, or five years hence and/or to prepare blind or visually handicapped persons to meet these needs. We were and had been "tagalongs" rather than being ready when the demands hit. Fortunately, we now seem to have learned how to deal with this problem. The Office for the Blind and Visually Handicapped of the Rehabilitaion Services Administration has done much to help us through many projects and grants to study occupations in depth and to keep abreast of the changing labor market and the ongoing competition for jobs. We are not really confronted with the scarcity of job opportunities for our clients; rather, the new jobs in our changing social and economic way of life are such that people are ill-prepared for them. There are many who still feel that the weakest link in the rehabilitation process is in the vocational training aspect—the preparation of the blind person to keep up with the changing world of technology and job demands.

Diversity of Jobs Available

Today, the job seeker has a wide choice of jobs and job conditions. More Americans had jobs this past year than ever in our history. One clear benefit of mechanization and automation has been the elimination of many menial, dull, low-paying, undesirable jobs, thus adding new dimensions to man-capacity. However, these new dimensions also entail challenges that can be met only by a better prepared work force. More education and more skills will be the chief prerequisites for a job in 1975. The fast-changing world of work is demanding brains, not brawn, and versatility, not narrowed skills, with the most substantial increase in employment opportunities coming in the professional and technical fields.

Just a few years ago, the vast majority of blind persons graduating from college were limited to professional opportunities in the field of work for the blind (hometeachers, counselors, and instructors at centers). Now, this situation is reversed and not only are more blind persons graduating from college, but most are finding professional careers dealing with the working world of the sighted. This fall, more than 2500 blind persons are enrolled in over 450 colleges and universities. They are majoring in almost every subject area offered. As these individuals move through college in a wide range of vocational fields, they will have an increasingly better chance to expect employment commensurate with their training. This is not to say that all the problems of placement or employment opportunities for the trained and qualified blind persons in professional occupations have been solved. We still have some way to go. First, there are still skeptics. Second, the nature of most professional pursuits is rapidly changing and totally new careers are opening. It is imperative that we continue to press forward through education and demonstration to lessen the effect of negative public attitudes, and it is equally important to plan training programs to meet the demands of new professional opportunities. Concurrently, we must continue to expand the number and kind of careers in which blind persons are now and can be employed.

Each year the number of blind and visually handicapped persons rehabilitated through the state-federal program has established new record highs. And the important part in this is the widening range and scope of occupations which blind persons are entering.

Factors in Career Choice

What then are some of the ingredients that make up good career choice and job selection? It has been said that there are four basic factors of suitability of work, all of which must be involved for a successful and happy worklife. First, the job must be reasonably consistent with the individual's physical condition; in rehabilitation, we must be concerned also that the disability does not interfere with ability to do the job nor should the job aggravate the disability. Second, the job or career must be consistent with the individual's mental ability. Intellectual demands must not be too low or too high. Third, the worker must gain some rewards other than money or prestige; the job must meet some value, need or goal. Last, the job must be in keeping with the individual's temperment and personality.

It is often helpful to have some procedure or criteria to evaluate how realistic a particular occupational choice is for a given client. A procedure I have found helpful for this purpose is described somewhat in a list of criteria for determining job readiness. These criteria are as follows:

A. Physical readiness
   1. Is the client at his maximum level of physical capacity?
   2. Can the client travel to and from a job?
   3. Can the client meet the physical demands of the kind of work sought?

B. Psychological readiness
   1. Do the client and his family accept his limitations?
   2. Do the client and his family recognize his capabilities?
   3. Is the client sincerely motivated toward employment?
   4. Can he adjust to the strains and pressure of a work environment?

C. Occupational readiness
   1. Are the client's aptitudes, skills, knowledge, and experience commensurate with job requirements, current and future?
   2. Is the client really interested in the job under consideration?
   3. Are the job's nonmonetary, psychological rewards in keeping with client's needs, values, and long-range goals?
   4. Is the client aware of opportunities and requirements for entrance into this field?
   5. Has the client's preparation been flexible enough for reassignment to other jobs or tasks?

D. Placement readiness
   1. To what extent can the client participate in the job-finding process?
   2. Does the client know sources of job leads?
   3. Can he develop a personal information packet?
   4. Can he satisfactorily complete an application?
   5. Can he present himself adequately in a job interview?

Problem Areas in Placement

Basically, there are four problem areas in placement. First, there is the employer with negative ideas. Examples are that (1) blind people have lower production rates and greater absenteeism; (2) they can perform only a limited number of jobs, leading to inflexibility of personnel; (3) fellow workers do not like to be "around" blind persons while others resent special consideration and generate feelings of concern which interfere with dismissal policies.

Second, the attitudes of the community and society often are such that employment for the blind person is rendered difficult in certain areas. Placement can be better facilitated when the community is made aware of the potentialities of the blind and when all community resources, public and private, accept responsibility for changing negative attitudes towards the employment of the blind.

Third, we must have a product to sell—a blind person brought to employers with qualifications of high motivation and good training as basic fundamentals, an individual who is carefully prepared to fulfill a contributing role in industry and society.

Last, but by no means least, is the attitude of the counselors who may not be completely convinced that the client he is trying to place can perform well on the job. When the counselor realizes that he has a fine product to offer in the form of rehabilitated personnel, his job of placement will become easier and more pleasant and rewarding. Placement in remunerative employment is simply the final step in the process of career planning and is thus a primary reason for evolving a plan in the first place. In other words, the real test of the effectiveness of the rehabilitation plan evolved jointly by counselor and client is to be found in the degree to which it produces satisfactory employment in the selected occupation.

Since this is the case, it seems logical to assume that the counselor should be heavily involved in helping a client to complete his career plan by assisting in obtaining for him the kind of employment the plan was designed to produce. With respect to jobs in industrial, service and clerical occupations, this means that the counselor will intercede directly with the employer on the client's behalf; in the case of a professional occupation, although the client must ultimately "sell himself," the counselor will demonstrate his interest and involvement by discussing with the client important aspects of the interview, helping in the preparation of a resumé, suggest appropriate contacts with employers and professional associations and generally be available for consultation. The counselor, viewing placement from this perspective, will be more effective in working with the client to develop a realistic employment plan.

Selective Placement

Much has been said about selective placement, about knowing the client and going out to get a specific job for a specific client —the old cliche, "Fit the man to the job or the job to the man." Others have said to approach an employer only for a specific job and only for a specific client. I am sure many clients have been placed in this manner, but I believe more effective programs of placement can be implemented through the broader concept of building and maintaining employment resources in which blind persons can be placed. This can be done best in a two-phase approach wherein the counselor incorporates into his work schedule specific plans for calling on employers and selling them on the proposition that qualified blind persons properly placed can compete safely and efficiently in the world of work. This means not waiting until a client is ready for work but calling on employers and selling a concept about blindness and about what blind people can do in the world of work. In approaching an employer the counselor should have not one but several clients in mind who are candidates for employment. The counselor must then proceed to facilitate the development of a receptive attitude toward the abilities of blind persons and bring to the employer's attention jobs in his own company which may lend themselves to being performed efficiently without vision. It would seem that if we sell the concept that there are a number of jobs that can be performed without sight, a blind person who is used to performing tasks without vision should certainly be able to handle such a job as well as or better than a seeing person.

There seem to be at least two ways to promote this concept and to sell the abilities of blind persons. We can show the employer that there are a number of things we do each day without sight from sheer habit. Examples are tieing neckties, shaving, tieing shoes, and typing. Also, we can sell or promote jobs for people without sight through showing an employer pictures, slides and filmstrips of blind persons working competitively on a variety of jobs ranging from machine operation to computer programming.

As a phase of placement, the counselor should help the employer resolve his fears and questions about what blindness does to an individual and to point out positive features such as loyalty, dependability and improvement of morale which a qualified blind employee can provide. The counselor also must go into the plant with the employer to realistically assess the visual requirements and thereby determine jobs that can be done without sight. During this phase, the counselor must help the employer come to understand that blind individuals can perform safely and can meet production standards. The counselor must see the types of jobs involved and do a job analysis on selected jobs. Through job analysis, he and the employer should reach an agreement that the selected job can be performed without sight and that since there are no visual requirements, why not employ a blind person for that particular job?

The counselor must then match the needs of the employer and the requirements of the job with appropriate skills of qualified clients. The use of these procedures will increase the counselor's chances of developing appropriate job opportunities, thus decreasing the length of time a client will have to wait for placement after becoming job-ready.

Placement and the development of an employment program

can best be achieved in a five-step process. The first step is called *precontact planning.* During this step the counselor is developing working relationships with community agencies such as the Chamber of Commerce, State Employment Office, civic clubs, apprenticeship councils, employer associations, labor unions, and so forth in order to get information about prospective employers which will help him to plan a more effective sales presentation. The counselor must plan for the interview so that he can get the attention and interest of the employer, and strive to meet some need of the employer. Some of the information needed about employers includes product or service, kinds of jobs, seasonal trends, turnover, size of plant, location, hiring practices, type of ownership, management structure, flexibility required, union, job openings, person responsible for the hiring, and anything else that will help in the planning or drawing up of a "plan of action" to meet the employer's needs.

The *approach,* then, is the actual sales presentation designed to convince the prospective employer of the advantages accruing to his organization by employing a qualified blind person. Sales people say that there are five stages through which we must move a customer for a successful sale. First, we must get his attention. Second, we must create interest. Third, we must create desire. Fourth, we must develop conviction. Fifth, we must promote action. The approach, then, is presenting logical reasons why an employer should work with the counselor and the agency for effective and selective placement.

The *demonstration* includes going into the plant or business to see the type of jobs in the flow of material. During this step, the counselor conducts a plant survey and completes job analyses on selected jobs. The plant survey, when properly conducted, can demonstrate that there are many jobs which can be performed safely and efficiently without sight. In addition, the plant survey can help the counselor answer questions about safety and flexibility that often are concerns of the employer in hiring the blind person. Job analysis in this step should be divided into two phases. The first is the standard four-part job analysis formula: what the worker does, how he does it, why he does it, and the skills required to do it. The second phase is composed of discovering how else each task can be performed, what extra skills are required in doing them, and what safety patterns can be established in performing each task. It is important to note here that a job can be performed without sight only if a four-point safety pattern can be established. This includes the following: (1) There must be a safe approach to the machine; (2) he must be able to safely determine if the machine is in a state of rest or motion; (3) there must be a safe path to the controls and back; and (4) there must be ways to follow the progress of the machine.

The fourth step in the placement process covers *putting the blind individual on the selected job* after agreement has been reached that a job can be performed without sight. The counselor *must* go with the blind individual and make himself available to assist both the worker and the supervisor in the process of orientation to the job. Many employers and many sighted coworkers are still concerned about how to communicate with a blind person; therefore, for successful adjustment, the counselor must make himself available for counseling during this crucial period.

The fifth step in the process is *follow-up*. Follow-up is the guarantee that the placement will be successful. In this step the counselor assures the employer that the services of the counselor and the agency always will be available to him in order to develop a good worker. During follow-up, the counselor should determine if adjustment is needed. Also, the counselor should provide the client with necessary information and support. From an employer's standpoint, follow-up evidences interest in the employee's welfare and in the ultimate satisfaction of the employer. Follow-up guards against the three main concerns or questions employers have today—safety, flexibility, and what to do if the blind person does not turn out to be a good employee. Even in slow economic periods, employers are interested in *good* workers; thus, if the counselor is successful in persuading the employer that a qualified blind person will be a good employee, job opportunities will be developed and blind persons will fill them.

REFERENCES

Bauman, Mary K. and Yoder, Norman M.: *Placing the Blind and Visually Handicapped in Professional Occupations.* Washington,

D. C., Office of Vocational Rehabilitation, Dept. of HEW, 1962.

Bauman, Mary K. and Yoder, Norman M.: *Placing the Blind and Visually Handicapped in Clerical, Industrial and Service Fields.* Harrisburg, Pa., Pennsylvania Office for the Blind, 1963.

Borow, Henry (Ed.): *Man in a World at Work.* Boston, Houghton, 1964.

Carroll, Rev. Thomas J.: *Blindness: What It Is, What It Does and How to Live With It.* Boston, Little, 1961.

Crawford, Fred L.: *Career Planning for the Blind.* New York, Farrar, Straus, 1966.

Hardy, Richard E.: Counseling physically handicapped college students. *New Outlook for Blind, 59*:5:182-183, 1965.

Hardy, Richard E.: Relating psychological data and job analysis information in vocational counseling. *New Outlook for Blind, 63*: 7:202-204, 1969.

Hoppock, Robert: *Occupational Information.* New York, McGraw-Hill, 1963.

Magers, George A.: *New Careers for the Blind.* Contemporary papers, vol. 4, American Association of Workers for the Blind, Inc. Washington, D. C., October 1969.

Oberman, C. Esco: *A History of Vocational Rehabilitation in America,* Minneapolis, Denison, 1965.

Peters, Herman J. and Hansen, James C. (Eds.): *Vocational Guidance and Career Development.* New York, MacMillan, 1966.

Sinick, Daniel (prep.): *Placement Training Handbook.* Washington, D. C. Office of Vocational Rehabilitation, 1962.

Thomason, Bruce and Barrett, Albert: *The Placement Process in Vocational Rehabilitation Counseling.* U. S. Department of Health Education, and Welfare, Vocational Rehabilitation Administration, Washington, D. C. 1960.

17

Vocational Placement and Blindness

Richard E. Hardy

There are many commonalities between approaches to the placement of the generally handicapped and those persons who are visually handicapped. Many persons who have visual problems also have a second handicap. The purpose of this chapter is to provide general information which will be useful in vocational placement.

One of the most substantial contributions a rehabilitation counselor can make which affects his client's overall mental and physical adjustment is the placement of the individual on a job that is well suited to his abilities and interests. Vocational placement is underrated by many rehabilitation counselors and others who do not understand the full effects of its outcome. Helping the client find employment is often relegated to scanning newspaper want ads in search of opportunities or responding to a call from an employer who happens to have a job available. Certainly, occupational opportunities can be located through these means; however, the matching of the individual and the job is a complicated process which requires careful study and evaluation through interrelating all casework data on the individual with all information that can be secured relating to job requirements and job settings.

VOCATIONAL PLACEMENT OF BLIND PERSONS

Blindness is a severe disability, and the counselor concerned with the placement of blind persons must be certain that the placement program is carefully planned. No magic is involved in the placement of the blind in competitive employment; however, a great deal of hard work and effective public relations are necessary.

There are many special considerations and much pertinent information with which the placement counselor must be very familiar. For instance, he should have some understanding of the physiological aspects of loss of sight. Such information can be obtained through the study of the medical aspects of blindness. The counselor will need to have answers readily available to many questions concerning the client's adjustment, his ability to communicate with others, to get to his work station, and to get to and from work. The better the counselor understands his client, the more effective he will be in vocational placement. One of the most important concepts for the counselor to remember in working with blind persons is that blind persons are people first and blind second. There are varying levels of potential according to the individual's personality and general intelligence.

A very important aspect of the placement of blind persons concerns getting the client psychologically ready for employment. He must believe in his own ability to do the work which is necessary and he must have confidence in the counselor's judgment concerning the types of jobs he can perform.

Blind workers have proven themselves over the years to be safe, dedicated, loyal, and low in absenteeism (American Mutual Insurance Alliance). Job opportunities for blind persons cover a very wide range and no list of jobs that blind people can perform is ever appropriate or complete. When he is helping the blind person decide on his vocational future, the counselor should remember that key sources of information for counseling are the client himself and his family. Counselors must move away from stereotyping jobs for blind persons and toward innovative placement. A great deal of information must be acquired about the client through interviews and counseling sessions with him and his family. It can be highly effective in counseling and phychological evaluation of blind persons to ask about the types of job fields they would be most interested in if they were fully sighted. This allows a broad vocational exploration which brings out many possible areas for consideration. Often, jobs in the suggested fields or in closely related ones are feasible.

The counselor concerned with the placement of blind persons will find that many industrial jobs do not require sight. Some of the jobs which do not require sight are the very ones which employers and counselors have thought definitely required sight. Blind persons, according to the legal definition, may have various amounts of vision up to 20/200 in the best eye with best correction or a visual field not exceeding an angle greater than 20 degrees (Jones, 1962). The counselor will have to know his client physically, psychologically, and socially and proceed with the placement plan after all information has been carefully studied and interrelated. Jobs can be evaluated with specific clients in mind or the counselor can approach the evaluation of jobs with various levels of required vision in mind. Again, the key to successful placement is careful planning. The counselor must think of various contingent possibilities. It is most helpful to observe workers performing jobs and to talk with them concerning all aspects of the jobs under observation, including whether they continue to do the job under consideration hour after hour, day after day without modification during all periods and seasons. This approach is often necessary in evaluating the job for a blind worker.

Generally speaking, blind persons continue to need the rehabilitation counselor in a salesmanship capacity. Most blind persons need help in selling their abilities to perspective employers. This is another reason why the work of vocational placement in rehabilitation counseling of blind persons has great importance.

The remaining sections of this chapter will offer various types of information which will be useful to the rehabilitation counselor serving blind individuals.

A Science of Vocational Behavior

Lofquist and Davis (1969) discussed a "science of vocational behavior" which they see as essentially vocational psychology. Whether one agrees or not that the science of vocational behavior is actually vocational psychology, the necessity for the full development of vocational behavior study as a science cannot be over stressed. The substantial growth during recent years of interest in the Vocational Evaluation and Work Adjustment Division of the National Rehabilitation Association and the subsequent publication of the *Vocational Evaluation and Work Adjustment Bulletin* have done a great deal to stimulate thinking and research on vocational behavior and practical problems of the individual and groups in the world of work. Certainly, in the future, vocational adjustment studies and work evaluation will take an even more prominent place in the rehabilitation counselor's work and in rehabilitation counselor education within university settings.

Above all, the rehabilitation counselor must be able to understand the "work personality" of his client. The "work personality profile" consists of such factors as vocational and avocational interests; abilities, needs, work habits; psychological maturity; and interaction with on-the-job factors including job hierarchies, communication, and health factors.

The rehabilitation counselor interested in developing expertise in placement should become familiar with available research on work adjustment. Studies done in vocational rehabilitation at the University of Minnesota (Lofquist, 1957) since 1957 offer a great deal of useful information.

Client-Centered Placement

Rehabilitationists have heard much about "client-centered counseling" over the years. Because placement is an important part of the rehabilitation process, counselors should think of "client-centered placement." Job placement is a major client service which has helped rehabilitation agencies in getting substantial amounts of federal and state funds for program operations. The goal of work is one of the unique characteristics of rehabilitation. The placement of individuals on jobs through which they can find methods to maintain themselves is the concept which has allowed rehabilitation counseling to gain in stature as a social service profession with a substantial contribution to make to the individual and to society. In fact, most laymen would probably say that the location of appropriate jobs for clients is the main function of the rehabilitation counselor. It is interesting that rehabilitation counselors downplay the importance of placement in their jobs when they describe their activities to their friends and colleagues. Counselors might reflect more seriously upon their placement responsibilities if clients were thought of as consumers of their services and were given an opportunity to actually evaluate the jobs which they have obtained with the help of the counselor.

In fact, the use of the phrase "PLACE in employment" is one which misleads the rehabilitation counselor trainee and others concerning the method which should be used. The client and counselor must work together in order for the client to reach a decision concerning the type of job he wishes to have. After this decision is made and the rehabilitation counselor helps the client secure information about various jobs that exist in the geographical area where he wants to be employed, the client himself should take some initiative whenever possible to get employment with the assistance of the counselor. Once a feasible job is located, the client should be given the opportunity to evaluate it as the source of his future livelihood.

Quite often, when considering placement, the counselor is confronted with the dilemma of determining to whom he owes basic loyalty, the client or the employer; that is, should he be protective of the client when dealing with an employer or protective of the employer. How much of the client's problems and disability should the counselor relate to the employer? Should he obscure the client's disability in discussion with the employer?

If the professional relationship was bilateral and concerned only the client and counselor, the answer to the dilemma would be immediately obvious; however, the relationship is trilateral.

Client
↗↙ ↖↘
Counselor ⟷ Employer

As such, the counselor owes equal professional responsibility to both the client and prospective employer. Therefore, the counselor should communicate with the employer in a basic, forthright manner. The counselor is professionally obligated to be honest in his dealings with the employer.

If the counselor fails to be completely honest and forthright with the employer, he not only jeopardizes his professional relationship with this employer, thereby obviating any possibility of placing clients in this area in the future, but he also takes a great chance of jeopardizing the client-employer relationship later when the employer becomes more aware of the client's attributes which the counselor chose to hide or misrepresent. Consequently, I feel rather strongly that the counselor should discuss with the client what he is planning to relate to the employer. If the client refuses to allow the counselor to discuss his assets, liabilities and disability with the employer, the counselor should modify his role in the placement process. His role should be one of providing placement information to the client, but he should not enter actively into the placement process with the client.

There are two limits to this interchange between the counselor and employer relative to the client and they are the following:

1. The counselor and employer should discuss thoroughly those aspects and only those aspects of the client's background which have a direct relation with the job.

2. The counselor should communicate with the employer on a level at which both are comfortable in the exchange of information.

Quite often a counselor approaches a prospective employer regarding a specific client and as the conversation progresses, the counselor finds himself relating information which, while highly pertinent in the rehabilitation process, has little to do with the client as an employee. In each instance in which the counselor makes an employee contact for placement purposes, the counselor should have previously summarized all material in the case folder which is directly related to the client's proficiency in a particular position—both his assets and liabilities. After reviewing this summary, the counselor should refrain from relating any other information he may have derived from counseling sessions, training evaluations, or diagnostic work-ups. A mark of professionalism is the ability to communicate the essential factors relating to the client and still respect the client's fundamental right to confidentiality of case material.

The second limitation to communication between the counselor and employer requires the counselor to assess the sophistication of the employer and to communicate with him on that level. As a general rule, the counselor should avoid using terminology which, though descriptive, is highly laden with emotional connotations. The most effective approach the counselor can take in discussing the client's assets and liabilities is to describe behavior rather than categorizing behavior with diagnostic labels. It is much more effective to relate to an employer that a client experienced learning difficulties in the academic areas rather early and is slow in learning new procedures, is ineffective in dealing with abstract concepts and carrying out complex, oral instructions and should not be placed in a situation requiring independent judgments in changing conditions but that he is very adept in performing concrete forms of tasks and is capable of making routine, repetitive judgments, than to relate to the employer merely that the client is a mental retardate and assume the employer is sophisticated enough to translate this diagnostic label into behavioristic terms as described above rather than stereotyping the client immediately with a diagnostic label.

Developing an Employment Program

Counselors who are involved with placement should be familiar with information offered in the publication, *Workers Worth Their Hire* (American Mutual Insurance Alliance), which is available through the President's Committee on Employment of the Physically Handicapped. Myths concerning employment of the handicapped are dispelled by information given in this publication. Counselors will find that discussions of the excellent record of handicapped persons in such areas as safety, absenteeism, production, and motivation to work are of considerable help to them in their discussion with employers, union leaders, and work supervisors. The counselor should be certain that he not only talks about these factors with top agency employment officials, but also that he manages, at the appropriate time, to mention these subjects to supervisors within the work area. The degree of acceptance which supervisors give to handicapped clients is often highly influential in not only helping them "get off to a good start" but also in maintaining their work at a level commensurate with the supervisor's expectations.

Some rehabilitation counselors have felt that the counselor should not have a specific client in mind when talking with an employer, but that he should sell the concept of hiring the handicapped to the employer and later get into the work setting in order to locate the types of jobs which would be available to handicapped individuals. This concept can be extremely useful and can help open many doors to blind employees; however, after convincing the employer of the value of hiring blind persons, the counselor often will be asked to refer a prospective employee immediately if a particular opening exists in the work setting. If a counselor is unable to meet this request, his public relations and sales program can be substantially damaged in terms of future placements with the employer.

Each rehabilitation counselor should constantly evaluate his efforts in placement to make certain that he is moving clients toward jobs in line with their overall adjustment and ability. One of the key sources of learning about job opportunities for any client is often the client's past experiences and previous job responsibilities. In many cases, clients will wish to return to the type of employment held prior to the onset of the employment handicap. In fact, many former employers will feel a responsibility for injured employees and wish again to offer them employment after they have received rehabilitation services. The client will offer many insights about himself to the counselor who then has the responsibility to match abilities, needs, and interests of the client with requirements and offerings of the job. One of the primary sources, then, of information about types of employment for the client is the client himself. This information can be gained by a study of his background and from interest inventories and interviews with him and his family.

The counselor will also wish to use the services of the state employment agency which maintains local offices throughout the United States. Many prospective employers inform the employment service of job openings. This agency also offers counseling, placement, and evaluation services for handicapped job applicants. The Vocational Rehabilitation Act, Public Law 89-565, stipulates that the vocational rehabilitation state plan shall "provide for entering into cooperative agreements with the system of public employment offices in the state and the maximum utilization of the job placement and employment counseling services and other services and facilities of such offices."

Questions Counselors Must Be Able to Answer

Of course, many different problem areas can arise when the counselor is discussing hiring handicapped workers with an employer. Questions range from "How will the person get to the place of employment?" to "What will he do in case of fire?" Incidentally, these two questions usually can be answered with the same responses which any employee would give (in the first case, "By bus or car," and in the second, "Get the hell out like everyone else.")

The first basic question which usually arises is that of increased insurance rates if handicapped workers are employed. This is most often an honest employer reaction to the question concerning employment of handicapped workers. Insurance rates would rise if individuals were employed in an agency which tended to have more accidents; however, handicapped workers have been proven to be as safe in the performance of their duties as other workers. In fact, some handicapped persons such as the blind have actually shown better records of safety than nonhandicapped workers. The counselor should have this information readily available and indicate to the prospective employer that indeed, workmen's compensation insurance rates are determined, in part, according to the relative hazards of the work done by the industry in question. Yearly rates also are determined according to the industry's record of accidents and insurance claims. These are good reasons for hiring handicapped workers. If an employer persists in believing that his insurance rates will increase, the counselor should ask him to contact his insurance agent or read again his insurance contract.

A second question which often arises is this: "Why should I hire a handicapped individual when I can employ normal persons whom I can count on for employment without difficulty?"

The counselor will have to answer this question according to his own philosophy and training. Some helpful responses might include the following:

1. Asking why he should not employ individuals whose em-

ployment records have been proven and who are well known and highly recommended by rehabilitation employment specialists.

2. Describing the medical, social, and psychiatric evaluations completed on all clients (not being specific or violating confidentiality). In other words, why not hire an individual who comes to the employer in a sense "certified" as ready for employment?

3. Reminding him that he is actually supporting what he, as a taxpayer, has already invested some money in—an employment program for the handicapped which has proven to be highly successful.

Another question which frequently is raised in employment interviews concerns the firing or dismissal of the employee and the employer's reluctance to treat the rehabilitant in the same manner as he would treat other employees. The counselor again will have to rely on his own resources; however, an analogy may be helpful here: If a salesman were selling refrigerators and the employer bought one which later malfunctioned, the salesman would stand by his product and attempt to get it in good working order. The counselor could briefly discuss follow-up procedures with the employer at this time. He might also indicate that once the handicapped employee has worked for the employer for a time, the employer will feel that he is a fully functioning, well-adjusted employee who should be treated just as all other employees are. The counselor should assure the employer of his confidence in the client.

A fourth question which counselors must be ready to answer concerns architectural barriers and physical limitations of the work setting. Counselors should be frank in their responses to questions concerning limitations of the client and restrictions imposed by the work setting. The counselor should be the first to indicate that certain jobs are infeasible for many of his clients. He should be certain to get across to the employer the fact that he is not going to place a blind person on an unsafe job or on a job which he cannot handle.

A fifth question which often arises concerning employment of the handicapped is that of the "second injury" which might result in total disability and affect the workmen's compensation payments made by the employer. In a vast majority of states and the

District of Columbia and Puerto Rico, "second injury" funds or equivalent arrangements have been established. In these localities, the employer is responsible only for the last injury and the employee is compensated for the disability which results from combined injuries.

Some Guidelines and Tools in Locating Employment Opportunities

The following are some suggestions:

1. The counselor should be aware of industrial developments within the area that he serves and in adjacent areas.

2. The three volumes of the *Dictionary of Occupational Titles* (1965) offer a wealth of useful information for rehabilitation counselors. Much emphasis is given to descriptions of physical and personality requirements for various jobs. In addition, these volumes can help expand the counselor's concepts about various types of jobs which are related to the general interest area of the rehabilitation client.

3. Employers with whom former clients have been placed can be important sources of information.

4. Previously rehabilitated clients can offer many sound ideas about existing employment opportunities.

5. Local chambers of commerce usually provide an industrial index which lists types of work available in their communities. Counselors also should coordinate their efforts with those of the state employment service since the mutual sharing of job information can be valuable to both employment service counselors and rehabilitation counselors.

6. When placing persons on jobs in rural areas, the worker should consider enlisting the support of local community leaders such as doctors, city councilmen, postmasters, and religious leaders as well as Rotary, Kiwanis, Ruitan and other civic groups.

7. If the counselor is interested in assisting individuals in becoming small business managers and operators, he should get in touch with the Small Business Administration office serving his local area.

Professional Placement

In rehabilitation jargon, "professional placement" generally means developing client employment opportunities which require at least a college education. Bauman and Yoder (1962) offer excellent coverage of this area of placement as it pertains to work for the blind. Professional placement is "facilitative" work for the counselor. The counselor can help his client in terms of giving advice and information; however, he must be certain not to take the place of the client in securing actual jobs. The client must be ready to meet with the employer without the counselor in order to discuss his professional qualifications for work. When he has a particular problem, the counselor should be able to assist him with information which could be helpful during the employer interview. For example, he should be coached on how to present himself most favorably. The counselor might help his client develop a resume or portfolio which would outline his training and give examples of any previous work done in the job field in which he wants employment. Other procedures usually followed in placement may or may not be appropriate according to the judgment of the counselor.

A worker in charge of professional placement may want to organize pre-college orientation groups for clients. It will be necessary also for the counselor who is dealing with persons in training to inform them about services available while they are in training and away from their home area. If, for instance, clients are attending college, the rehabilitation counselor should help them become acquainted with college counseling center services at the institution they attend (Hardy, 1965).

Effective professional placement requires long-range planning on the part of both counselor and client. Two years before placement (in training cases) is not too early for the client to begin planning with his counselor in order to solve problems related to his securing the type of employment he wants. The counselor will need to prepare by knowing who the prospective employers are and the requirements of the job.

Getting the Client Ready for Employment

Planning for placement does not begin once the client has

had vocational training and is ready "skillwise" for employment, but when the counselor first reads the client's rehabilitation referral form. The rehabilitation worker must constantly learn about his client in order to effectively help him secure the type of employment he needs. Jeffrey (1969) has developed a job readiness test which helps in the evaluation of job preparedness of clients. While the total instrument is not applicable to all rehabilitation clients, certain questions are quite helpful with most rehabilitation clients.

Role playing is an excellent method to use in preparing a client for employment interviews. After going through a mock interview which includes a variety of questions, the counselor can give suggestions concerning how the client might improve the impression he makes with the employer. In role playing, it is helpful for the counselor as well as the client to play the role of the employer. Once this is tried, counselors will immediately realize the usefulness of this procedure. The client should realize that getting a job is not an easy task and that he, to the best of his ability, should participate in the job-securing aspects of placement. In some cases, it is an indicator of effective rehabilitation procedures when the client is able to, in fact, "get his own job," assuming of course that he is ready for employment. The ability with which the client will be able to do this will vary with his motivation and the severity of his social, mental, or physical handicap.

The rehabilitation counselor must stress "training" as a partial answer to many of the problems of the handicapped worker. Overtraining a worker for a job which will affect his personal and family adjustment for many years to come is seldom done. In each case, the counselor must take an individual approach to helping his client. In the case of those who are educationally or socially retarded, various remedial programs may be necessary before actual work training programs can begin. In each case, the counselor must exercise considerable judgment concerning what his client needs in order to be totally ready for employment.

On-the-job training can be a very effective arrangement for client training. In many of these cases, the state rehabilitation agency will make "tuition" payments to the employer-trainer in order that the rehabilitation counselor may get the employer interested in training a client and evaluating his work. It may be necessary for the counselor to help the employer arrange the appropriate payment schedule for the client since he is not a trained employee and would not receive an amount equal to a regularly salaried employee.

Bridges (1946) offered four major factors which are involved in successful employment of handicapped workers. These remain as highly important considerations for the counselor and are listed below:

1. The worker should have the ability to accomplish the task efficiently, i.e. to be able to meet the physical demands of the job.
2. The worker should not be a hazard to himself.
3. The worker must not jeopardize the safety of others.
4. The job should not aggravate the disability or handicap of the worker.

Common Misconceptions about Vocational Placement

Misconceptions about vocational placement are as follows:

1. Because placement occurs toward the end of the rehabilitation process, the counselor's responsibility to the client diminishes.
2. Placement is an activity which requires no counselor training and is a matter of matching an available client with an available job.
3. Client location of his job ("self-placement") cannot be effective rehabilitation work.
4. When a client is ready for vocational placement, the information in his case folder is no longer of value to his counselor since the client has been, in a sense, readied for employment.
5. Follow-up after placement always can be handled easily by phone or mail communications with the employer or client.
6. Labor market trends and job information and analysis are the responsibilities of placement specialists and employment service counselors, not of general rehabilitation counselors.
7. An employer will notify the counselor and the rehabilitation agency when he is dissatisfied with a client placement.
8. An employer will automatically call upon the rehabilitation

agency to furnish him with additional employees when he needs them.

Rehabilitation counselors should be certain that their clients understand that it is not necessarily bad to be turned down for a job. Counselors should understand that experience has shown that nine or ten employer contacts often must be made before the counselor makes a placement.

Job Analysis

Every rehabilitation counselor should be thoroughly familiar with the techniques of job analysis for use in selective placement. The rehabilitation counselor has to be able to match the prospective worker's social, mental, and physical qualifications with requirements of the job. Factors such as judgment, initiative, alertness, and general health and capability must always be taken into consideration as well as the individual's social and economic background.

Job analysis should answer certain questions concerning the job. *What* does the worker do in terms of physical and mental effort that goes into the work situation? How is the work done? In other words, does this job involve the use of equipment, mathematics, or does it require travel. *Why* does the worker perform the job? This component of the job analysis answers the question concerning the overall purpose or the sum total of the task and is the reason for doing the job. The worker also should understand the relationship of his task to other tasks that make up the total job.

Generally, the rehabilitation counselor should attempt to place clients on jobs which they can "handle" and which do not require modification. In some cases, however, minor modifications can be made with little or no reengineering effort. The counselor will have to be careful in suggesting reengineering of a job, since this can be a costly undertaking in many instances. The major objective should be that of helping handicapped workers integrate effectively into the total work force without major modification or change in the work situation.

The following outline can be used in evaluating a job which is to be performed by a handicapped worker:

1. Name used for position surveyed:
   a. D.O.T. title:
   b. Alternate titles:
   c. D.O.T. definitions:
   d. Items worked on in plant surveyed:
2. Usual operator:
   a. Sex:
   b. General characteristics:
3. Physical and psychological demands:
   a. Activities:
   b. Working conditions:
   c. Skill required:
   d. Intelligence:
   e. Temperament:
   f. Other:
4. Description of physical activities:
5. Description of working conditions:
6. Description of hazards:
7. Steps required to accomplish the goal of the work:
   a.
   b.
   c.
   d.
   e.
8. Equipment found in the particular plant surveyed:
   a. Identification:
   b. Set-up and maintenance:
   c. Modification (if required for blind persons):
9. Equipment variations which may be found in other plants:
10. Pre-employment training required:
11. Training procedure:
12. Production:
    a. Full production definition:
    b. Time to reach normal efficiency:
13. Interrelation with preceding and succeeding jobs:

Relating Psychological Data to Job Analysis Information in Vocational Placement

As a first step in getting to know clients well, the counselor should make arrangements to secure appropriate psychological information about them. He should either complete job analyses or use available job evaluation data to make decisions about types of information which will be of value to his clients in the job selection and placement procedure. In many instances, however, the counselor fails to synthesize information obtained from two of his most important sources: the psychological evaluation and the job analysis.

The counselor should take five basic steps, as described by Hardy (1969), in developing a successful procedure for interrelating and using important information. He should do the following:

1. Study the needs of the client and the types of satisfaction meaningful to him.

2. Make certain that valid psychological and job analysis data have been gathered.

3. Review the requirements of the job and evaluate the individual traits needed to meet job requirements.

4. Consider the environmental pressures with which the individual must interact.

5. Discuss the job analysis and psychological evaluation with the client so that he will understand what the work will require of him and what it will offer.

Both client and counselor need to have an understanding of job requirements in order to make realistic decisions. One important move should be structuring a set of goals—a guide to help the client avoid useless foundering that gets him nowhere. What satisfactions is he seeking? What is important to him in the long run and what types of work or work settings will provide these satisfactions? These are questions which the counselor must help the client answer.

Maslow (1954) has suggested a hierararchy of the individual needs which the counselor must understand in order to evaluate a client's psychological status—his satisfactions and frustrations. In the usual order of prepotency these needs are for the following:

1. Physiological satisfaction.
2. Safety.
3. Belongingness and love.
4. Importance, respect, self-esteem, independence.
5. Information.
6. Understanding.
7. Beauty.
8. Self-actualization.

In our society, there is no single situation which is potentially more capable of giving satisfaction at all levels of these needs than a person's work, and it is the responsibility of the counselor to help his counselee plan for future happiness through adjustment on the job.

The worker needs to help his client become fully aware of the social pressures of the job, because these are as important to the individual as the actual job pressures. A client's ability to adapt to the social interactions of the work environment will directly affect his job performance.

The counselor always must ask himself what the requirements of the job are. This questions can be answered superficially or in considerable detail. A lay job analysist can give superficial requirements, but the responsibility for an in-depth job description belongs to the expert—the counselor who will often have to give direct advice to the client.

Effective placement requires effective planning. Planning cannot be really useful unless appropriate information has been obtained, interrelated, and skillfully utilized so that the client and the counselor have a clear understanding of possible problems and possible solutions.

Follow-up after Placement

A rehabilitation counselor often is tempted to consider his job completed when the client is placed on a job which appears suitable for him; however, the phase of rehabilitation which begins immediately after the person has been placed in employment is one of the most complex. Follow-up involves the counselor's ability to work as a middleman between employer and client in order to help the client solve problems related to his handicap which may arise after being hired. The counselor must be diplomatic and resourceful in maintaining the employer's confidence in his client's ability to do the job. At the same time, he must let the client know that he has full faith in him. The counselor, however, must somehow evaluate how his client is performing on the job and make certain that he is available to help if problems arise which the client cannot solve.

In addition to the worker's service to the client during follow-up, this period can offer real public relations opportunities for the counselor, especially when the employer notes the interest with which the counselor "follows" his client. The frequency of follow-up varies according to the counselor's judgment of the client's job ability and adjustment.

Agency regulations usually require that a final follow-up be done after 30 days in order to make certain that placement is successful before a "case" can be closed as rehabilitated. Counselors should also consider follow-up periods of 60 to 80 days after placement. Again, this helps reassure the client of the interest of the agency and the counselor in his success and can be of value to the counselor in further developing employment opportunities for handicapped persons.

In follow-up after professional placement, however, the counselor must increase the 60- to 90-day period which is usually adequate in the placement of clients in nonprofessional jobs. A longer period will be necessary and this period will vary with job complications and severity of the client's handicap. Bauman and Yoder (1962) have recommended six months to a year for follow-up in most cases where blind persons have been placed in professional work.

Counselors will probably wish to schedule specific days for follow-up in the field. Generally, the period of follow-up is a time when the counselor sees the efforts of the entire rehabilitation process coming to fruition. If the job has been well analyzed and the client well evaluated and placed, follow-up will be a pleasurable experience for the counselor.

Summary

The counselor's responsibility in vocational placement must not be underrated. The decisions made at this stage in the rehabilitation process not only affect the client's immediate feelings of satisfaction and achievement but also, of course, his long-term physical and mental health. The counselor has a real responsibility to "ready" the client for employment by giving him the type of information that he needs about the job and about holding employment once it is achieved. Placement should be "client-centered" with strong emphasis given to the client's opinions about work and how it will affect him and his family. Counselors must be ready to answer the questions that employers will ask about hiring handicapped persons and about the rehabilitation program. Vocational placement is high level public relations work.

The counselor must be knowledgeable about job analysis and must interrelate all medical, psychological, and social data with job analysis information in order to be successful in client-centered placement. Once placement has been achieved, the counselor must follow-up the client in order to make certain that he is doing well on the job. The client should have an opportunity to evaluate his job and also the efforts of his counselor in helping him decide on and obtain the job. Effective placement requires effective planning, and counselors must constantly evaluate their knowledge of the world of work and their ability to interrelate information in order to assure real placement success.

REFERENCES

American Mutual Insurance Alliance: *Workers Worth Their Hire.* Chicago, Illinois.

Bauman, M. K. and Yoder, N. M.: *Placing The Blind and Visually Handicapped in Professional Occupations.* Office of Vocational Rehabilitation, Department of Health, Education and Welfare, Washington, D. C., 1962.

Bridges, C. C.: *Job Placement of the Physically Handicapped.* New York, McGraw-Hill, 1946.

Department of Veterans' Benefits, Veterans' Administration: *They Return to Work.* Washington, D. C., U. S. Government Printing Office, 1963.

Hardy, R. E.: Counseling physically handicapped college students. *New Outlook for Blind, 59*:5:182-183, 1965.

Hardy, R. E.: Relating psychological data to job analysis information in vocational counseling. *New Outlook for Blind, 63*:7:202-204, 1969.

International Society for the Welfare of Cripples: *Selective Placement of the Handicapped.* New York, 1955.

Jeffrey, David L.: Pertinent points on placement. *Clearing House,* Oklahoma State U., November 1969.

Jones, J. W.: Problems in defining and classifying blindness. *New Outlook for Blind, 56*:4:115-121, 1962.

Lofquist, L. H. and Davis, R. V.: *Adjustment to Work—A Psychological View of Man's Problems in Work-Oriented Society.* New York, Appleton, 1969.

McGowan, J. F. and Porter, T. L.: *An Introduction to the Vocational Rehabilitation Process.* Rehabilitation Services Administration, July, 1967.

McNamee, H. T. and Jeffrey, R. P.: *Service to the Handicapped 1960.* Phoenix, Arizona, Arizona State Employment Service, 1960.

Maslow, A. H.: A theory of human motivation. *Psychol. Rev., 50*:370-396, 1954.

Office of Vocational Rehabilitation. *Training Personnel for the State Vocational Rehabilitation Programs—A Guide for Administrators.* Washington, D. C., U. S. Government Printing Office, 1957.

Sinick, D.: *Placement Training Handbook.* Washington, D. C., Office of Vocational Rehabilitation, 1962.

Stalnaker, W. O., Wright, K. C., and Johnston, L. T.: *Small Business Enterprises in Vocational Rehabilitation.* U. S. Department of Health, Education, and Welfare, Vocational Rehabilitation Administration, Rehabilitation Services Series No. 63-47, 1963.

Thomason, B. and Barrett, A.: *The Placement Process in Vocational Rehabilitation Counseling.* U. S. Department of Health, Education, and Welfare, Office of Vocational Rehabilitation, GTP Bull. No. 2, Rehabilitation Services Series No. 545, 1960.

U. S. Employment Service: *Dictionary of Occupational Titles.* Washington, D. C., U. S. Government Printing Office, 1965.

U. S. Employment Service: *Selected Placement for the Handicapped* (Revised ed.), Washington, D. C., 1945.

Weiss, D. J., Davis, R. V., Lofquist, L. H., and England, G. W.: *Minnesota Studies in Vocational Rehabilitation.* University of Minnesota, Industrial Realtions Center. (Series published since 1954.)

18

Special Problems of the Blind in Rural Areas

William T. Coppage

This chapter will focus on some of the unique problems that are related to rehabilitation in its broadest sense; that is, not only vocational rehabilitation, but social rehabilitation and various other aspects of the complete rehabilitation process. "Habilitation" is part of the picture because those who work with congenitally visually handicapped children usually refer to their efforts as habilitation rather than rehabilitation.

LOCATING RURAL CLIENTS

Before any type of rehabilitation can begin, however, these individuals have to be found; we have to know about them. Once the referral is made, we do make initial contact. Often, contact is made in the individual's home rather than by his coming to the rehabilitation office. It is wise for counselors, particularly if they are not familiar with the part of the country in which they are going to visit their clients, to determine before they go where the individual lives and have some idea about how to get to his home. Otherwise, most of the workday can be spent finding his home.

Regardless of what the worker's profession might be—rehabilitation counselor or social welfare worker—it is always helpful to talk with the local welfare department caseworker who perhaps has known about the client or has been working with him previously. Another possible contact prior to the first visit is the referral source, assuming that some other community agency or some other individual in the community has made the referral to the agency. Certainly this individual or agency would be in a position to give helpful background information.

Because the client does live in a rural setting, statistics will bear out the fact that on the average he has probably had his disability longer and has been without services longer than the individual who lives in the city. The length of time between the event of disability and referral for services is quite likely to be longer for those in rural settings. This, in itself, can have some implications for workers in providing services, because if the individual has been isolated longer, his patterns of dependency are likely to be more "set" than those of a person referred earlier. Therefore, we will have this additional factor to take into account in planning an approach with these individuals. Of course, there are usually some things that may be on our side with individuals from a rural setting. Rural people and mountain folk are known to be independent by nature; but certainly, as with all individuals, when a traumatic condition is involved the family tends to be overprotective. This pattern can change, but the author's experience is that the nature of these individuals is pretty much toward independence, and this makes the rehabilitation job easier.

An important point to consider is the relationship which the individual has had with the family. Another characteristic of rural people is that families tend to be closer together and more interdependent so that we can develop within the family constellation some assets in our work with the individual. Not only is it important to work with the client in assessing his needs, but this cannot be done as successfully if carried on independently of the other family members.

Providing Services in a Rural Setting

If the counselor is working toward vocational rehabilitation of the individual, he must realize that the job opportunities in a rural area normally are not as diverse as they are in a less rural segment of the state, and therefore a number of factors will have to be taken into consideration as he makes his plans for the individual. First of all, how much adjustment training does the individual need and how can this need best be met? Depending again on the individual family circumstances, it may or may not be possible for the client to go to a rehabilitation center to receive adjustment training. If he has a wife and children, he is going to feel more obligation and more reason not to leave this type of family circumstance than if, perhaps, he is living with his parents. So, we have to discuss very early not only vocational potential and job opportunities with the individual, but we also have to relate these to the family situation.

If for some combination of circumstances it is not feasible for the individual to go to a rehabilitation center within his state or elsewhere, then the counselor is obliged to make some arrangements for needed vocational training or personal adjustment training. This can be done in a variety of ways, depending on the agency setting. In most agencies, the services are available from rehabilitation teachers who are trained in the skills of providing adjustment training within the client's home. This is an important resource, in addition to other resources available.

There are two basic patterns in providing adjustment training, and in some agencies in the country a third has more recently begun to develop. I have mentioned the rehabilitation center approach and the itinerant approach, which often is the label given to the rehabilitation teacher or team which might go into the home and provide the services there. A third approach which has been used quite successfully is that of local community adjustment training classes which are set up on a short-term basis.

In this approach, the mobility instructor, several rehabilitation teachers, and perhaps a rehabilitation counselor or two go into a community as a team. They "set up shop" in some local community setting—a recreation center, a church building, or some rented space—and operate a training program of short duration, perhaps two to three or four weeks. In this way it is possible to speed up the personal adjustment training process beyond what it would be if the client had to depend on individual lessons once or twice a week.

In these community classes there could be as many as eight or ten clients being served five days a week and having a variety of services provided in one setting. This approach is an improvement over having the rehabilitation teacher go in one day, the mobility instructor another day, and the counselor another day. Certainly the community adjustment training classes approach is preferable when it can be worked out and is of more benefit to the client than the lesson-by-lesson approach on an individual basis. This latter process is not as fast or complete as the training which can be provided in the rehabilitation center. But even though there are many more rehabilitation centers now (up to one in every state) there are still some individuals who, because of a combination of circumstances, will not leave their home communities to go away to the center to get needed services. So, in this respect perhaps, the rural client's problems are not too different from those of the individual who lives in the city or a more urban area of the state.

In thinking about rehabilitation counseling in the rural area, it might be well to cover types of jobs and the other aspects that have to be considered in the actual planning for vocational training, job placement, and so forth. A realistic goal must be selected with the individual. The client, after all, does live in the rural community, and in most rural communities his job opportunities are rather limited. Not only are job opportunities limited, but also the types of jobs available are more limited than they are in the urban areas of the state. Therefore, a counselor has to make a realistic assessment of the prevailing job market in the rural area. With a thorough knowledge of the job market, a counselor's assessment of the client's placement opportunities in that area is going to be easier as the rehabilitation process proceeds.

Farming is one natural vocation that we think of in relation to rural areas, and it is not an unrealistic job objective for the blind person. In Virginia's state program, successful placements have been made in quite a number of farm operations and farm endeavors for blind persons. Eight years ago in Virginia, we had a special project to demonstrate the feasibility of blind individuals being placed in a variety of farming operations, and this was quite successfully done.

Several projects have proved to be particularly well suited for blind individuals. One was the egg production business utilizing mobile trailers. Quite a profitable business can be established in the selling of eggs produced through this type of farm operation. Another successful project was called the "Pig Parlour." This, of course, consisted of raising and marketing hogs. Also, several blind clients were quite successfully placed or set up in business in beef operations or cattle raising. Few if any counselors are knowledgeable enough to know how to establish these businesses with a client, but there are experts available in all rural communities, specialists in the area of farming and in the area of livestock production. A booklet printed as a result of the Virginia project, entitled *Correlating Services Available to Farmers,* goes into some detail on each of the various areas of farm operations. This publication could be most helpful to counselors and to the community agricultural extension agent or other experts working on the case.

The labor market today embraces many employment opportunities in service occupations. Approximately 60 percent of all jobs in the labor market today are in this category. This percentage is much higher than it has been in the past, and I feel confident that as leisure time grows and there is more demand for leisure-type activities, the demand for workers in the service-type occupations will increase. These occupations represent an important area to be explored for possible job placement of the visually handicapped.

Because there are more job opportunities where more people are located and where there are more demands for services, it is not unusual—in fact it is quite common—for sighted people or people without an obvious disability to leave the rural area and go to the city to seek job opportunities. So, if it is not possible to place an individual or find a realistic job opportunity for him in his home community after completion of adjustment training and other training, then the counselor should look to the urban area for job placement possibilities.

Again, the importance of family counseling cannot be overemphasized because the success of any plan which we might develop for an individual is going to depend, in large measure, upon how the plan has been worked out with the other family members. The counselor has offered no service to the client if he has made him enthusiastic about leaving for training or for job placement when his wife or children may not be interested in leaving. We have to work with the family unit. If an individual lives with his parents, then again we have to work with the family but perhaps the problems are not quite of the same scope as they are when there is a family unit of husband, wife and children. Certainly, the same would be true of the client who is a housewife.

In evaluating the client's mobility, usually I have considered the male member of the family first. It is natural to think of the male as the breadwinner and he usually is, but certainly the client might sometimes be a housewife. In such instances, job placement often involves problems different from or in addition to those just mentioned. After the counselor has exhausted the possible placement opportunities in the home area and before he begins to plan for job opportunities outside the home area, he should objectively assess the family situation. He should be sure that the other family members are in accord with the objectives, for if the other family members are not sold on the plan, such planning might be unrealistic.

Educational services are another particular area in which we may have to approach the problems of a rural blind person somewhat differently. First, we have the basic assessment of the needs of the family, but beyond that, we need to know what services are available in the community for educating the blind child. In assessing the available schools and facilities, it is important to know—and the counselor can find out only by contacting the school officials—what programs, if any, are available in the area of special education. Do these programs in any way meet the needs of blind children? Have teachers been trained in the education of the visually handicapped? Have they previously had blind students in the classroom? We need to know to what extent the schools are prepared to teach blind children, and in some cases, we need to know whether the schools are willing to do so. Often, school personnel are willing to accept help from available resources such as the state department of education or the state agency for the blind and visually handicapped. This assistance usually provides an opportunity to learn from educational consultants how to work with these children in the classroom. But often, even in today's society, school officials will not entertain the idea of having a blind child in the classroom. We have a selling job to do. In spite of our best efforts, we still are not going to always be successful in gaining immediate acceptance of the thought of serving a blind child in the local public school. This may be particularly true in rural areas. The specialist would make a mistake in trying to place a child in a school where local school officials have to be forced to take the child. In that case, I would suspect that the state's residential school for the blind would probably offer the best opportunity to meet the needs of the particular child. I will not permit myself to be drawn into the argument, if there is one, about the advantages of the residential school over the public school or vice versa. I think each still has its place and can meet the needs of particular individuals. I think that there will be a need for both types of educational opportunities for blind children in the foreseeable future.

I feet strongly that when good "schooling" is not available to the child in his home community, placement in a residential school should be considered. As difficult as it might be for the specialist to encourage the parents who are faced with the prospect of the child leaving home for practically nine months out of the year, it is to the child's benefit for him to do so. This is certainly preferable to having the child stay at home and not receive needed educational services.

Many rehabilitation teachers work with children of school age who have not been successfully placed in an educational program. Some teachers work with children who are actually placed in a local school setting because there are proportionately so few children in the rural area. The teacher in whose classroom the child is placed is not likely to have the special skills and knowledge that a teacher specially trained in work with the visually handicapped would have. So, the rehabilitation teacher might be called upon to provide lessons in braille for these children. This often is the only source of braille instruction for the children since the classroom teacher does not know how to teach braille reading and writing. Later on, in junior and senior high school, the mobility instructor will no doubt be called upon to provide basic instruction in mobility skills and orientation techniques.

Certainly, proficiency in all of the travel techniques needed to cross busy city streets is different from the skills that one must have to go from the barn to the pasture, back to the house and so forth. There are thus some basic differences employed in travel training in the two settings.

It is absolutely necessary to remember that rehabilitation is always a team effort. In remote areas, the rehabilitation specialist —whether he is a rehabilitation teacher, counselor, or social worker—will have to call upon various other professional persons in the field of rehabilitation as well as those outside of rehabilitation. In the latter category are county agents, home demonstration agents, agricultural and home economics teachers and rehabilitation's usual allies: public health and social service personnel, ministers and other concerned community leaders.

In summary, when we attempt to rehabilitate any client we must take into consideration whatever special problems or assets he has in terms of his own personality characteristics, his family and their reaction to his disability, and the geographic area in which he lives. Because handicapped persons who live in rural areas often wish to remain in these areas, special problems frequently confront rehabilitation specialists. However, by working cooperatively with local resource people and by selling the concept of rehabilitation and productivity, the counselor will often find working with rural clients a most rewarding experience.

19

Community Resources and Services Available to Blind Persons

Keith C. Wright

The newly employed rehabilitation worker for the blind soon realizes that neither he nor his agency are able to solve all of the problems of blindness. The problems of one individual or of one family often require services from several professional persons and agencies. Within a very short time he learns that problems of disability and problems accompanying disability cannot be dealt with within one system, one agency, or one profession.

The community houses a wide variety of agencies and programs for its citizens, and it soon becomes apparent to the newly employed rehabilitation worker that his community is organized in some fashion to help the handicapped. He discovers that he is in the midst of several communities. Examples of such are the medical community, the academic community, the social service community, and others.

One of the major problems which the newly employed rehabilitation worker encounters is that of becoming acquainted with the wide variety of agencies and services available in his community. Governmental agencies with their national, state, and local counterparts function alongside citizen groups and voluntary agencies. Scores of agencies and associations exist, and within these have developed hundreds of programs aimed toward meeting the needs of people.

With this proliferation of agencies and services, problems for the rehabilitation worker for the blind become apparent. He must first determine what services are available in his own agency, and then become acquainted with other available community services. Even more important, he must develop a system for getting his clients into the service systems of other agencies.

Generally speaking, delivery systems in most communities are not well thought out, well organized, or well developed. Most do not have clear-cut lines of responsibilities and congruent goals. There are a variety of reasons for this such as the mere fact of the proliferation of professional disciplines, volunteer personnel, and vested interest groups.

The newly employed rehabilitation worker soon learns that rehabilitation concepts and principles are based on teamwork. He also realizes at the same time that teamwork is more often preached than practiced, and that however proficient an agency or institution may be in fulfilling its purpose, it cannot meet all human needs and cannot serve all human beings equally well. He recognizes the fact that the needs of people are too many and diverse. This leads him to recognize the multiplicity of problems which develop due to blindness and the interrelationships of these problems. With this recognizition, he then develops an understanding of the need for coordinated and cooperative efforts to solve them. The multiple problems induced by blindness clearly demonstrate the "clustering principle." The effect of the clustering of such problems as loss of sight, limitation of mobility, loss of communication skills, problems in the general areas of daily living, marital problems, emotional problems, and unemployment problems is indeed profound. Furthermore, it has been demonstrated and observed that serious illness or behavioral problems in one member of a family invariably are reflected in the health and the well-being of the entire family unit.

Understanding the clustering principle is important if the rehabilitation worker is to provide comprehensive and meaningful services to his blind clients and their families. Recognition of this principle also should give more meaning to the importance of developing an effective community resource utilization program. The development of such a community resource program means that the counselor or rehabilitation worker must not be bound to his desk or his office. It means that he must get out into the community and become acquainted with other people in other agencies. He must interpret his agency services and develop a relationship between the various community service systems. Professional isolationism must become tabu and a smooth merging of many professional skills becomes a necessity for comprehensive and meaningful services. No one professional worker nor a series of professionals working one at a time can accomplish the necessary rehabilitation task. People must work together, all at once, if they are to come up with the best answers for their handicapped clients. Community resource utilization means effective interagency cooperation and interdisciplinary teamwork.

Newly employed rehabilitation workers for the blind will need a considerable amount of time in order to get acquainted with all of the available resources in the community. It takes time and personal contact to establish effective working relationships with the variety of resources and persons in any community. It is imperative, therefore, that the rehabilitation worker develop an itinerary which will afford the opportunity for the development of necessary contacts.

Rehabilitation workers for the blind should set aside each week a specified amount of time for community relations and community contact work. Perhaps this amount of time should be the equivalent of one day per week. The itinerary should be well developed with scheduled appointments and names of persons to contact. It is through this itinerary that the rehabilitation worker for the blind can develop a community teamwork approach to services for the blind.

The establishment of community teamwork is essentially a process in itself which can begin with the preparation of a well-organized regularly scheduled itinerary. Getting acquainted is the first step in establishing effective community resource utilization. Once the formalities of introduction are achieved, the rehabilitation worker can then move toward the exchange of information and with this exchange he can establish the relationship between the community resource and the rehabilitation program which he represents. At that point the rehabilitation worker can move toward the establishment of referral action which would be followed by joint planning and coordination with concurrent cooperative services.

There are, however, several problems inherent in developing effective community resource activities. One of the major problems centers around the lack of knowledge. Agencies and professionals in these agencies often become so involved in their "own little world" that they fail to establish effective working relationships outside agency bounds. It is necessary to keep in mind that the rehabilitation worker basically coordinates and supplements community services to the disabled.

Another barrier to effective resource utilization centers around personnel turnover within agencies. This fact, incidentally, indicates that maintenance of effective community relationships is an on-going activity.

Another barrier to teamwork is the stereotyping of professionals and agencies. We could, of course, add problems of vested interest, professional jealousies, and so forth. Effective community resource utilization necessitates an understanding and acceptance of differences among ourselves as professional persons to the same extent that we try to do this with our clients.

A typical day's itinerary for community service development might include one or two regularly scheduled weekly meetings with the rehabilitation worker's counterpart in the welfare office and the employment service office. It might include one or two visits to local physicians and ophthalmologists as well as a scheduled visit to a plant or job survey. Time should be scheduled for follow-up purposes with employers who have employed rehabilitated clients. It would be appropriate for this itinerary to include at least one new employer or business, one or more employers for follow-up and one or more visits to cooperating agencies who serve people in the community. The wide variety of community resources available in most communities would assure that this one-day itinerary would not be static but would offer a variety of visits each week, and would provide the opportunity to meet with clients who have been placed as well as the opportunity to find new clients within the community.

Generally speaking, the rehabilitation worker for the blind utilizes the same community resources as the general rehabilitation counselor. There is, of course, some modification due to the disability itself. For instance, the rehabilitation worker for the blind must necessarily know the ophthalmologist in his area and the otologist and audiologist. Quite often he utilizes the services of the adjustment center.

Although the rehabilitation worker utilizes the same general community services, it soon becomes apparent that he must become more involved in interpretation of abilities of the blind. Many people in the general public as well as employers are fearful of associating or working with the blind. Many people actually believe that the majority of blind persons must settle for sheltered work environments. Therefore, with public attitudes and fears in mind, the rehabilitation worker for the blind may have to deal with more severe problems than those of the general rehabilitation worker.

SOME SELECTED COMMUNITY RESOURCES FOR THE REHABILITATION WORKER

The *state employment service* should serve as a good source of referral for rehabilitation, and the rehabilitation worker should recognize the employment service for its special abilities in placement. The employment service is more familiar with job openings and job requirements than any other organization. Each employment service office has designated a person to serve as a counselor for the disabled, and the rehabilitation worker for the blind should know this person in his own locality.

State welfare departments provide a variety of services which could be of help to the rehabilitation worker. This department can provide assistance to family members when the rehabilitation worker has entered into the rehabilitation program with the family breadwinner. Family assistance by this department during this time could enhance the rehabilitation plan of the client. The welfare department also provides aid-to-the-blind benefits and a good source for cooperative programming. Most state welfare departments have entered into written agreements with the state vocational rehabilitation agency and agencies serving the blind, and these agreements describe the contributions of each in a typical cooperative program.

Most communities have a *family and children's service society* which provides a variety of services which might be of help to the blind client. This agency generally provides for marital counseling, legal aid assistance, and short-term financial assistance as well as budget counseling for families on a limited income. In some instances, the service provides for homemaker services also. The family and children's service generally provides a variety of services concerning various types of family and individual social and emotional problems.

Sheltered workshops can serve the agency for the blind and the rehabilitation worker in a number of ways. In addition to job tryout and job training, many workshops provide for prevocational evaluation, development of work tolerance, development of work habits, personal adjustment training, as well as interim employment and terminal employment. Many workshops have developed effective work evaluation units where the worker can evaluate his client through reality testing. This involves the use of actual job samples and real work under real work conditions. The client is evaluated, in addition to aptitudes and performance, for a variety of other reasons such as work habits, work tolerance, ability to take supervision, ability to follow instructions, and ability to get along with his fellow worker. These work evaluation units can actually evaluate clients along those lines in which employers are usually interested. Sheltered workshops can often provide for prescription services for the counselor and his client. Some workshops utilize a vending stand training program at the workshop while others, in contract shops, utilize opportunities provided for by the Wagner-O'Day Act and are affiliated with the National Industries for the Blind.

The rehabilitation counselor often has available at the *medical and/or dental schools* a variety of services which might help him in serving his client. Many of these schools operate a wide variety of clinics which offer more extensive evaluation than may be available elsewhere. Many of them offer a number of special clinics which the counselor might use. For instance, prosthetic clinics, seizure control clinics, diabetic control clinics, etc. Since many rehabilitation agencies frown somewhat upon the purchase of dentures or tooth extraction and filling, the dental school can provide these services for the rehabilitation counselor without the necessity of extensive use of his case service funds.

Most communities include a number of *voluntary organizations* that are usually concerned with specific disabilities and problems. Some of these organizations operate loan closets whereby the rehabilitation worker might secure a wheelchair, crutches, and other equipment which might be necessary on a temporary basis. Some of these organizations provide for transportation services and homemaker services; some, such as the YMCA, Salvation Army, American Red Cross, and Travelers Aid might provide for temporary lodging, meals, and emergency assistance. Many times these services are of a crisis intervention type and are needed immediately. Voluntary agencies are often able to handle such emergency situations. Flexibility is a keynote of voluntary agency work.

Part Four

Social and Educational Services for the Blind

20

Aid to the Blind

William T. Coppage

Aid to the Blind is one of the categories of public assistance which was created by the passage of the federal Social Security Act in 1935. The act was passed in that year but not implemented; programs were not developed in the states for about three years. At the time congress passed the Social Security Act, the public assistance program was administered by the Social Security Board. A few years later, the name of that agency was changed at the federal level to the Federal Security Board and later to the Federal Security Agency. Finally, in 1953, the programs were transferred to the newly created Department of Health, Education and Welfare. These public assistance programs remain under that agency today, administered by the Social and Rehabilitation Service Administration. The other related categories of public assistance are Old Age Assistance and Aid to the Permanently and Totally Disabled, these, plus Aid to the Blind, form the adult categories while Title IV of the Act created Aid to Dependent Children.

LEGAL ASPECTS OF AID TO THE BLIND

Legal aspects of Aid to the Blind, like those affecting other welfare programs and public assistance, remain subject to continued change. Changes can result from amendments to the Social Security Act; through new federal and state regulations; and through Supreme Court rulings on existing laws and guidelines. Therefore, rather than dwell on the technical and legal aspects of the program, this chapter will instead develop a general overview of the purpose of the program as it is administered around the country today and will present some generally accepted professional philosophy regarding public assistance.

At the end of the fiscal year 1970 there were approximately 80,000 individuals in the country who were receiving Aid to the Blind payments in varying amounts. The average payment was approximately $99 per month. Of course, the number of individuals who are eligible for Aid to the Blind and the number actually receiving it are not the same figure. There are quite a few individuals who receive public funds through other categories.

An individual who is eligible for Old Age Assistance or Aid to the Permanently and Totally Disabled also may be blind and may be placed in one of these other categories. However, we encourage the local department of welfare to place all individuals who are blind and eligible for public assistance in the Aid to the Blind category.

Program Administration

Another point of interest, and certainly of importance to social service workers locally, concerns how to work with recipients of Aid to the Blind. The administration of this program varies from state to state. Some programs are administered by state agencies which have district offices or branch offices scattered throughout the state to serve individuals in their own localities. And in many states, the program is supervised at the state level but administered by local boards of public welfare with staff hired by these boards for local administration of the program. For example, Virginia has 128 local departments of welfare and social service bureaus, all of which are under a city or county board of welfare. West Virginia has a state administered program while Virginia's is locally administered. In four of the states, there are two agencies which administer public assistance programs; these are North Carolina, Virginia, Massachusetts and Delaware. The Aid to the Blind program is supervised at the state level and the other categories are supervised by the state welfare agency. It is important to know who is responsible for the actual administration of the program in the state in order to know where the contact or referral source is.

Government statistics reveal a great deal about the evolving philosophies of public assistance. In Virginia for example, 72 percent of the recipients of Aid to the Blind are over the age of 50. This is significant because it indicates that many of the people who should be working and who are capable of working are being served through rehabilitation programs or programs which assist individuals in staying off welfare and in engaging in gainful activity. This approach to cooperative efforts between rehabilitation and welfare programs is one of our major national priorities. The Department of HEW is now encouraging vocational rehabilitation agencies to work with recipients of public assistance to try to end the cycle of dependency in which many of these persons find themselves. Blind individuals, therefore, who are on welfare but who have work potential are now being given attention in the priorities scheme.

Eligibility Factors

Many working individuals are on public assistance, particularly Aid to the Blind. An amendment to the federal act several years ago made it possible, in determining the formula for payment, for a blind person to earn $85 a month plus one half of any additional amount above $85 which is not counted toward his need or toward a resource. As a result, a number of recipients of Aid to the Blind are allowed to be employed in workshops or in other work activities to supplement their incomes and are thereby encouraged to become fully employed and independent.

Eligibility for Aid to the Blind is very basic, with again some variation from state to state. One basic requirement, of course, is that an individual be legally blind. A person must be in need of assistance, and the standards of need will vary from state to state because of the lack of a federal standard. The "responsible relative" provision must also be taken into consideration in some states. An individual does not have to be a resident of the state in which he applies. Some states had residency requirements, but a recent Supreme Court ruling overturned that restriction, and now the individual must be in the state with the intent to reside there when he applies. Visual eligibility has to be approved by a medical specialist hired by the state agency that is responsible for the program in the state—the welfare department of one of the commissions for the blind, for example. There are other criteria which must be taken into consideration in establishing need. In some states, a lien must be placed on the property of the individual. In most states, Aid to the Blind is not a pension. This is a question or an assumption that often is misunderstood. Two states did have a pension for the blind until very recently. Thinking of aid as a pension creates some real problems in the workshop, particularly because these pensions, after certain levels of earnings, can either be cut off or reduced. As a result, many of the individuals who are employed, particularly in workshops, will work a certain number of hours a day or a certain number of days a week and then not come back until they can earn more without their payments being threatened. This probably happens in states other than the two pension states, and it is certainly a factor that has to be considered when working in a program of rehabilitation or placement within a workshop program.

Funding the Program

The financing of the Aid to the Blind program also varies in amounts of funds and sources of funds. Roughly 55 to 65 percent of the aid comes from federal funding. The balance is financed by the state government or by the state government in conjunction with the local government, depending on the particular state. Nationally, the latest figures were 57 percent federal, 35.3 percent state and 7.7 percent local. There are various kinds of formulas that are used in different categories of the program. For example, one percentage is used for prescribed social services, another percentage is used for money payments. However, averages come out roughly to the percentages listed above.

Another development of recent years is the separation of money payments from social services. Most states are now reorganizing their administrative structures to enable one division of the welfare agency to be responsible for the provision of the money payments. The agency division is responsible for making a determination of financial needs and issuing the check. Another group of professional staff is responsible for seeing that needed social services are provided to the recipients. Included in the broad range of social services are emergency services, legal assistance, help with housing, mobility and orientation and assistance with the whole gamut of daily living needs. In fact, the "social services" concept includes all those services which meet an individual's needs so that he can become less dependent and more involved in a program of vocational rehabilitation leading to employment. Funds are available to local agencies to purchase these services where they have to be purchased. This is an encouraging recent development in the whole program of public funding, particularly the program of assistance for the blind.

We are not trying to sell, as a philosophy, the dependence of a blind person on public assistance or on Aid to the Blind. Certainly, every effort should be made through a program of rehabilitation or through the provision of other social services when a person is perhaps beyond the age of feasible consideration for vocational rehabilitation. Also, every effort should be made to provide other programs which would help meet the needs of these individuals and which will help them become as independent as possible. But, in spite of our best efforts, some individuals for various reasons will continue to be dependent on public assistance for their basic livelihood. It is necessary that agencies serving blind people also provide as many support services as they can for those persons and do whatever they can to enable even those who must remain in public dependency to live out their lives with as much self-respect as possible.

21

Communications

Robert S. Bray

The thoughts expressed in this chapter are predicted on a belief which I, as a librarian, share with those who are professionals in the field of rehabilitation services: namely, that our common goal is to rehabilitate the whole person, and to sustain and develop this condition in the individual in his everyday life at work, at home and as a member of the community. It is not enough to return the visually or physically handicapped person to his home and to place him in the work force, commendable and difficult through these achievements may be. He must also communicate with his friends and associates and with his country and its culture. Since communication means receiving as well as sending, then reading becomes an essential aspect of this continuing process. When the individual can read or handle regular printed material, even though he may require low vision aids, then the problem is simplified substantially. When he can no longer use or read print, special library services are required and special instruction and counseling are necessary for reading and communication skills.

SERVICE FOR THE HANDICAPPED

The Library of Congress program is designed and intended for persons who can no longer read or communicate in the world of regular print forms. These individuals, therefore, become readers of talking-books in either phonograph record or magnetic tape form, or rely on books in large print. Their use of braille, or reading by touch, while included in the free national program of the Library of Congress will be presented in detail in the next chapter. Notice that we are going to drop the labels that set people apart as blind, visually impaired or whatever and consider them as individual library users requiring particular communication services and materials. Everybody wants to read and has to read and everybody can read (or communicate) if we apply as much effort and professional skill to this aspect of the problem as we do to all other aspects of rehabilitation and library services.

The Division for the Blind and Physically Handicapped is responsible for carrying out the Library of Congress program first established by a law approved by the President on March 3, 1931. Recent expansion of the library program resulted from the passage in July 1966 of Public Law 89-522, which authorized the Library of Congress to extend its free books-for-the-blind program to people who are unable to read conventional print materials because of physical limitations.

Since reading or communicating normally involves the ability to hold a book or magazine, to turn pages, and to see the print clearly and comfortably for a reasonable length of time without special aids or devices other than regular eyeglasses, the degree to which a person's vision or manual dexterity is impaired will determine his eligibility. The following are examples of physical handicaps where muscle or nerve deterioration or paralysis might be present: cerebral palsy, multiple sclerosis, muscular dystrophy, arthritis, infantile paralysis, myasthenia gravis, and quadraplegia. The program is available to residents of the United States and American citizens temporarily abroad.

To qualify for this library service, an individual should secure a brief statement describing the characteristics of his physical disability and certifying his eligibility for such competent authority as a doctor, optometrist, registered nurse, professional staff member of a hospital or other institution or agency, or in the absence of any of these, from a professional librarian. In cases of total blindness a statement signed by a responsible member of the community is accepted. Library service to an individual may begin when the regional library serving the area where he resides receives the certification of disability.

Located in public and private institutions, regional libraries for the blind and physically handicapped distribute recorded and embossed books provided under the federal program. They furnish the housing, supplies, and equipment necessary for their functions within the program, and the library staff of each maintains records of the needs and preferences of its borrowers. As area requirements for additional service become evident, new regional libraries are established. Books and other materials are mailed free of charge to the reader who returns them by mail to the sending library, also without cost.

By placing books from its collection in other libraries in the area, a regional library may make it possible for readers to browse and receive personal attention in their own community.

Books selected for the blind and physically handicapped range from titles of current and popular interest to classics and vocational and practical materials—the type of reading offered sighted persons using an average public library. Selections are made for all age levels. Magazines also reflect a wide variety of tastes and needs and include such well-known titles as *American Heritage, Good Housekeeping, Look, Sports Illustrated, Newsweek,* and *Reader's Digest.*

Talking Books

Most widely used of the media provided by the program, talking-book records are significant in providing a new and easy avenue to continued reading. Record players especially designed for operation by blind persons are lent to readers free of charge by the Library of Congress through more than 50 lending agencies. Research is under way to produce talking-book machines that immobile handicapped readers can operate.

Talking-books produced in several hundred copies are now recorded on 10-inch discs at 16⅔ rpm, giving 45 minutes of playing time on each side of a record. All magazines are recorded at the 9⅓ rpm speed. Materials selected by the Library are produced professionally at the American Foundation for the Blind in New York and the American Printing House for the Blind in Louisville and are distributed simultaneously to all the regional libraries.

The tape collection which supplements talking-book records includes materials of special interest for a growing audience of blind and handicapped persons. A limited number of tape cassette players are available and veterans, students and employed persons receive priority in the assignment of these new devices. Selection of titles is often based on requests by individual readers.

The contributions of volunteers throughout the nation have always been a vital element in the Library's books-for-the-blind program. Through its long-established program for certifying braille transcribers, the Library has set standards and trained volunteers to produce hand-copy braille for the regional libraries and for individuals. More recently, the Library has encouraged the growth and improvement of the volunteer program of recording books on tape for either national or local use. Books required by persons seeking employment or employed in special fields can be assigned for reading.

Two bimonthly publications, *Talking Book Topics* and *Braille Book Review,* are mailed free of charge to blind and physically handicapped persons who borrow books from the regional libraries and their branches and to other interested individuals and organizations. In addition to announcing book titles, these magazines include reviews and feature articles on books, authors, and library services. Cumulative catalogs list books previously announced. Pamphlets describing all aspects of the program are available on request. Lists of titles of interest to people in various fields of employment will be prepared upon request.

The Library also offers a national reference and referral service on all aspects of blindness and other physical handicaps by working closely with organizations which are sources of information and statistics on those subjects. Local, regional, and national associations working with or interested in physically handicapped people help governmental agencies in both publicizing the service and evaluating its effectiveness. The Library also attempts to reach its potential public through program participation and exhibits at conferences, magazine articles and mass mailings of publications.

Copies of all of the division's publications are available for individual readers or for rehabilitation personnel for use in counseling. Kits of publications and special reading lists can be assembled in multiple sets for use in conferences and workshops.

The nationwide network of libraries cooperating with the

Library of Congress is growing. At this writing all but seven of the states have at least one so-called regional library for the blind and physically handicapped within their borders. These seven states are served by their neighbors. The nation's public libraries are steadily becoming more knowledgeable of services available to blind readers. The number of volunteers, both individuals and those operating in groups is increasing. All this augurs well for rehabilitation counselors and their clients in need of increased reading resources and more efficient communication skills. Rehabilitation personnel are urged to visit their regional library and to maintain an active liaison with their regional library. Clients should be reminded that once they become established as a reader anywhere in the system, they can continue to use the service wherever they may live without the inconvenience of recertification of eligibility.

Users of the library service throughout the country, borrowing from the 48 regional libraries or from a limited number of public library branches, hospitals, institutions and other small deposits of Library of Congress materials, now number at least 220,000. About 10 percent of these are braille readers and most of these prefer braille reading almost exclusively. Braille, of course, is something that has to be taught. We librarians are increasingly convinced that good listening habits have to be taught, too, although one can listen by simply paying attention. The number of users of tape is increasing rapidly and is restrained only by the relative scarcity of tape books and players as compared to the more traditional talking-book records. We have no accurate measure of the number of readers of books in large print much less how many are able to read virtually any printed material with the use of magnifiers and low vision aids. The number of people using our program of brailled musical scores and texts approaches 2,000.

The talking-book record has been developing and improving ever since it ushered in the familiar long-playing record in the middle 1930's in its initial 33⅓ rpm, microgroove configuration. Since 1963, our books have been recorded at 16⅔ rpm. By the early 1970's, the whole talking-book program in disc recording form will stabilize on 8⅓ rpm records. This is made possible largely by the acceptability of voice recording frequencies when played at this slow speed, and by technological improvements in the talking-book machine, the materials from which records are made and other advances. Records at 4 rpm and even 2 rpm are possible and have been produced in the laboratory. But there is such a thing as too much engineering for everyday use. These excessively slow speeds would require such fine grooves in the records that the slightest vibration would cause the needle to skip or would place more reading on one side of a record than would be desirable. The so-called "flimsy" record or sound sheet holds great promise for the future. We ponder the potential advantages of a throw-away talking-book comparable to the paperback book in the print field. But the talking-book in phonograph record form is a one-way street in the sense that it can be read but it cannot be used to originate a communication. It is manufactured in quantity, used until it wears out and is then discarded. Its strong points are rapidity of duplication (almost as rapidly and inexpensively per unit as a page of print), its ease of use and its familiarity as a household appliance encountered at an early age by nearly everyone.

Taped Books

Tape is another proposition and for a number of reasons must be considered an additional medium of reading and communication, not a competitor with disc recordings destined to replace the discs in the immediate future. Of prime importance is the capacity of tape to serve not only as a reading method but as a two-way communications method. Multiple copies, though tedious and expensive to obtain, can be produced and placed in libraries. In addition, a single copy of a book magazine or any portion thereof can be produced rather quickly and inexpensively for a single reader. Further, this specific tape, having served its purpose, can be reused for a similar specialized and transitory need.

Each year only 700 books are reproduced on talking-books for readers of all ages together with 275 in press braille. These are deposited on a quota basis with the 48 cooperating regional libraries. Several hundred books are recorded on open reel tape and less than 300 in cassettes as this new medium emerges; problems in multiple-copy duplication are still substantial. In view of the annual production in printed form of well over twenty thousand books of all kinds in English, it is apparent how much material must be omitted altogether or produced on a one-copy for one-requestor basis.

Large Print Books

Books in large print—14 point or larger—are not a part of the regular program of the Division for the Blind and Physically Handicapped of the Library of Congress. They can be obtained from a limited number of standard book publishers and are available in very small numbers from most of the regional libraries as a result of independent purchase by the several administering agencies. An increasing number of books are being produced in large type by volunteers using photoenlarging techniques or direct copying with special large-print typewriters.

There is a great need for closer cooperation between the professions. The rehabilitation counselor, the optometrist or ophthalmologist, and the librarian should work closely as a matter of standard procedure to advise the low-vision reader on the optical reading aids that are available, to prescribe and demonstrate the proper aids and magnifiers to each visually handicapped reader, and to assure regular and comfortable use of these aids under optimum reading conditions of good lighting and interesting reading. It is a fact that a great many visually handicapped and legally blinded persons could be reading at will from the world of books. These same people could be communicating more effectively to those around them if we combine forces to make the best use of available resources.

REFERENCES

Blind and physically handicapped library service. In *Encyclopedia of Library and Information Science,* vol. 2, 1969.

Books for the Blind and Physically Handicapped, A Postscript and an Appreciation, 3rd ed. Washington, D. C., Library of Congress, Division for the Blind and Physically Handicapped, 1962.

Braille Book Review. Published for the Library of Congress by the American Foundation for the Blind, *39*:6, 1970.

Bray, Robert S. and Staffen, Edward S.: Aural reading by blind persons. In *AAWB Blindness Annual.* Washington, D. C., American Association for the Blind, 1968.

Magazines Braille and Recorded. Washington, D. C., Library of Congress, Division for the Blind and Physically Handicapped, 1968.

Publications. Washington, D. C., Library of Congress, Division for the Blind and Physically Handicapped, (annual).

Reference Circular. Washington, D. C., Library of Congress, Division for the Blind and Physical Handicapped, August, 1970.

Reference Circular. Washington, D. C., Library of Congress, Division for the Blind and Physically Handicapped, February, 1970.

Sources of Reading Materials for the Visually and Physically Handicapped. Washington, D. C., Library of Congress, Division for the Blind and Physically Handicapped, 1970.

Standards for Production of Reading Materials for the Blind and Visually Handicapped. New York, National Accreditation Council for Agencies Serving the Blind and Visually Handicapped, 1970.

Talking Book Topics. Washington, D. C., published for the Library of Congress by the American Foundation for the Blind, January-February, 1971.

Volunteers Who Produce Books, Braille—Large Type—Tape. Washington, D. C., Library of Congress, Division for the Blind and Physically Handicapped, 1970.

22

REHABILITATION TEACHING

Roy J. Ward

As most people are aware, the total absence or loss of vision or a severe restriction in usable vision causes many problems for the individual. For the person who is blind from birth or very early childhood, these problems necessitate adjustments in his preschool training, in his academic education, and in his overall training and preparation for adult life. For the person who becomes blind as an adult, many adjustments, modifications, and substitutions in the sighted way of life must be accomplished before he can function effectively as a blind individual. In most instances the person who becomes blind as an adult will need considerable assistance from trained professionals in order to make successful adjustments, both in attitude and in daily living activities, which will enable him to lead a full and meaningful life. One of the key professionals who is trained to assist blind persons in their personal adjustment is the rehabilitation teacher.

ORIGINS OF REHABILITATION TEACHING

The history of blindness and services to blind persons reveals that in the mid-1800's there were particularly competent blind persons in England who took it upon themselves to work as volunteers toward helping less competent blind persons improve their attitudes toward blindness and learn how to function more adequately as blind persons. In the latter 1800's there were similar evidences of this type activity in the United States. In the early 1900's the activities of these volunteers became increasingly evident, and their services led to the founding of several well-known agencies for the blind. The interest and the services provided by these volunteers were obviously important to the individuals whom they helped to become more self-sufficient and independent, but perhaps the greatest contribution which they made was to demonstrate the fact that specialized training could help blind persons to become more capable. At the same time, through their contacts with blind persons, they helped to bring to public attention the fact that blind persons living in the community needed and wanted help and needed and wanted to become self-sufficient and contributing members of society.

Many of these volunteers eventually became employed in small organizations or agencies which tried to develop service programs for blind persons. The workers became identified as home teachers because they went to the homes of blind persons and taught them many skills which compensated for or substituted for the lack of sight. These home teachers were initially untrained, but worked on the basis of their experience and their own capability. Their efforts, therefore, produced varying degrees of success. In many instances there was a noticeable tendency to do many things for the blind person, rather than devoting full attention toward assisting the blind person to learn to do things for himself.

Over the years, however, home teachers throughout the country have become better trained, have developed more standardized methods of teaching clients, and have restricted their activities to the area of adjustment counseling and instruction instead of being generalists who were called upon by their employers to perform a wide variety of tasks ranging all the way from their present area of activity to fund raising, public relations, job placement, and casework counseling.

FUNCTION OF REHABILITATION TEACHERS

The home teacher in today's agency for blind persons is a true specialist and a valuable member of the agency service team. The teacher works not only in the home, but in the community in which the blind person lives and also focuses attention not only on the needs of the blind person, but on the need, the attitudes, the lack of understandings of family members and friends. In this respect the teacher is a true and meaningful contributor to the total rehabilitation of blind persons and it is total rehabilitation which we are all endeavoring to assist blind persons to achieve. Rehabilitation once meant merely training a person for a job and placing him in employment, but now we recognize that the true total rehabilitation of a blind person must go a great deal further. It must not only provide training for employment and placement in employment, but it must offer the basic preparation of the individual in terms of attitudes and performance skills. Rehabilitation must prepare the persons to lead a full and well-adjusted life, not only on the job but in all his activities, as a member of his family and community and in his leisure time. It is in these areas that the rehabilitation teacher specializes.

Communications as they relate to blind persons must be thought of not only in terms of special equipment and special techniques but also in a much broader sense. We must think of the need for communication between the blind person and the professional specialist who will assist him in his adjustment to blindness and in his relearning toward the ultimate objective of a more productive personal life. We, therefore, must think of communications as the interpersonal relationships between the blind person and agency service staff, as well as between the blind person and members of his family and community. Effective interpersonal relationships are the key to the successful rehabilitation of the blind person. The rehabilitation teacher must be effective at such interpersonal relationships in order to establish rapport with his client; in order to convince the client that through proper training he can learn to become at least reasonably self-sufficient and independent; in order to provide the instruction and services which will assist the blind person in achieving this independence; in order to inform the blind person of available services which will be helpful and meaningful to him; and in order to understand the attitudes of the blind person, of his family members, and of people within the community in which the blind person lives.

In working with clients or trainees, rehabilitation teachers interlace adjustment counseling with instruction in communication skills, daily living activities, home management (including kitchen activities of all types, homemaking, and simple household repair), recreation, crafts and games, and orientation to the home and its immediate vicinity. All instruction is related to the needs and the basic capabilities of the individual client.

COMMUNICATIONS ASPECTS OF REHABILITATION TEACHING

I should like to place particular emphasis on the communication aspect of rehabilitation teacher instruction. We must keep in mind that the communications problem which faces blind persons is primarily communications in the form of reading or writing. The instruction which the rehabilitation teachers provide in order to help the blind person overcome this problem in reading and writing can be broken down into six areas: braille, typing, handwriting or script, dialing the telephone, special problems as exemplified by the person who is both deaf and blind, and optical aids.

Braille is a system of raised dots based on the braille cell which contains six positions. All the letters of the alphabet, the punctuation marks, numbers, and the contractions which speed up braille reading and writing are worked out by using combinations of dots in different positions within the braille cell or, as is the case with some contractions, by using two cells in combination. The blind person who is not able to see enough to read print can learn to identify the various braille characters by touching them with his fingertips, and in this way is able to read. He can also be taught to use either a pocket slate and stylus, a board slate and stylus, or a braille writer, to write braille for his own use or for use in communication with other blind individuals. The entire braille system contains approximately 225 characters and can be learned by the average adult in three to six months. It must be emphasized, however, that it will require a considerably longer period of time with regular practice for the adult to develop enough speed and facility for braille to be used effectively.

In this respect, learning braille for adults is a lot different from the case of blind children who usually are able to read considerably faster because they learn at an earlier age. Nevertheless, braille can be and is effective and useful for adults and is to be encouraged wherever it is needed. It is important to note that braille instruction now is geared to the specific needs of the individual. It was accepted practice 25 years ago to expect every newly blinded person to learn the entire braille system; if the individual failed to do so, he was considered to be an unsuccessful student. Today it is recognized that not every adult is going to sit down and read entire books in braille. Many wish to learn enough only to play cards, to mark canned goods and medicines, to identify clothing, to be able to write out and read recipes and telephone numbers, or to handle certain other limited reading and writing needs. If this is the case, it is not always necessary for the individual to learn the entire braille system, and the teacher will gear instruction accordingly.

In providing braille instruction there are a number of accepted textbooks used by rehabilitation teachers, and information on these is available through reference material and lists of teaching supplies and materials to which all the agencies have access.

While braille is a very effective means by which the blind person can read and write for his own benefit and can communicate with other blind persons, it is important for many blind persons to be able to communicate in writing with sighted persons. One of the best ways to accomplish this is through typing; for the blind person who has reasonable dexterity and fairly good verbal skills, typing is not too difficult to learn. The standard system for teaching touch typing is applicable to instruction to blind persons. A recorded text, *Touch Typing in Ten Lessons,* is used extensively by rehabilitation teachers to assist them in providing typing instructions to blind persons. These records make it possible for the blind person to practice typing between lessons given by the teacher. Since many rehabilitation teachers are blind themselves, it is frequently asked how such teachers can actually instruct blind persons. The basic instruction can be provided by the teacher by keeping contact with the fingers of the blind person while he is learning the typewriter keyboard. As the student progresses and begins to use the records or other assigned materials provided by the teachers and types out practice pages, the blind rehabilitation teacher can use members of the family, volunteers, or sometimes clerical staff of the agency to inspect the practice material which the student has prepared. Over a period of several months the average adult can learn to type accurately and with reasonable speed. While most students will use typing for purposes of correspondence or other personal needs, there are some who are of an employable age and who become competent enough so that they can undertake specialized training which will ultimately lead to employment as a transcription typist.

Another means of helping a blind person communicate with sighted persons is through script writing. It is important to note here that the potential for effective writing by persons blinded at birth and those who lose their sight in adult life is considerably different. In using braille, it is usually the blind child who becomes much more facile than the average adult. In script writing it is the reverse. The congenitally blind child must be painstakingly taught the shape of each letter, both script and printed. Usually, the blind child does not progress beyond the point of learning to sign his or her name, or perhaps to do very limited additional script writing. In the case of the adult who has been able to write throughout his life and who already knows the formation of letters, the potential for extensive writing is much better. Through the use of signature guides and writing devices, the average adult not only can sign his name very legibly, but can be taught to write checks and write letters. It is interesting to note that one bank system in Virginia provides check guides for blind persons and maintains braille checking accounts which include providing the blind person with a braille statement of his account each month.

Another useful communication skill for blind persons is that of dialing the telephone. While a blind person wishing to contact someone by telephone might be able to dial the operator and have her dial the number for him, it is something which the telephone company does not like and something which is not necessary. There are a number of different touch systems or modifications of systems which can be taught to blind persons so that they can effectively dial telephone numbers for themselves. The systems usualy are based on having the blind person memorize at least certain positions, numbers and letters on the telephone dial, and then use a fingering system which enables him to keep contact with the dial from the time he dials the first digit until he completes dialing the number. The rehabilitation teacher can effectively provide this instruction using the regular telephone in the client's home or by using instructional telephones which usually can be borrowed from the local telephone company. The ability to dial telephone numbers without having to depend on someone else can be an important means of assisting a blind person to improve his self-sufficiency and independence.

It is not uncommon for blindness to occur in association with other disabilities such as deafness, cerebral palsy, brain damage, mental retardation, and physical illnesses such as diabetes and heart trouble. Oftentimes the existence of other disabilities creates problems in providing instruction in the four communication areas already described. In such instances the rehabilitation teacher uses modifications of standard instruction where they can be applied and in other instances uses either special equipment or special instruction in order to help the multihandicapped blind person achieve whatever degree of competency with communication skills he is capable of achieving. In working with deaf-blind persons, for example, it is helpful for the rehabilitation teacher to know the one-hand manual alphabet for the deaf and at times to be able to teach this to clients. It is also helpful to be able to trace letters in the palm of a deaf-blind person's hand or to write them on his shoulder or back. As an alternate to the manual alphabet, if the deaf-blind person knows braille it can be used as a communications medium. A particular device which is helpful in such instances is the telatouch machine. In working with diabetics it is not uncommon to find that the sense of touch is inhibited to the extent that the diabetic cannot feel the braille characters too accurately. In such instances it may be necessary to use a large dot braille slate and stylus or to forego braille completely and to use more identifiable markings to enable the diabetic person to recognize medicines, canned goods, etc. In all instances when working with multihandicapped persons, the teacher must be resourceful and attempt to find methods and equipment which will be of particular benefit in helping such clients to meet their individual needs.

In considering the communication needs of blind persons, it

is important to recognize that not all clients are totally without sight. Many do have residual vision and where such is the case, every attempt should be made to help them to learn to function to maximum efficiency using this residual vision. It is not the function of the rehabilitation teacher to be a low vision or optical aids specialist, but it is important for the teacher to know that such devices do exist and that they frequently can provide the potential for enabling partially sighted persons to read regular print. In such instances the teachers should make referrals to specialized examination sources which can recommend and prescribe appropriate aids. The teachers can then frequently be helpful by encouraging clients to practice—in some instances, even to assist them in practicing—until they learn how to use the optical aid which has been prescribed for them.

ACTIVITIES OF DAILY LIVING

Instruction in the various communication skills which previously have been described can be blended by the rehabilitation teacher into effective instruction in other skill areas which also are the responsibility of the rehabilitation teacher. In meeting daily living needs such as personal grooming, personal hygiene, identifying clothing, identifying money, and so forth the sense of touch and a knowledge of even a limited amount of braille can be extremely helpful. Therefore, the teacher, while providing instruction in communication skills, can at the same time be working with clients in the many areas of meeting his daily living needs and associating the instruction in communication skills to the instruction in many aspects of daily living activities. In so doing, the instruction in both areas is made much more meaningful to the blind person. The same can be said for instruction in home management where the client can learn to write down recipes, identify canned goods, and write down telephone messages, names and addresses, etc. He can use communication skills to further his competency in carrying out his responsibilities in keeping house, in cooking and working around the kitchen and in performing simple household repairs. Also, the development of manipulative skill as can be accomplished through instruction in recreation, crafts and games can be very much related to having a basic knowledge of communication skills.

The important point to keep in mind is that in all areas of instruction provided by rehabilitation teachers including orienting the client to his home and getting around in it and in its immediate vicinity, the instruction can be and should be associated and interrelated. The objective of course is to assist the blind person in developing knowledge and competency which will enable him to carry on his daily living responsibilities in a self-sufficient and independent manner.

Over the years most instruction by rehabilitation teachers has been provided on a person-to-person basis in the home and in the community. There have been some exceptions to this, particularly where rehabilitation teachers have gotten groups of blind persons in large cities together and provided group instruction, usually on an informal basis centered around instruction in crafts and games. More recently, the Commission for the Visually Handicapped in Virginia has undertaken a new type of group instruction as a cooperative venture between its rehabilitation teachers and vocational rehabilitation counselors. In this new program activity the teachers and counselors work together and select a group of from 10 to 12 trainees. These trainees are gathered together in a community of moderate size and housed in a local hotel or motel. Training facilities are found in a local church and a two-week program of intensive instruction is offered to the trainees. The areas of instruction include communication skills, cooking and kitchen activities, homemaking, simple household repair, recreation crafts and games, and orientation and mobility. A staff of five instructors and two mobility specialists, plus a part-time counselor who conducts group counseling sessions, form the faculty. The students receive instruction in each of the skill areas every day during the two-week period. In addition, staff has an opportunity to observe them at mealtime and in leisure time activity. These programs have proven to be extremely valuable. They provide a comprehensive evaluation of the needs and capabilities of clients, and thus enable the rehabilitation teachers and rehabilitation counselors to join forces in developing follow-up instructional and training programs to best meet the needs of each individual. It is to be emphasized that these programs are essentially evaluation tools with concentrated instruction built into them. They have additional beneficial elements in that they provide an opportunity to instruct and evaluate in a group setting, and the fact that the programs are carried on in a neutral setting, rather than the client's own home, provides another beneficial ingredient. The programs have been so productive that plans are already being developed for additional programs throughout the next few years.

In conclusion, may I emphasize the fact that effective and qualitative services to blind persons will require good communications. These communications include not only the specific materials and services available through regional libraries as has been described previously, and include not only instruction in the various specific communication skills such as I have described, but in a much broader and much more fundamental way include communications in the form of effective interpersonal relationships through which trained professional personnel working for agencies serving blind persons can establish the necessary rapport with clients which will open the door to an effective rehabilitation program. In order to provide comprehensive and total rehabilitation services, a team of well-trained professionals representing various disciplines including education, vocational rehabilitation, rehabilitation teaching and social work must be blended together. I have attempted to describe the role that the rehabilitation teacher plays as a member of the agency service team.

23

Social Work and Blindness

William F. Gallagher

I am very pleased that there are many new workers coming into the field of blindness. With new workers come new ideas, fresh concepts in approaching problems, and stimulating and thought-provoking questions to be studied and answered.

The field of rehabilitation of the blind at times has been quite staid and set in its practices. Until recently, working with blind persons has had a touch of ingrown traditional concepts because of a degree of success with some persons, and these practices have been handed down to the incoming workers for the blind. Only in the last decade have a variety of professional disciplines been well represented in schools and agencies for the blind.

As social workers and rehabilitation counselors, we do have a body of knowledge, and it is the responsibility of directors of programs to get professional persons to utilize this knowledge and adapt it to the understanding of blindness. The skills and techniques of professional persons will be effective only after these persons understand what blindness is and what it means to the individual who does not have sight. As is well known, human relationship is an attitude. The professional worker's attitude toward the client and the client's attitude toward (and confidence in) the worker are important.

Developing Philosophy of Service

If the professional does not have some insight into his own positive or negative feelings about blindness, he may very easily transfer these feelings to the client in counseling. Without some insight the worker could very easily overidentify with or set up a dependency role for his client by trying to make all decisions for him. We must learn what is right for the individuals to whom we offer services, and we must develop understanding of what the individuals believe they need from us. This can be done by meaningful communication.

It is important for new professionals, to read material that will help not only by just having the information about blindness and agencies serving blind persons, but also will help in gaining a better understanding of our own feelings toward blindness. I should like to recommend three books that will help gain the understanding and the proper attitude toward blindness: Chevigny, 1950; Cholden, 1958; Carroll, 1961. These three men made intensive studies and wrote their material so that new workers would have some understanding of their findings and could make good application of this knowledge in working with blind persons.

Carroll's definition of the adventitiously blinded person is "one who has acquired blindness." By understanding the adventitiously blinded person, he felt that the worker would have a better concept and understanding of a congenitally blind person. As new workers, it is important to make a distinction in counseling practices between the congenitally and the adventitiously blind person. In counseling, it is important to know what total blindness means to the congenitally blind person, and what it means and what it has done to the self-image of the adventitiously blinded person.

The counselor also should study partial sight, the difficulties encountered, and different reactions to situations by partially sighted persons. So many times, the partially sighted person is frightened by total blindness, and at times he has difficulty in discussing the fact that he has a visual problem. In many situations, the partially sighted person, by his denial, appears to have more problems in his social and business relationships than the person who is totally blind.

The social worker or the counselor in interviewing should explore his client's feelings about being congenitally blind or recently blinded, taking into consideration the self-imposed limitations and capabilities set by the client. He should find out whether these stem from fear or lack of self-confidence in learning new adaptations in skills and techniques to restore or find substitutions for his deprivation or loss.

Blindness affects people in different ways. Newly blinded persons react differently, depending upon their original concepts of blindness. Whether they felt blind persons were odd, different, freakish, geniuses gifted with extrasensory qualifications, or wholly dependent upon other individuals or upon society, affects their reaction to loss of sight.

Adjustment to Blindness

Cholden states that the newly blinded person should and must go through a shock period, or a mourning period for his loss, and that we, as workers, should allow this person his mourning time. Too often, we jump in and give the person false hopes and do not allow him to express his desperateness. It is always a good sign when the newly blinded person can use the word "blind" without biting his lip, shedding tears, or trembling when he discusses his "blind" situation. Many times, when he is able to use the word "blind" it is a real sign of starting his adjustment. He is beginning to adapt to a stress situation. It is important to allow him to reveal his true feelings, whether in outbursts of anger or in quiet despair. The newly blinded person with the exuberant facade and joking manner could be showing real signs of denial in hiding his true feelings and, therefore, his progress in adjustment could be hindered.

It is the role of the ophthalmologist to inform the patient when it is determined that he is blind and that all which could be done medically has been done. If the patient is not made cognizant of this fact, then he will retain hopes of gaining his vision and will be unable to recognize his need for a rehabilitation program. The ophthalmologist also should inform the patient with residual vision for whom nothing can be done further medically. When optical aids may be prescribed, all efforts should be made in a rehabilitation program to train the patient to use the mechanical visual aids to maximal benefit, whether these are for reading, traveling, everyday chores, or on-the-job efficiency.

A rehabilitation program should be suggested to all patients within the legal definition of blindness to increase their independence of activity and decrease the restrictions imposed by their visual impairment so that there is no diminution in self-respect and dignity of self-support.

Acceptance of Blindness

It is at this stage that a counselor or a social worker can help the client accept his blindness and recognize the reality of the situation. To accept does not necessarily mean to like the prognosis, but it can mean that the person now thoroughly dislikes the fact that he has to live without his sight for the rest of his life. The counselor can help the patient realize that he can still have a very useful and active life. The patient is the same person now —but without sight—and he must use other techniques and make stronger use of his other senses to perform daily activities, whether they are associated with his work or with his social life.

The early stages of blindness are traumatic and trying times for the person. He may feel helpless and sorry for himself (and rightfully so). He feels that now he is a burden to his family and community and is insecure about his vocational future. Now that he is blind, he feels he is unable to return to work and to support his family. This has a degrading influence upon his self-image. During this time, he is unable to express his feelings with family members or fellow employees; therefore, supportive counseling is the only avenue of relief for him.

It is too early to discuss vocational plans because he does not realize how he can function independently as a blind person. Before discussing his vocational plans, he must regain confidence in himself. This can be done by his recognition that by using other senses, he is able to handle techniques of daily living skills such as shaving, pouring coffee, cutting meat, lighting a cigarette, assembling his clothes for the day, and so on. Once he is able to do these daily routine tasks, he then can give thought to more complicated tasks, e.g. independent travel and communication skills such as writing and reading braille.

Counseling

Counseling can help the person with his attitudes toward learning and performing new skills, at the same time maintaining his social relationships. In his quiet apartment, he may feel comfortable doing the daily routine chores, but he still may feel extremely conspicuous in public places such as church, restaurants, or theatres. If a student in school, he may feel uncomfortable with his peer group. Supportive counseling can help him to overcome his frustration in handling daily routine skills.

There are two skills that are hard for the newly blinded person to accept and learn because of their strong association with blindness. These are the proper use of the cane and the writing and reading in braille. It is only when the person is able to work through his feelings about blindness that he will gain the motivation to learn to travel independently and to learn braille.

Many reasons may be given why he does not need mobility lessons. "The cane is too long." "The neighbors will be watching." "My wife or friend will always take me places." "It is not safe; the motorists never look where they are going." There are also excuses for not taking braille. "I have poor circulation in my fingers." "I never read much when I had my sight." "I am a poor speller." "It is too complicated, and I never was a good student in school."

Once the person has decided upon the mobility device best suited for his purposes, whether it be a cane, guide-dog, or human guide; once he has learned and is comfortable in using new communication tools, such as braille, typing, handwriting; and once he has gained real insight into what blindness has done to his image and his relationships with other people then, and then only, is he ready for vocational counseling. Oftentimes, newly blinded persons are asked to make decisions about work when they have not come to grips with their blindness.

We have in the past set up stereotype jobs for blind persons, mainly ones with hand skills. The trend these days is to determine and use the capabilities of the mind as well as the hands. The social worker and the newly blinded person should explore educational qualifications, work experience, and knowledge of his profession or trade in order to assist the blind person in returning to his previous level of employment if possible. We also must be very realistic and practical. A truck driver or surgeon who has lost sight cannot return to his previous position. But, the truck driver possibly can work for the same company as a dispatcher, using his knowledge of routes, rates, etc. The surgeon, having the benefit of a medical degree, can possibly pursue other vocational opportunities in the medical profession that do not require sight such as a consultant or professor.

It is important to the blind person's self-esteem to be able to return to work on the same level as before, with the same challenges of giving of his knowledge in his respective competitive field. He may have many different feelings about returning to work as a blind person and especially in competing with sighted fellow employees; therefore, he may need some counseling to overcome these frustrations. The counseling should be so directed that the person is able to regain confidence in himself in order to apply for his own job and not depend upon his counselor to act as the go-between. However, the social worker or counselor may help the person in returning to work by assisting with the resumé, suggesting the manner in which to handle possible questions asked by the employer and checking to see that mobility, communication, and personal management skills are adequate for maintaining the position.

A person returning to work too soon without coming to grips with his blindness may regress in his attitude, become very tense and uncomfortable on the job, and decide to quit. He must be emotionally ready for work and socially adjusted. It is the person's attitude toward himself and toward his family that emerges in his entire attitude toward participation in the community. This is why I place such emphasis on effective counseling with the individual and his family to insure that the person has a realistic insight to his situation and feels comfortable with his blindness so that it will not interfere with his social and vocational activities.

REFERENCES

Carroll, Rev. Thomas J.: *Blindness—What It Is, What It Does, and How to Live with It.* Boston, Little, 1961.

Chevigny, H.: *The Adjustment of the Blind.* New Haven, Yale, 1950.

Cholden, L. S.: *A Psychiatrist Works with Blindness.* New York, American Foundation for the Blind, 1958.

24

Social Services and Blindness

Douglas C. Mac Farland

Social services to blind persons, as we envision them, might currently be classed in the area of hopes and dreams for the future. We in social and rehabilitation services believe that we have an understanding of the needs and can develop a program to meet these needs. Requisite to this, however, is the demonstration of benefits that will accrue from such a program and the proper method or methods for obtaining the financial support that is vital to its implementation.

During the past few years we have witnessed the greatest influx of social legislation that this or any other nation has ever known. Without attempting an exact count, I know of 27 bills which have been enacted into law that will have a revolutionary effect on our department alone. Of course, these are familiar to me because they will have a profound bearing in one way or another on those who work in the various components of the Social and Rehabilitation Service.

Legislation is vital to social change because in most instances, without a legislative base we have no foundation on which to build a program. Important though the foundation is, however, the way the house is constructed and the purposes for which it is to be used are even more important. It will, therefore, take a considerable amount of time to design programs that will make maximum use of all the legislation available to us. Concurrent with the many legislative changes, and perhaps as a result of them, vocational rehabilitation and other welfare services within the Department of Health, Education, and Welfare underwent a major reorganization—a change aimed at welding those services together that were most concerned with serving people and regrouping in a more logical manner to get the greatest program impact for our tax dollar.

Obviously we are still very much in the testing period and greatly concerned with fashioning the most effective tools to deliver the services needed by all the people we serve. With this background in mind, then, plus an understanding that much of what will follow is concerned with plans for the future, I will attempt to define some of the problems and indicate avenues of approach to solving these problems.

BASIC SOCIAL SERVICES

In spite of some significant successes, our provision of social services to blind persons is tragically inadequate. This is especially true for our older blind citizens, who constitute more than 50 percent of the total blind population. Perhaps the greatest obstacle to service delivery is a misunderstanding on the part of both the professional and lay public. Too often they confuse a social need with the disability or treat both as inseparable.

It is comparatively easy to demonstrate special training needs or comprehensive rehabilitation services for a newly blinded person. These call for special techniques and professionally trained personnel who cannot be obtained from normal channels in a community. Most of the social needs of blind persons, however, are identical with those of their sighted peers, and it is a distinct disadvantage to blind persons to assume that their needs can or should be provided in a segregated environment.

Many of the older agencies for the blind were founded on the premise of providing services from "the cradle to the grave." This concept eventually established deep roots in our society—nurtured on one hand by a well-intentioned but ignorant community and sustained on the other by agencies that began to believe this was the best way to get the job done. Agency attitudes were strengthened by bitter experiences of some blind persons who attempted to break the social barrier.

It is only within the last few decades that we have come to

recognize that segregation as a way of life disadvantages the majority of blind persons in a community in two ways. The blind person receiving services is usually forced by circumstances to live within narrow confines. What is even more tragic, however, is that there is neither time nor available facilities within the agency to provide special services for the majority of blind persons who may need them.

The answer to the problem cannot be found in a fruitless debate regarding the relative merits of special services versus a generic approach. Obviously, there are clearly identifiable services that require the skills of specially trained professional personnel. Most of the social needs, however, can be obtained from already existing community resources. In order to make use of these resources, we must have individuals who are capable of interpreting the problems of blindness to the general public.

The following few examples are meant to illustrate how this is already being implemented in many communities. A blind person may need special assistance in locating suitable housing. His need is not for a special segregated development for the blind. In fact, this arrangement might pose many problems that he would not otherwise encounter. His real need involves assistance in locating suitable convenient quarters in keeping with his financial status. It may also involve a factual explanation to building management that will allay any fears that he may not be a desirable or safe tenant. In spite of several validated studies, many home owners still believe that blind persons present unusual fire risks or that they are incapable of keeping the premises clean. A second example is the blind parent who wishes to refer a child to a guidance clinic. Unless blindness is understood by the persons providing this service, it may have a profound effect on the outcome. This is not to say that blindness may not be a contributing factor, but it should be put in proper perspective.

There are social services where blindness definitely is the focal point and here the services of a specially trained person are vital—for example, counseling with a newly blinded person to make certain that he is aware of all services available to achieve his maximum potential within the confines of his disability. Professional services are also required to counsel with members of the family, anticipating problems and helping with solutions. There is a great need for specialists in this area. The only way we can hope to overcome this shortage is by redirecting the focus of the private agency with a view toward purchasing the services when necessary.

The greatest problem we face today is that of providing social services for the older blind person. We have only begun to demonstrate in a few areas of the country how the social needs of this large group can be met (Service Needs, 1967). The services are relatively simple: regular social visiting for the person living alone; reading mail and writing essential correspondence when necessary; accompanying the blind person on special shopping tours; orienting the blind person to immediate surroundings so that he can find restaurants, laundry, and other essential facilities; making certain that the person receives special training in home management if desired; and obtaining assistance to help the blind person make full use of recreational facilities that may be available to him. In order to implement these services to any great degree and have an appreciable impact on the total population that can profit from them, state and private agencies must recruit, train, and supervise vast numbers of volunteers. Models of such programs already exist (*Annual Report,* 1969/70; Annual Report Braille Institute, 1969), but these must be replicated on a much larger scale.

Our studies in the early 1960's, which led to the introduction of a formalized university training program for mobility instructors, clearly indicated that the vast majority of blind persons in the United States are unable to travel independently. While we have made some impact through the training of special mobility instructors and the development of comprehensive rehabilitation centers for the blind, it is still a fact that the majority of blind persons—due to age and other factors which have precluded them from vocational rehabilitation services—are unable to move about independently. Thus far, no one has developed an action program to deal with this pressing problem. If we use the current prevalence statistics available (*Estimated Statistics, 1966;* Hurlin, 1962) and measure these against the backdrop of our own experience, it would seem conservative indeed to estimate that there are probably 100,000 blind persons in this country today who could profit from a modicum of travel instruction plus some training in activities of daily living. These services alone could mean the difference between continuance in the family constellation and custodial care.

In this area, special consultation is needed to work with state and private agencies to design new techniques in training that can be taught to the blind person in his home environment. We cannot hope to accomplish this task through training of special personnel for state agency staffs. The problem must be solved through a combination of state staffing, purchase of specialized services from private agencies, and, most important of all, the development of a volunteer corps working in conjunction with either a state or private agency.

In order to be effective, the program should have a three-pronged attack. One, it should be designed to make the blind person as independent of the services of others as possible. No one can achieve self-fulfillment and self-satisfaction without this vital link in the chain. Two, the program should be aimed at freeing others in the constellation immediately surrounding the blind person for activities other than catering to his immediate needs. In the family, this would mean that the person ordinarily assigned to stay home with the blind relative would be free to engage in other activities, including productive work . In hospital and nursing home settings, it would mean that service personnel assigned to feed and assist in activities of daily living of blind patients would no longer be needed for this work, and therefore could be used to extend other vital services within the facility.

A third goal accruing from the provision of self-help and self-care services relates in part to point number two. In most nursing home facilities, care for blind patients is considerably more expensive than for services rendered to nonblind patients in the same facility. The increased cost is based on the erroneous assumption that all blind patients will need to be led around, to be given intense assistance in coping with routine activities, and, in the majority of cases, to be fed by attendants. If all this were true, the 25 percent increase would be justified. However, in the few demonstration projects in which we have engaged it has been conclusively proved that a proper training program designed to make the person independent of others in daily activities can be given in a very short period of time.

For reference, we would cite the research (Smith, 1966) conducted by the Minneapolis Society for the Blind. The objective here was to close a segregated home for the blind and train the residents to get along in nonsegregated environments. From the results presently available, it is obvious that the project has not only been a success from the standpoint of ability to train older blind persons in self-help and self-care, but the success is further enhanced by the positive attitude of blind residents, who now seem much happier in their new environment and newfound independence. There are many voluntary agencies throughout the country like the Minneapolis Society for the Blind that can provide the much-needed services, and wherever, possible, this would seem a desirable approach rather than attempting to expand professional staffs of the state agencies.

Recreation for the Older Blind Citizen

Ours is a work-oriented culture and, therefore, it is extremely difficult to inculcate an acceptance of the proper use of leisure time. If this is true for the general public, certainly it is that much more difficult for the older blind person whose employment possibilities are nil and whose social outlets are likewise nonexistent. For the vast majority of older, blind citizens, social isolation has become a bitter way of life.

Barriers can be broken, but in order to do so a grass-roots program must be stimulated, not to develop special activities for the blind, but to introduce already known techniques that will make it possible for the blind person to take advantage of the many social events which could be meaningful to him in his own community. This program has the following two-fold objective:

1. Helping the blind person bridge the social chasm.

2. Consulting with social organizations to develop a climate of understanding that properly oriented blind persons can contribute to social events without placing special burdens on their staffs.

Integration of blind persons into ongoing recreational facilities in the community will seldom be completely successful unless the activities are coordinated by a specialist who is well aware of what is needed and knows how to bring about a smooth integration. The coordinator must also be able to assess the recreational needs of a blind person and, working in concert with the client, determine the specific services needed to prepare him for the extent of integration he wishes.

Judging from the many private agencies now in operation, it would seem that most professional services needed in this area could be purchased. Obviously, if we are to serve the many blind persons now requiring help, it will be necessary for voluntary agencies to expand their personnel and to make maximum utilization of volunteers in the communities. State agencies should only be encouraged to provide the services where they are not obtainable otherwise. In large states the state agencies may wish to consider the use of one or two consultants who will be responsible for organizing the program in an orderly fashion, identifying caseloads, and evaluating the strengths and weaknesses of private agencies from whom the state may purchase extensive services. There will always be a need for such evaluation to make certain that the client is attaining his objectives rather than being forced to fit into an existing pattern arbitrarily decided by the private organization.

Services to the Multihandicapped Blind

Some of the most difficult problems we will face will be concerned with the solution to the provision of services to multihandicapped blind persons, including older blind citizens. One solution would be to develop a program in cooperation with the Department of Agriculture and the Department of the Interior to take advantage of the burgeoning opportunities in the field of recreation. Fairly simple centers could be set up and staffed to teach blind persons how to operate boat rental and repair shops successfully; how to operate riding stables; how to stock fish ponds or trout streams manually; how to manage and care for hunting preserves; and hundreds of similar jobs that would absorb millions of workers in coming decades.

Another attack geared for particular problems of older blind citizens living in the urban area is the development of unique workshops (Service Needs, 1967). Production would be arranged to meet the worker's needs. Work scheduling would be so designed that an employee might work at least two hours a day or whatever seemed practical at peak performance. Under these circumstances, the worker could justifiably feel he was making his contribution to society as well as earning a supplement to retirement benefits. It is our suggestion that this experiment take maximum advantage of the limited talent now available. The shop could be staffed with older supervisors and managers because persons drawn from this group would have a much better understanding of the problems facing the worker; furthermore, it is a well-established fact that effective managerial and supervisory talent is available in the retired age group.

Services to Children

Nearly all of the separate agencies serving the blind—independent commissions and agencies within welfare organizations—bear the total cost of major services for blind children without federal support. The primary reason for this situation is omissions and deficiencies in state and federal laws and narrow interpretation of existing laws which limit the use of federal funds. Most of the services provided are financially supported by the states; even surgery and other corrective therapy normally cared for by the Crippled Children's Commission are not covered in many states for blind or severely visually handicapped children. Nevertheless, the services have been provided by the states and are usually under the auspices of the special agency designed to serve the blind.

In view of the new Social and Rehabilitation Service organization, it would seem an appropriate time to develop federal assistance to broaden these programs. In many instances, simply increasing the funding of the Crippled Children's Commission would not provide the desired effect without extensive changes in state legislation, and even if this were accomplished, it would ignore important segments of the children's program which are absolutely essential for their future success. In order to get an action program moving immediately, it is essential as an initial demonstration that the larger special agencies for the blind be given federal support to provide all necessary services to children other than those that fall within the purview of special education. The SRS functions would include eye surgery and treatment; personal adjustment services which might be provided during the summer; mobility instruction as needed; examination, prescription, fitting, and training in the use of special optical aids (microscopic and telescopic lenses); prevocational and vocational counseling; precollege preparation; and a similar course for preemployment or orientation for those who are not planning to attend college.

Much of the rehabilitation success depends on how early the agency is able to begin work with the potential client. This is especially true with the multihandicapped blind youngster. For purposes of illustration, we only need review the tragic lack of facilities provided for the mentally retarded blind child. There is no question that the blind person's chances for maximum vocational success can be greatly enhanced by treating him as an individual and recognizing and helping to solve major problems that occur in childhood and during the formative school years.

Services for Blind Persons of All Ages Who Are Now Residing in Mental Institutions

There are literally thousands of blind persons who are now being held in mental institutions and in facilities for the mentally retarded (Eichorn). With the provision of good diagnostic evaluation, plus a modicum of self-help and self-care training, most of these persons could return to living arrangements with their families and in certain instances might even be trainable for self-support in a workshop or other employment situation. The techniques for dealing with this pitiful dilemma are well established.

In facilities for the custodial care of the mentally retarded as well as in hospitals for the chronically disabled, only a few efforts have been made to identify blind persons who may be under custodial care without any reasonable basis other than that the person is blind, has been committed, and there is no one willing to take the responsibility for his release. Preliminary information brought to our attention in RSA is sufficient to indicate that there are eight to ten thousand persons now so incarcerated. We believe our estimates are conservative. These persons need all our services to prepare for self-help and self-care, recreational services and other services. There is a great need for the establishment of teams to visit institutions in question, identify blind persons now being retained by these institutions, assess their mental and physical capacities, and recommend an action program which can be put into effect immediately.

Because little has been done in the area, it may not be practical to remove all blind persons who apparently do not need custodial care from the facilities. In most instances, intensive training will be necessary before the patient can return to his family or to independent living. For these individuals we are recommending that halfway houses be constructed in a few selected areas to demonstrate how such a program can be instrumental in providing the help blind persons need to bridge the gap between custodial care and life within a family constellation. The program is experimental in nature and should be tried cautiously. The halfway house should also be made responsible for providing self-help and self-care services to individual blind persons within the community and consultation to recreational facilities where blind persons will be enrolled. Once the current backlog is identified and services provided, the essential component of a residential facility can be deleted. Due to the length of time the condition has existed, however, it seems obvious that the residential portion will be essential for several years.

Eye Health Care and Prevention of Blindness

Most of the separate agencies serving the blind have prevention of blindness programs. In fact, many of them have been in operation for a number of years. In spite of the excellent quality of work and the great need for such services, they have remained small because of inadequate funding. Some are funded solely from state appropriations, with the remainder of the financing coming from the welfare departments. Many persons who were medically indigent were unable to secure services or did not wish to apply because of the stigma they attach to being considered a welfare recipient. Eye health care and prevention programs have tremendous potential growth, and with our broader concept plus cooperative agreements, this potential could be realized and prove to be one of the most beneficial services we could render to visually impaired persons.

Certainly, no one would refute the benefits and desirability of operating a prevention of blindness program. Since the passage of the Vocational Rehabilitation Act Amendments in 1943, we have spent millions of dollars in rehabilitation services with excellent dividends accruing to the program. During the same period, however, we have neglected to recognize the most significant contribution of rehabilitation—that is the prevention of disability wherever possible.

It would be wasteful to present a series of contentious arguments in favor of supporting prevention of blindness services; we need only cite the figures from two small programs now in operation in our state agencies for the blind. The first is Hawaii (Program Highlights, 1968) where 4,296 persons were examined in one year. Second—and even perhaps more significant—is the program of prevention conducted by the Utah agency (Glaucoma) where in excess of 60,000 persons were provided special glaucoma and amblyopia examinations at little or no cost. Utah's program also includes unique preventive services for an isolated Indian population (Preliminary Observations). These are only two of many outstanding programs that could be cited, but they will centainly serve to illustrate what can be done with a minimum of staff time and budget.

Organized Volunteer Activities

Although this entire discussion is designed to indicate needs of blind people and what can be done with a total SRS approach, and while it is obvious that much of the program outlined cannot become effective without a substantial amount of funding, we believe that the program is entirely feasible and that the mechanisms to make it work are already available. The real test of success or failure will rest on how well we are able to make use —not of funds for purchasing new staff for state agencies and not necessarily of extra funding for purchase of services from private agencies (although this does constitute one of the major thrusts to get the job underway quickly). Rather, final and continued success will depend on how well we are able to take advantage of the vast amount of energy now available through proper and efficient use of volunteers.

Thus far, agencies for the blind have demonstrated success in this area. They can justifiably boast that they are far ahead of most other social service agencies in this regard, and yet an honest appraisal of the situation, viewed against the background of the great need, would suffice to indicate that we have hardly scratched the surface. Recruitment, training, and supervision of volunteer workers will ultimately provide the answer to whether we are indeed able to provide a great society that all can take part in. Voluntary workers represent one of the greatest untapped sources of energy in this nation, and it is only through skillful use of this work force that we can do the many vast and complex jobs that must be done in so short a period of time. Work for the blind provides an excellent small experimental working area to test many of the theories which must be put into practice with respect to volunteer work if social services are to become a reality.

As indicated at the outset, the ideas set forth in this chapter formulate our design for the future. They are presented here to stimulate imagination and to elicit much-needed comments and suggestions. We need help in devising a sound program for the many thousands of blind persons that will receive services as a result of our current planning.

REFERENCES

Annual Report 1969/70. Recording for the Blind, Inc. 215 East 58th Street, New York, N. Y., p. 6.

Annual Report of Braille Institute of America, 741 Vermont Avenue, Los Angeles, California, 1969.

Eichorn, John R.: Unpublished survey. Department of Special Education and Rehabilitation, Boston College, 96 College Road, Chestnut Hill, Massachusetts 02167 (copy available upon request).

Estimated Statistics on Blindness and Vision Problems. The National Society for the Prevention of Blindness, Inc., 16 East 40th Street, New York, N. Y., 1966.

Glaucoma and Amblyopia Detection. Survey conducted by Services for the Visually Handicapped, Sight Conservation Unit, Salt Lake City, Utah.

Hurlin, Ralph G.: Estimated prevalence of blindness in the United States and in individual states, 1960. *Sight-Saving Rev., 32*:1, Spring, 1962.

Preliminary Observations and Fact-Finding Directed toward Prevention of Blindness Program Planning among Navajo Indians Residing in San Juan County, Utah. J. Fred Whitney, Coordinator, Prevention of Blindness, Services for the Visually Handicapped, Salt Lake City, Utah.

Program Highlights Fiscal Year 1968. Services for the Blind, Division of Vocational Rehabilitation, Department of Social Services, Honolulu, Hawaii.

Service Needs of Aged Persons with Severe Vision Impairment or Blindness. Research Conference on Geriatric Blindness and Severe Visual Impairment sponsored by the American Foundation for the Blind and the Administration on Aging, Washington, D. C., Mayflower Hotel, Pan American Room, September 7-8, 1967.

Smith, Byron M.: To Demonstrate the Significant Achievements in the Vocational Adjustment of Blind Persons Through the Provision of Specialized Services. RD-1956. Minneapolis Society for the Blind, 1936 Lyndale Avenue, South, Minneapolis, Minnesota, 1966.

25

Educational Services

Dennis L. Holmes

For the purpose of this chapter, the discussion of educational services for visually impaired children is based upon Virginia's state program and deals with those children attending nonresidential public, private, and parochial schools. The format of the chapter gives attention to the following topics: the visually impaired student; the state program; the services to visually impaired students; the local school program; and a brief summary. The attention given to each of these topics can provide, if not a guide to those entering the field, at least a point of departure for the planning and development of a sound educational program for our children.

The Visually Impaired Student

To repeat an overused phrase, "The visually impaired child is more like than unlike his sighted peers." This is particularly true if one looks at the growth and development patterns of children in general rather than keying on the deviations which occur as a result of an impairment. The existence of an impairment cannot and should not be eliminated from the considerations one brings to the evaluation of a child, but it must be given appropriate importance. It is entirely possible that much of the overt behavior symbolic or typical of visually impaired children may be due, not to the impairment itself, but to the stereotypes, preconceptions and expectations of those who come into and become a part of the child's life.

Most will agree that man, regardless of age or physical and mental capacity, has basic needs which are common to all and that he is in fact the result of his ability to satisfy these needs. Further, his actions will be directed toward need fulfillment.

For purposes of discussion, let us look at visually impaired children at various growth and developmental levels and at how the basic needs for love and affection, acceptance, recognition, and adventure can affect what the children become.

Preschool years (Halliday, 1970) are terribly important for the visually impaired child, his parents and siblings. It is during this period that the child and family establish initial patterns of interaction concerning the development and satisfaction of the needs for love and affection. It is unnecessary to belabor the "guilt feelings and overprotection syndromes" which have been widely recognized and expounded upon in the past, except to reinforce the fact that they do exist and that behavior of the visually impaired child is often a result of his ability to meet the love need at this point. The important consideration here is *not* that the visually impaired youngster cannot see the expression of love by his family, but rather that he must feel love that is real because he is an important person in the life of the family. The youngster cannot experience success in fulfillment of the love need alone. It must be between him and other family members and it must be felt by him among others in his family. The high incidence of divorce and separation among families of visually impaired children and the retardation of skill development and lack of expectation of visually impaired children by many parents point out that not the child's impairment but the attitude of the family members toward the impairment can be a determining factor in his ability to satisfy the love need. It further can be an underlying cause for the child's deviate overt behavior.

By the time the young, visually impaired child enters school, he is well on the way to developing his own need patterns and means of meeting those needs even if the means are deviate and not fully satisfying. Through contact with a new environment (school) and new people (the teacher and his peers) he behaves in a manner that was reinforced in the past. Due to the nature of the new situation the overt behavior is subjectively evaluated and attempts at modifying unusual behavior are carried out. As the young child attempts to handle a new reaction to his behavior, he finds the need for acceptance of even greater importance to him. This dimension of a youngster's life is crucial in the lower elementary grades. Attitudes and interests of the youngster are modified by those of other children to whom he looks for his acceptance. Common interests and group identification develop with a striving for peer approval or acceptance by each of the individuals in the group. Parents of children in this stage see their children elated one day and depressed the next simply on the basis of how they have been accepted by their peers. Competing for the "center ring" can be particularly frustrating for the visually impaired youngster, who of necessity takes a little longer to accomplish tasks or who does not participate at all because of the impairment or the attitude of the person in the leadership role (teacher) toward the impairment.

As acceptance continues to be a primary goal of these children, success in school subjects becomes a vehicle for measurement. The reading groups, no matter by what names they are called, can and do affect adversely those youngsters in the lower groups. Reading, being a visual task, or a tactual one if the student is totally blind, places the visually impaired child in an undesirable position. The implications of braille and large print materials will be discussed later in the chapter. What must be recognized, however, is that participating in physical activities and success in reading and other schoolwork will enhance the visually impaired student's chances for acceptance if the teacher's attitude concerning visual impairment is sound.

The need for love and acceptance is keen during the preadolescent years, grades five through eight. During this period when children undo the past to get ready for the future, peer groups and peer approval almost completely dictate the youngster's life. This is a difficult period for all children, for it is the time when girls are larger than boys, pimples appear, sex organs develop, and everyone is awkward. This is also a time when visually impaired students (partially seeing) will reject the use of large print or special aids in favor of being like their friends. A teacher who does not understand can interfere significantly with the youngster's feeling of acceptance by forcing the use of these materials without alternatives. It is important for us to understand that a visually impaired or otherwise handicapped person, unless he feels he is accepted by his peer group or family, in essence is not.

The needs for recognition and adventure, though evident as a part of the maturation process up to this point, became much more important to the adolescent. The desire for a position of leadership, individual importance, and recognition as a unique person as he participates in school activities, extracurricular events, dating, driving, and vocational planning can affect deeply the visually impaired student's attitude about himself.

Heavy lenses, scars, or divergent eyes cause apperance to be oftentimes less attractive; therefore, the self-image is lessened and normal girl-boy relationships are difficult at best. While dating is a critical concern of the visually impaired girl, not being able to participate in sports and not being able to drive are realities with which the boys struggle. Together, the uncertainty of their vocational future brings about some rather significant anxieties.

With some of these thoughts in mind regarding visually handicapped children, let us now consider what of necessity should make up a state program for them.

The State Program

Each of our states has established within its governmental agency structure a program to provide for the educational needs of handicapped children. Most frequently, these programs are housed in the state educational agency. Some are housed in agencies providing services to persons with a particular handicap. Obviously, the philosophy of the program is far more important than is its location in the state agency structure. A state program whose orientation is toward services to handicapped children is much more appropriate than is one whose orientation is rule-making and regulatory.

Educators have continued to take the position that the operation of our schools should remain with the local citizenry. This is as it should be. However, serious question arises as to who is most capable and equipped to establish and coordinate educational programs for handicapped children in our public schools. We are wrong to assume that localities are capable of providing for the special needs of all of their children or to expect it of them. A high school with one blind child or a school system with ten visually impaired children lacks the necessary resources to provide for its visually impaired charges. The above description is fairly representative of the visually impaired population in most school systems which need special services, excluding, of course, the larger city systems. The concept of a state educational program for handicapped children, the blind and visually impaired in particular, is not new. Until the 1900's the state residential school was all that was available for them.

Today, there is absolutely no good reason why public education should not accept the idea of a state educational program for visually impaired children who attend the local public schools.

In Virginia, after three years of evaluation and identification of visually impaired children in public, private and parochial schools, it was found that about 650 out of over 1500 were in need of educational services.

This figure of 650 youngsters is equal to the enrollment of an average neighborhood elementary school in most communities. Unfortunately, not all of the visually impaired children are located in one school, but rather are distributed throughout the state. For this reason, the specific educational services needed by visually impaired students can best be provided by a service oriented state program.

Legislation written for the purpose of establishing authority with the responsible state agency is absolutely necessary in order to draw distinct lines of authority and communication between the state agency and the local school. Without specific legislation, confusion will exist with regard to responsibilities for hiring and supervising personnel and procurement and ownership of equipment and materials. It will also hold those accountable for their responsibilities, insuring that visually impaired children receive appropriate services.

The Services to Visually Impaired

Of all the services available, the consultative service is by far the most important. It is through the consultant that children are identified and evaluated, that counseling and information programs are carried out, and that other appropriate services are initiated. An adequate number of consultants is necessary to provide for preparation in advance of actual need of the students. The educational consultant plays a specific and important role with regard to the services to be discussed later. So that he can be effective, he must understand his role and how others see him. It is important for the consultant to evaluate how he is expected to behave with regard to those with whom he comes into contact. Communication will not exist unless the consultant is aware of how the other person sees him. A person in this role can be seen as an expert, as a demonstrator, or as a consultant. If a school administrator considers the consultant to be an expert, then he will expect him to come in and evaluate, recommend, and remediate the problem. If the consultant is seen as a demonstrator, he will want him to come in and take charge of the class or activity and demonstrate how to do it. The consultant would be expected to come in, be assessed of the problem or situation, and together with school personnel seek alternative solutions. Though the latter is preferable, there are times when the expert or demonstrator can do the job more easily. The critical point is that the effective consultant will assume the role expected of him and from that point will work toward modifying the expectation of the administrator or teacher regarding his role as consultant. Only in this way can communication exist and rapport be established so that attention to the youngsters' needs can take place.

Preschool services, along with identification and evaluation, are oftentimes the bringing together of medical and social services with the family of the visually impaired child. Counseling plays a tremendously important role at this level, from helping parents to better understand and accept their visually impaired youngster, to recommending toys, exercises, games, and so on. Much effort is needed at the preschool level in this counseling situation, for it is during this period, as was stated in the beginning of this chapter, that the fulfillment of the acceptance needs are so vital to normal adjustment and behavior of the child.

The provision of learning materials for visually impaired children is usually recognized as the major educational service provided by state departments of education. Not only is this an inappropriate assumption, but it also is a function inadequately performed by many of those who have responsibility. No specific or single learning medium should be recommended or provided simply on the basis of a classroom teacher's or a doctor's recommendation. Large print, in particular, has been felt to be a panacea for the visually impaired youngster without regard to what his impairment was. How often are visually impaired children, whose correction in their glasses is for distance, forced to wear their glasses and read large print? How often do doctors recommend large print without knowing the implications of the medium?

The educational consultant has as one of his responsibilities the duty of determining the learning material needs of the youngsters. Then, additionally, he initiates the request for specific kinds of material. It is ridiculous to expect that one person at the state level can evaluate the specific learning material needs of all the visually impaired children in his state. It is ridiculous for him to assume that because a youngster is 20/200 he must have large print. Yet, this is the rule rather than the exception in the United States. Further, unless visually impaired children meet the legal definition of blindness, they usually are neither identified nor do they qualify for educational services from their state departments of education.

The testing program is a very important part of the service program to visually impaired children. Though psychological testing is not administered by the education consultant, it is through his contact with the case and consultative service with the school officials and parents that initiation for and payment of service is made. Due to the nature of blindness, a special amount of expertise is required on the part of the tester to provide an adequate evaluation of the child. The state educational services program is in a position to provide for such a person's services while a local school system would lack both funds and knowledge of where to find such a person.

Of necessity, almost all tests for blind persons have been adapted in some way (vocational, personality, and achievement as well as intelligence). Access not only to the tester but to the materials and sources—if left to the local school system—would go undone. These tests are essential, for they help to guide the student and those working with him towards finding success, developing confidence, future planning, and goal setting.

Orientation and mobility is a particularly necessary service, especially for totally blind students, and one that requires specialized training beyond that which the educational consultant possesses. Except for very large cities, school systems cannot employ such a person, while a state program can have an adequate number of these professionals on staff to provide for all the students across the state. The educational consultant can and does provide instruction to school personnel, parents, etc. with regard to pre-cane skills, leaving instruction with the cane to a qualified person.

Evaluations of low vision aids are again a service coming through the educational consultant. Such evaluations are arranged and paid for through the state service agency. Careful control of the use of proper aids is as important as evaluation for possible usage. The low vision aid examination should always be made by a competent eye doctor who has an understanding of the particular or unusual situation that brings the child to the evaluation.

Vocational counseling is a critical area in service programs for visually impaired children and unfortunately often comes too late. As was mentioned earlier, visually impaired students need the advantage of special testing materials in addition to a person knowledgeable in blindness and visual impairment. Most public school counselors feel totally inadequate to work with blind students; unfortunately, because vocational rehabilitation establishes age 14 as a beginning referral age, the most critical planning and counseling stage that time prior to selection of a tentative high school program—has passed.

It must be the job of the educational consultant to bring together school guidance counselors and vocational rehabilitation counselors who together can deal with the young visually impaired child and his program at an appropriate time. In addition, the consultant can assist the guidance counselor in communication with laboratory teachers as to how visually impaired children can take part and be involved.

The educational consultant has primary responsibility for

bringing the aforementioned services together with the children, especially in those school systems where no specially trained teachers are available. A final service provided is the supervision of special teachers working within large or joint school systems. For further discussion of this function, let us review various local programs and their structure.

Local School Programs

The majority of visually impaired children, in all but several states, are in integrated classrooms with their sighted peers. These children receive no special instructional help other than that given by the classroom teacher. Any or all of the previously discussed educational services could be provided, however, by the service oriented state agency. For those students not requiring specific instruction in braille, orientation and mobility, or personal care skills, this integrated program is a superior arrangement.

Children who are in need of special instruction by specially trained personnel can benefit from the itinerant or resource room programs. These special personnel working in the local systems are supervised by the state educational consultants.

In those systems where special personnel are warranted, the special teacher can assume, along with his direct teaching responsibilities, a consultative role with regard to those children in the system enrolled in the integrated situation. The itinerant program lends itself more readily to this arrangement. The resource room program has other merits. For the multihandicapped blind and visually impaired, the special class can be a superior arrangement.

A state such as New Jersey can and does provide well for its visually impaired charges because the responsibility rests completely with their state commission for the blind. All of the specially trained teachers are employees of the state service oriented agency rather than of individual school systems. This arrangement allows for the assignment of specially trained personnel across school district boundries and brings the proper kind of attention and services to those children in need.

In summary, it is apparent that the number of visually impaired children who attend public schools will continue to grow. Through early identification, they will have an opportunity to receive necessary services in advance of enrollment in school.

A state program employing an adequate number of educational consultants and specially trained teachers will not only improve educational services but will allow for an opportunity to educate the educators in the public schools.

A greater emphasis on abilities and less attention to disabilities will most certainly improve our youngsters' opportunity for success in school and fulfillment of their basic needs. Well-adjusted young people, realistic about themselves and idealistic about their world, cannot help but be a great dividend to this society.

REFERENCES

Barker, R. G., et al.: *Adjustment to Physical Handicap and Illness: A Survey of the Social Psychology of Physique and Disability* (Rev. ed.). New York, Social Research Council, 1953.

Bruner, J.: *Learning about Learning: A Conference Report.* Superintendent of Documents, Cat. No. FS 5.212:12019, Washington, D. C., United States Government Printing Office, 1966.

Cholden, L. S.: *A Psychiatrist Works with Blindness.* New York, American Foundation for the Blind, 1958.

Cowen, E. L., Verillo, R. T., Underberg, R. P., and Berham, F. G.: *Adjustment to Visual Disability in Adolescence.* New York, American Foundation for the Blind, 1961.

Cruickshank, W. M. (Ed.): *Psychology of Exceptional Children and Youth.* Englewood Cliffs, New Jersey, Prentice-Hall, 1963.

Haimowitz and Haimowitz: *Human Development: Selected Readings.* New York, Crowell, 1966.

Halliday, C.: *The Visually Impaired Child: Growth, Learning, Development-Infancy to School Age.* Louisville, Ky., American Printing House for the Blind, 1970.

Jervis, F.: A comparison of self-concepts of blind and sighted children. In Davis, C. J., (Ed.): *Guidance Programs for Blind Adolescents.* Watertown, Mass.: Perkins School Publication No. 20, 1960.

Lucio, W. H. and McNeil, J. D.: *Supervision: A Synthesis of Thought and Action.* New York, McGrawHill, 1962.

Miller, W. H.: Manifest anxiety in visually impaired adolescents. *Education of the Visually Handicapped, 2*:3, 91-93, 1970.

Perspectives on Human Deprivation: Biological, Psychological, and Sociological. U. S. Department of Health, Education, and Welfare,

Public Health Service, National Institutes of Health, The National Institute of Child Health and Human Development, 1968.
Seidman, J. M. (Ed.): *Readings in Educational Psychology*. Boston, Houghton, 1965.
Somers, V. S.: *The Influence of Aparental Attitudes and Social Environment on the Personality Development of the Adolescent Blind*. New York, American Foundation for the Blind, 1954.

Index

I

J

K

L

Q

R